THE EYE AND NUTRITION

---MORPHOLOGICAL ASPECTS---

The Eye and Nutrition

---Morphological Aspects---

Tsugio Amemiya

Nova Biomedical Books
New York

For permission to use material from this book please contact us:
Telephone 631-231-7269; Fax 631-231-8175
Web Site: http://www.novapublishers.com

LIBRARY OF CONGRESS CATALOGING-IN-PUBLICATION DATA

The eye and nutrition : morphological aspects / Tsugio Amemiya, editor.
p. :cm.
Includes bibliographical references and index.
ISBN 978-1-59454-563-4
ISBN 1-59454-563-4
1. Eye—Physiology. 2. Nutrition. 3. Eye—Abnormalities—Nutritional aspects. I. Amemiya, T. (Tsugio)
[DNLM: 1. Ocular Physiology. 2. Nutrition. WW 103 E965 2005]

Published by Nova Science Publishers, Inc. ✦ New York

To Ikuko Amemiya, M.D.--- with affection and with appreciation for her critical support during my long life of research and the preparation of this book.

Ibaraki, Osaka
Tsugio Amemiya

CONTENTS

PREFACE

For forty years the author has studied the role of several micronutrients while working in two University Hospitals as an ophthalmologist. The micronutrients studied were five vitamins (A, B_2 (riboflavin), B_{12}, C (ascorbic acid) and E), and seven trace elements (Zn, Cu, Mn, Mg, Se, Cr and Al). The effects of both excess and deficiency were examined. Excessive nutrient studies are important to clarify intoxication, but the author thinks that studies of deficiency are more important and should be performed first, because they clearly demonstrate the significance of nutrients in the living body. Therefore, the author has paid attention mainly to deficiencies of micronutrients.

Symptomatological and biochemical studies of nutrition have progressed, but morphological studies have always been secondary. In spite of the development of electron microscopy and of histochemical and cytochemical techniques, morphological studies have been in the minority for the past 50 years at least. In the ophthalmological field there have been few symptomatological, biochemical and morphological studies of micronutrient except for several studies on the effect of vitamins A and E and Zn on the ocular surface and the retina.

Ocular tissue consists of neural cells, epithelial and endothelial cells, muscle cells, connective tissues, secretory gland cells, skin, mucous cells, etc. Thus studies of the nutritional aspect of ocular tissues may provide clues to the significance of the nutrients common to all organs. Since morphological studies of nutrients are scarce, this book may contribute to the understanding of nutrients in all organs. It may be unusual for one person to study five vitamins and seven trace elements continuously with only light and electron microscopes. This book describes the morphological results collected from the papers published by the author and his associates. Biochemical mechanisms and their significance are discussed by other researchers. Such discussion will always take place. Since the complete elucidation of a biochemical mechanism corresponding to each morphological change may be impossible, or take a long time, the author will describe only clear-cut morphological changes with a putative mechanical explanation.

The author studied the conjunctiva, cornea, retina, optic nerve, and sometimes rectus muscles, but not the lens. The lens is one of the most important ocular tissues, because cataract is one of the most common diseases in ophthalmology. However, the author could not study the lens morphologically, because he does not know at the present time the most suitable, reliable and reproducible morphological techniques for lens study. That is, the author is not able to differentiate the true images of the lens from artifacts in scanning and transmission electron microscopy. For this purpose, tissue fixation methods and slicing procedures must be improved. The author must wait for a while until such methodological problems can be solved.

A historical point of view, places nutrition as one of the world's most urgent and important problems. Since world war II, the developed countries have not worried about nutritional deficiency, but there is now great concern about excessive food intake which leads to diabetes mellitus etc. However, in under-developed and developing countries, lack of food is still a serious problem. Good nutrition can prevent disease, decrease signs and symptoms and even sometimes cure disease. Therefore, the study of nutrition should always be required as one of the main topics in medicine. In spite of this probably well-recognized concept, the study of nutrition actually seems to be out of date.

The author is grateful to Dr. Alice S Cary for her continual revising of English in many original papers the past 40 years. The author greatly appreciates Ms Chieko Hori, Department of Ophthalmology and Visual Sciences, Graduate School of Biomedical Sciences, Nagasaki University, for her secretarial assistance and Yumiko Takami BS of the same Department for her assistance with experiments and making all the photographs. The following doctors contributed to the studies described in this book: Drs Yoshinori Dake, Takashi Kitaoka, Junichiro Takano, Tsukihiko Ogawa, Naoki Imamura, Kazuaki Mishima, Huaqing Gong, Yoshiaki Hirayama, Imran Ahemd Bhutto, Yasuo Tsuda, Keisuke Oba, Noritake Miyamura, Suketaka Kanazawa, Yoshiko Ueda, Zhong-Yang Lu, Akinori Takehara and Azusa Fujikawa.

Chapter 1

MAGNESIUM

I. SIGNIFICANCE

Magnesium (Mg) is one of the essential trace elements in humans and animals. Mg has various physiological actions related to Mg-containing enzymes, growth factors, hormones, gene expression, fibrous proliferation, etc. (Shils, 1997).

Mg deficiency can lead to sudden death probably due to focal necrosis in the heart muscle (Elwood, Sweetnam, Beasley, 1980; Galle, Mohr, Lossnitzer et al, 1981), hypertension (McCarron, 1983), arteriosclerosis (Ito, Toda, Kummerrow et al, 1986), and edema (Bunce, Saacke and Mulins, 1980). However, few ocular diseases related to Mg deficiency are known. There is a hypothesis that retinopathy of prematurity may be related to Mg and Cu deficiencies which are found in premature infants (Caddell, 1988; Caddell, 1995). Although Mg-related enzymes are prominent in ocular tissues and have been widely investigated, most of the studies have been performed in vitro. To our knowledge, there have been no reports on the histopathologic aspects of Mg deficiency in ocular tissues. Most of the intercellular Mg is associated with organic compounds and particularly with ATP. Thus relatively small percentage changes in the amount of bound Mg may cause major changes in the amount of Mg^{2+}.

II. MG-DEFICIENT EXPERIMENT

Material and Methods

Normal 10-week-old female Wistar Kyoto rats were mated with normal male Wistar Kyoto rats with free access to usual commercial rat pellets containing 24mg Mg per 100g of diet and all other nutrients, obtained from Oriental Yeast Co. Ltd., Tokyo, Japan, along with distilled and deionized water. After delivery, mother rats with several litters were divided into three groups: control, Mg-deficient and pair-fed control groups. In the Mg-deficient group, mother rats were given free access to a Mg-deficient diet containing 0.1mg Mg per 100g of diet and all other nutrients obtained from Nippon Clea Incorporated, Tokyo, Japan and distilled and deionized water. Infant rats were suckled by these mother rats for 21days, and then fed the same Mg-deficient diet. Control mother rats were fed usual commercial rat pellets as described above, and infant rats were also fed the same diet starting 21 days after birth. The control rats developed and continued to survive until 6 weeks after birth.

In the pair-fed control group, infant rats were suckled by their normal mother rats for 3 weeks, then given the same amount of the usual diet that Mg-deficient rats had eaten on the previous day and distilled with deionized water. All the rats were killed at 6 weeks of age.

Clinical Features of the Mg-Deficient Animal

Most rats fed the Mg-deficient diet died suddenly after jumping high in response to a loud noise or even just after being placed on the experimental stage. Only one third of a litter can survive for 3 weeks after weaning, i.e. 6 weeks after birth.

The Mg-deficient rats exhibit characteristics typically seen in Mg-deficient animals, including growth retardation, edema of all four paws and scrotum (Fig. 1.2.1), frequent sudden death, slight coarsening of fur, and a jumping response to loud sound.

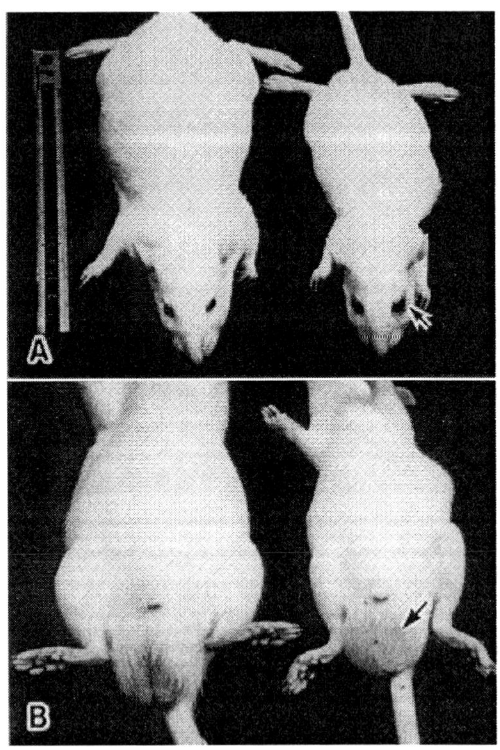

Figure 1.2.1. Left side, a control rat and right side, Mg-deficient rat in (A) and (B). A rat (B) fed a Mg-deficient diet for 3 weeks after being suckled by a mother fed the deficient diet after delivery is much smaller than the control rat (A) and shows conjunctival secretion [arrow in (A)]; edema in scrotum arrow in (B)].

Body weight: At 6 weeks of age the body weight of the Mg-deficient rats is significantly lower than that of the controls ($p<0.0001$): control rats: 283±15g, n=10, deficient rats 145±12.7g, n=10. The body weight of the pair-fed control rats is 106±18.2g, n=10, significantly lower than that of the controls.

Serum magnesium: At 6 weeks of age the serum Mg level is 4.3±0.7mEq l^{-1} in ten control rats and 1.2±0.2mEq l^{-1} in six Mg-deficient rats ($p=0.0018$), and that of serum Ca is 11.0±0.2mEq l^{-1} in ten controls and 14.1±0.6mEq l^{-1} in six Mg-deficient rats ($p=0.0022$). In pair-fed control rats the serum Mg level is 4.1±0.5mEq l^{-1}, n=10 and that of Ca level is 10.3±0.5mEq l^{-1}, n=10.

III. The Conjunctiva and Cornea

Results

The Conjunctiva

Transmission electron microscopic (TEM) findings

In the conjunctiva of rats fed a Mg-deficient diet for 6 weeks, microvilli and microplicae of the surface were decreased and goblet cells had scarce secretory granules (Fig. 1.3.1).

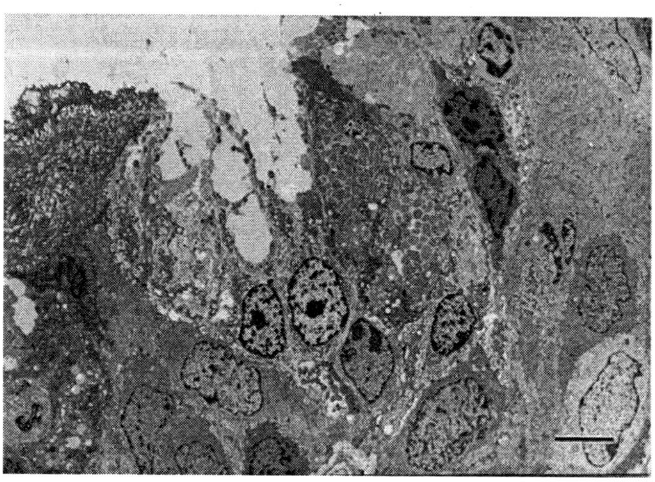

Figure 1.3.1. TEM micrograph of the conjunctiva of a rat fed a Mg-deficient diet for 6 weeks showing decreased microvilli and microplicae in the most superficial epithelial cells and decreased secretory granules in the goblet cells. Bar: 5μm.

Control Rat Cornea

Scanning Electron Microscopic (SEM) Findings

Epithelial cells were mostly light cells and had numerous microvilli and microplicae. Epithelial cells were hexagonal, all nearly the same size and arranged regularly resembling pavement.

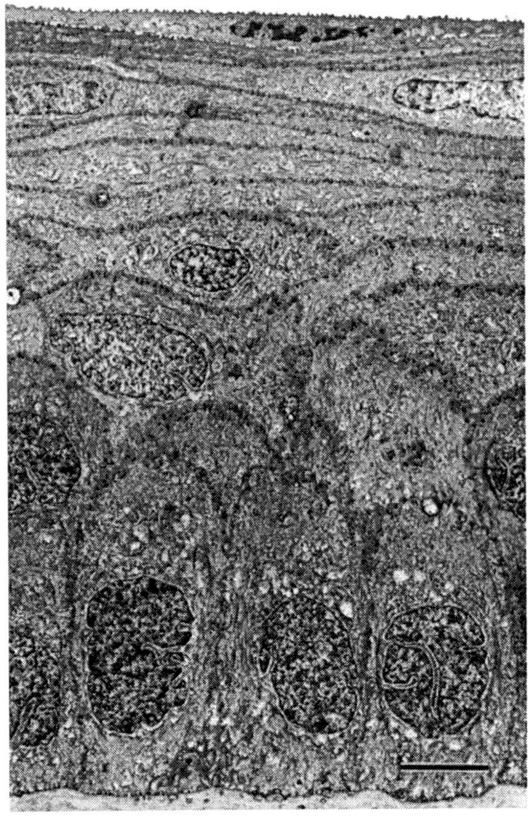

Figure 1.3.2. TEM micrographs of cornea of a control rat. The most superficial epithelial cells have many microvilli and epithelial cells have many desmosomes and fibrils. Basal epithelial cells have many hemidesmosomes and basement membrane. The subepithelial layer has no abnormal deposition. Bar: 5μm.

Transmission Electron Microscopic (TEM) Findings

Epithelial cells had many microvilli in the most superficial cells and well-developed fibrils and desmosomes (Fig. 1.3.2). The basal cells were tall and had vertical-oval nuclei (Fig. 1.3.2). There were no abnormal cells or deposition under the epithelium. In the stroma, numerous collagen fibers were tightly and regularly arranged. Keratocytes appeared normal as did Descemet's membrane. Endothelial cells were arranged a sheet.

Mg-Deficient Rat Cornea

SEM Findings

Dark cells were increased in the most superficial cell layer as compared with those in the control rat, and they had fewer microvilli and microplicae (Fig. 1.3.3). Endothelial cells had lost their hexagonal shape and formed an irregular pattern (Fig. 1.3.4). In some areas, epithelial cells were destroyed (Fig. 1.3.5).

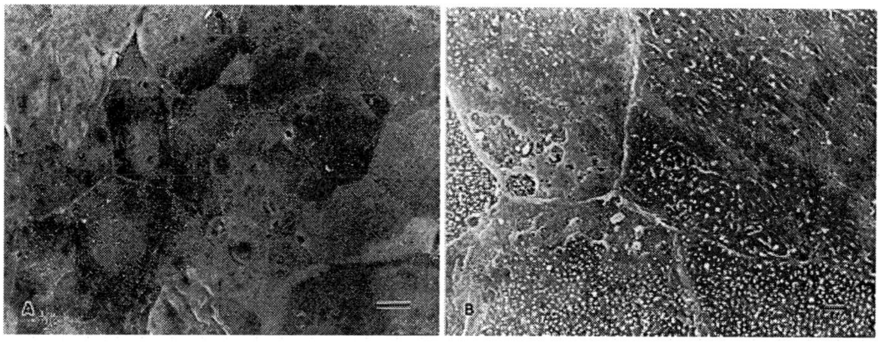

Figure 1.3.3. SEM micrographs of the corneal epithelium of a 6-week-old Mg-deficient rat. (A) There are many dark cells in the most superficial epithelial cell layer. Dark cells have less microvilli and microplicae. (B) Enlarged view of corneal surface. Microvilli and microplicae are scarce and the surface is rough. Bar: 10μm (A), 1μm (B).

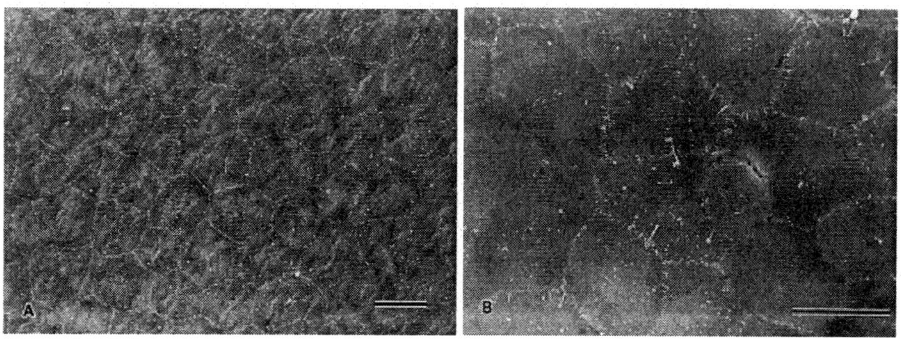

Figure 1.3.4. SEM micrographs of the endothelium of 6-week-old control (A) and Mg-deficient (B) rats. The control rat endothelial cells are almost the same in size and are hexagonal (A), while the endothelial cells of the Mg-deficient rat are square or pentagonal. Bar: 10μm (A,B).

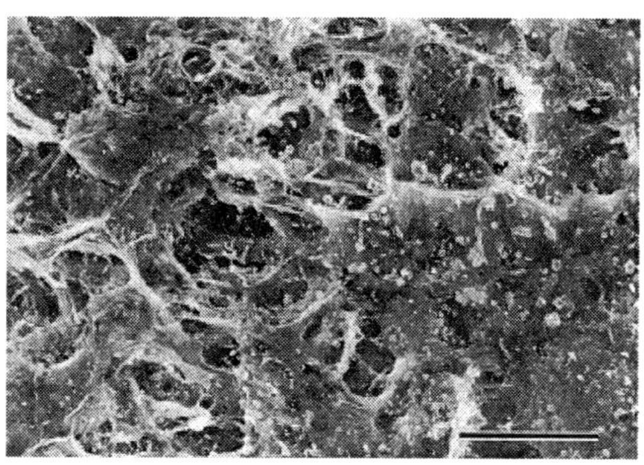

Figure 1.3.5. SEM micrograph of the endothelium of a 6-week-old Mg-deficient rat. Endothelial cells are partially destroyed. Bar: 10μm.

Table 1.3.1. The thickness of the whole cornea, the epithelial layer, and the Descemet membrane of the cornea in the control, Mg-deficient, and pair-fed control rats.

Groups	Whole thickness of cornea (μm)	Thickness of the epithelial layer (μm)	Thickness of Descemet membrane (μm)
Control	111.27±6.2(n=10)	36±2.4*(n=10)	1.6±0.08(n=10)
Mg-deficient	110.0±10.4(n=15)	23.6±3.9*, **(n=5)	1.6±0.14(n=15)
Pair-fed control	108.0±12 (n=9)	33±3.4**(n=9)	1.7±0.2(n=9)
P value	P>0.05	*P<0.001;**P=0.0072	P>0.05

n: the number of the specimens examined in the three groups. There are significant differences only among the epithelial layer in the three groups.

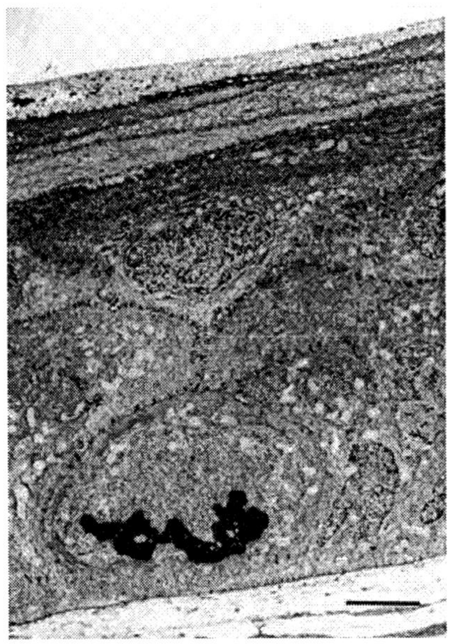

Figure 1.3.6. TEM micrograph of corneal epithelium of a rat fed a Mg-deficient diet for 6 weeks. The epithelium is thin. The most superficial epithelium has no microvilli. Many desmosomes still remain, but apoptosis-like chromatin condensation is seen in the nucleus of a basal cell. Bar: 5μm.

TEM Findings

There was no statistically significant difference in the total corneal thickness between the control and Mg-deficient groups. However, the thickness of corneal epithelial layer in the Mg-deficient rats was 23.6±3.9μm (n=15), while in the controls, it was 36±2.4μm (n=10) and 33±3.4μm (n=9) in the pair-fed controls, statistically significant differences between the control and Mg-deficient groups and between the pair-fed control and Mg-deficient groups (Table 1.3.1). Epithelial cells in the most superficial layer had reduced microvilli (Fig. 1.3.6). The basal cells were short and had many vacuolated mitochondria (Figs. 1.3.6, 7; 1.3.9B). Some nuclei were horizontally oval and had clumped chromatin masses (Fig. 1.3.7). Under the basal cells were dense bodies of cells of unknown origin containing dense bodies and crescent-like dense masses of chromatin in the nucleus (Fig. 1.3.8). The hemidesmosomes near the base of the basal cuboidal cells of the epithelium were significantly fewer in Mg-deficient rats than in the controls (p<0.0001) (Table 1.3.2) and had disappeared at some sites

(Fig. 1.3.8). Dense materials were present at the bottom of basal cells and subepithelium (Fig. 1.3.8,9). On the other hand, there was no significant difference from the controls in the number of ribosomes (Table 1.3.2). The thickness of Descemet's membrane was 1.6±0.14μm in Mg-deficient rats (n=15), 1.6±0.08μm in the controls (n=10) and 1.7±0.2μm in the pair-fed controls (n=9) (Table 1.3.1). There was no statistically significant difference in the thickness of Descemet's membrane between Mg-deficient and control rats ($p<0.05$) (Table 1.3.1). Endothelial cells showed vacuolated mitochondria and fragmented or detached cytoplasm (Fig. 1.3.10).

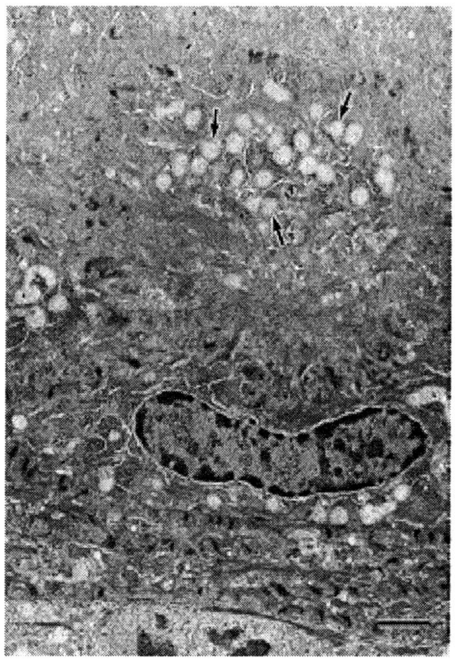

Figure 1.3.7. TEM micrograph of corneal epithelium of a Mg-deficient rat. The epithelial cell has numerous ribosomes and fibrils, but mitochondria (arrows) are destructed. Bar: 1μm.

Table 1.3.2. The number of hemidesmosomes and ribosomes located at the base of the basal cuboidal cells in the corneal epithelium.

Groups	Number of hemidesmosomes counted at 4-μm baseline/number of fields examined	Number of ribosomes counted in 8μm^2/number of fields examined
Control	10±5.1/119	246±63/35
Mg-deficient	7±2.1/164	231±82/79
Pair-fed control	9±3.1/114	256±73/65

The number of hemidesmosomes in the corneal epithelium in Mg-deficient rats is significantly lower ($P<0.0001$) than in controls, but the number of ribosomes is not significantly different among the three groups ($P=0.35$)

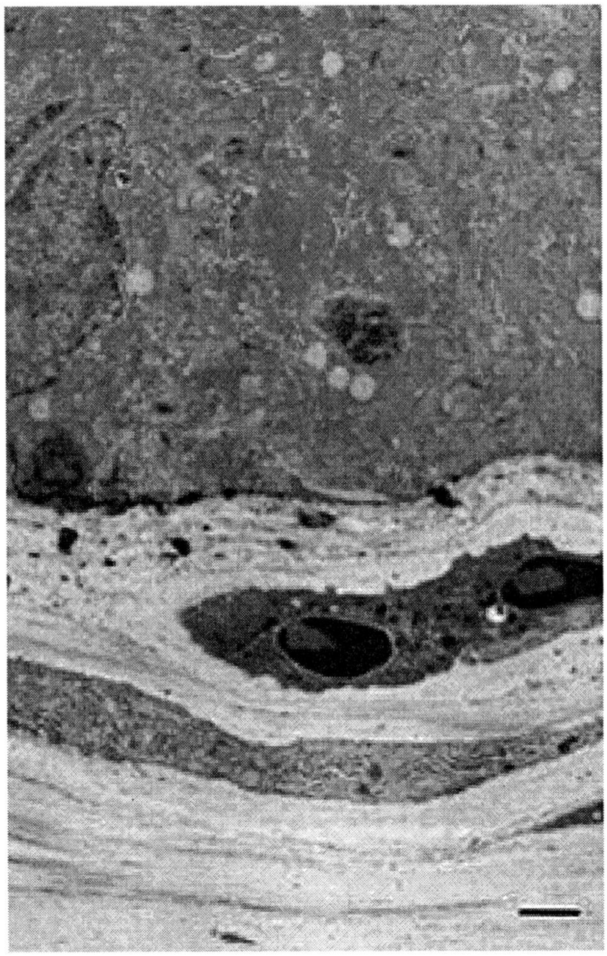

Figure 1.3.8. TEM micrograph of a 6-week-old Mg-deficient rat. There are various phases of dense materials in the subepithelial layer and cells with apoptotic crescent-shaped nuclei, and a probable fibrocyte near the abnormal deposits seems to phagocytize high density deposits. Bar: 1μm.

Pair-fed control rat cornea

There was no statistically significant change in the cornea thickness. The cornea consisted of eight to nine layers of epithelium, stroma, Descemet membrane, and one layer of endothelium (Table 1.3.1).

SEM Findings

The most superficial layer cell of the cornea had densely arranged microvilli and microplicae. The endothelial cells kept their hexagonal shape.

TEM Findings

The epithelial cells kept many desmosomes and normal intracytoplasmic organelles such as fibrils, tonofibrils, mitochondria, and ribosomes.

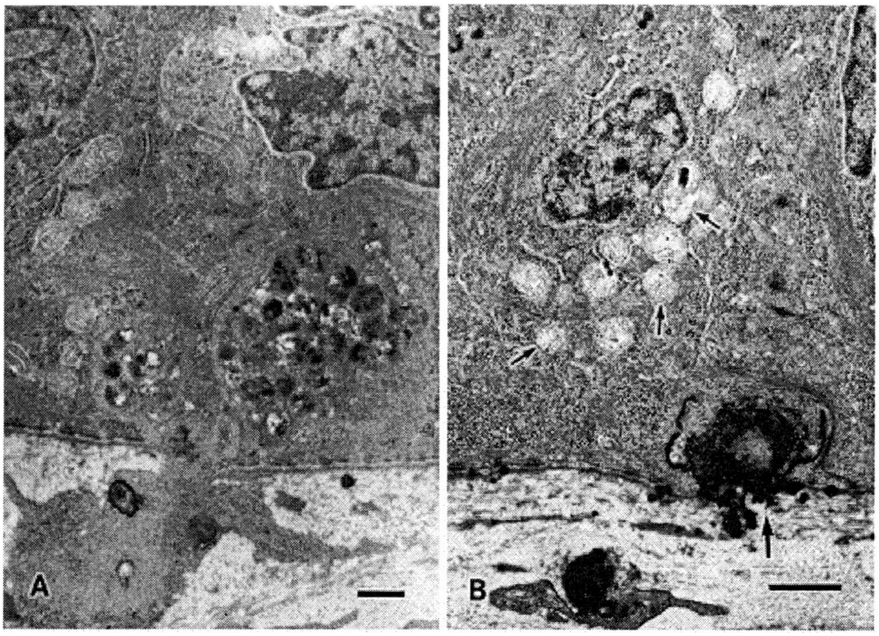

Figure 1.3.9. TEM micrographs of the basal cell and subepithelial layers of cornea of a Mg-deficient rat, showing various phases of releasing materials from the basal cell to the subepithelial layer. (A) Dense materials are on the basement membrane and break the basement membrane to protrude to the subepithelium. Some dense material is already in the stroma. (B) A part of a basal cell loses the basement membrane and hemidesmosomes and is indented with amorphous materials, dense granules and cellular debris. Basal cells contain dense materials and are present in the subepithelial stroma. A basal cell contains a cluster of destructed mitochondria (arrows). Some dense materials are about to release as a mass from the cytoplasm to the stroma. Bar: 500nm (A); 1μm (B).

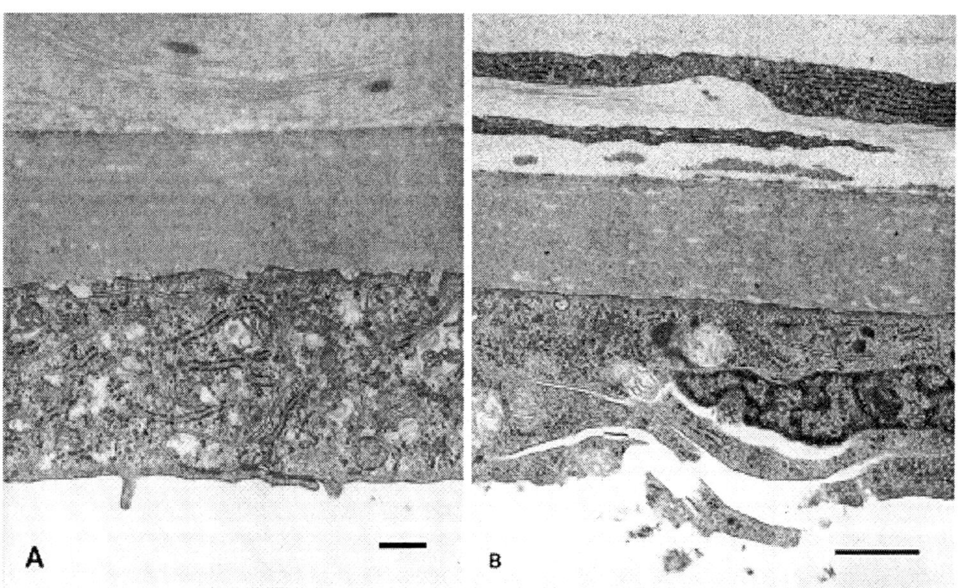

Figure 1.3.10. TEM micrograph of the corneal endothelium of a 6-week-old control rat (A). The corneal epithelium of a 6-week-old Mg-deficient rat (B) shows part of the cytoplasm of the endothelial cell which is destroyed at the anterior chamber side. Bar: 500nm (A); 1μm (B).

Nuclei were normal in appearance. Hemidesmosomes were present at the base of the basal cells. Neither deposits nor blood vessels were found in the subepithelial space and stroma. Endothelial cells had normal intracytoplasmic organelles and intercellular junctions.

Discussion

All enzymatic reactions that involve ATP absolutely require Mg^{2+}. Levels of Mg^{2+} seem closely linked to calcium, potassium, and sodium metabolism (Reinach and Holmberg, 1987). A Na^{+}, K^{+}-ATPase pump localized in the basolateral cell membrane of the corneal epithelium, and a Ca^{2+}-stimulated Mg^{2+}-dependent ATPase in the plasma membrane play important roles in the transport of Na^{+}, K^{+}, and Ca^{2+} (Reinach and Holmberg, 1987). In the corneal epithelium, plasma membrane-derived ATPase activity has a regulatory function in maintaining intracellular Ca^{2+} activity (Reinach and Holmberg, 1987). Although the balance between Mg^{2+}-ATPase and Na^{+}, K^{+}-ATPase is very different in in vivo experiments from that in in vitro experiments (Whikehart, Montaomery and Wells, 1989; Riley, 1971; Ottlecz, Garcia, Eichberg et al, 1993; Herse and Adams, 1995). Mg^{2+}-ATP and Na^{+}, K^{+}-ATPase activities appear to be linked in a biofeedback mechanism (Whikehart, Montaomery and Wells, 1989; Whikehart, Montaomery, Angelos et al, 1993). The fact that the epithelium behaves as a semipermeable membrane is experimentally confirmed by the use of solution containing $MgSO_4$ (Riley, 1971). It has been shown that the epithelial surface is maintained best with a buffered solution containing potassium, calcium, Mg, phosphate, bicarbonate, and sodium chloride (Bachman and Wilson, 1985). Thus such a buffered solution, tear film, may be affected by Mg deficiency. On the other hand, the endothelium has the function of pumping fluid out of the corneal stroma by a process of active transport. Herse and Adams (1995) suggested that corneal endothelial Mg^{2+}-ATPase and Na^{+}, K^{+}-ATPase activities have complex dynamic interactions with corneal thickness. Most of the intracellular Mg is associated with organic compounds and particularly with ATP. Thus, a relatively small amount of bound Mg may cause major damages in the amount of Mg^{2+}. Although it is still unknown what morphologic effects Mg has on the cornea, Mg deficiency may induce morphologic changes in the cornea through abnormal ATP activity and abnormal transport of Na^{+}, K^{+}, and Ca^{2+}.

The epithelium and stroma did not show edematous findings despite endothelial damage. The author and his associates cannot explain this discrepancy clearly. They assume that corneal edema did not appear because the damage was localized and morphologically intact endothelial cells were also seen in the SEM.

Magnesium-deficient rats showed abnormal cells with apoptotic nuclei in the epithelium and subepithelial stroma, although no apoptotic changes were found in those with Zn or Mn deficiency. The photoreceptor nuclei in Mg-deficient rats were apoptotic. Therefore, Mg deficiency may be involved in the induction of apoptosis due to disturbed topological modifications of DNA through topoisomerase, which is an Mg-dependent enzyme (Covacci, Bruzzese, Sgambato et al, 2000). However, further proof is necessary for this assumption, since it is not yet certain that the appearance of apoptotic cells in the cornea is specific for Mg deficiency. The corneal endothelial cells of Mg-deficient rats showed dense bodies in the cytoplasm and structural destruction. These changes were found only in Mg deficiency and not in Zn or Mn deficiency (Gong , Takami, Amemiya et al, 2004, Gong and Amemiya, 1999).

The appearance of many dark cells in the most superficial epithelial layer of the cornea is a common change in Zn, Mn, and Mg deficiencies (Table 1.3.3) (Gong, Amemiya and Takaya, 2001; Gong and Amemiya 2001; Gong and Amemiya, 1999). The dark cell phenomenon is usually seen in both normal and pathologic tissues and it is occasionally seen in poorly fixed tissues, immature cells such as embryonic and developing cells, technical artifacts, and dead, dying, dehydrated or degenerating cells. The dark cells in Mg, Zn, and Mn deficiencies may well be effete or dying cells because of their scarce microvilli and microplicae and reduced numbers of ribosomes and other intracytoplasmic organelles (Gong and Amemiya, 1999).

Table 1.3.3. Corneal changes in Mg, Zn, and Mn deficiencies.

Deficiency	Epithelium	Stroma	Endothelium
Mg	Scarce microvilli and tonofibrils, vacuolated mitochondria, increased dark cells, high-density deposits, apoptotic nuclei, decreased hemidesmosomes	Subepithelial abnormal cells with apoptotic nuclei	Irregular shape, destruction of cytoplasmic membrane, dense bodies, vacuolated mitochondria
Zn	Scarce microvilli, deformed and decreased epithelial hole, decreased tonofibrils, decreased ribosomes, increased dark cells		
Mn	Scarce microvilli and tonofibrils, abnormal mitochondria, increased dark cells	Thin stroma, irregular diameter of collagen fibers, irregular arrangement of collagen fibers, small diameter of collagen fibers	Irregular shape, abnormal cytoplasmic processes, thick Descemet membrane, pentagonal cells increased

Divalent Mg is the fourth most a bundant metal ion in cellular metabolism. Although approximately 90% of intracellular Mg^{2+} is bound to ribosomes or polynucleotides (Cowan, 1995), the current study could not confirm the decrease in ribosomes in the corneal epithelium of Mg-deficient rats. Mg^{2+} has other biologic functions, including structural stabilization of proteins, nucleic acids and cell membranes by general surface binding. Magnesium activates enzymes in pathways related to nucleic acid biochemistry, glycolysis, amino acid synthesis, photosynthesis, and the TCA cycle (Black and Cowan, 1995). The reduction of Mg activation of enzymes in Mg deficiency may lead to the maldevelopment of intracytoplasmic organelles. Magnesium plays a role in cell wall and cellular membrane stabilization (Shils, 1997). Since Mg-binding ATP is located in the membrane, components of the membrane such as microvilli, microplicae, cytoplasmic membrane, and mitochondrial cristae may easily be damaged by Mg deficiency. The decrease or loss of microvilli and microplicae may lead to changes of membrane stabilization and formation of the tear film.

These disturbances interfere with protection from infections, foreign bodies, dryness and direct exposure to the air. The nucleus is also affected in the Mg-deficient rat cornea. Magnesium deficiency is accompanied by a high Ca concentration, which may induce nitric oxide production (Roth, 1997). The current study showed high Ca and low Mg levels in the cornea. Magnesium deficiency never induces multifocal necrosis in the cornea as it does in the retina, optic nerve and heart muscle (Gong and Amemiya, 2001).

High density bodies in the subepithelial stroma were histochemically proven to be calcium deposits and may be due to a high level of Ca in the serum. The positive immunohistochemical staining for fibrocytes strongly suggests that certain cells in the subepithelial stroma were derived from fibrocytes.

Mg is suggested to play an important role in the development and maintenance of the corneal structure.

IV. The Retina

Results

Light microscopic findings

In the posterior part of the retina, Luveak-embedded semi-thin sections of the retina of the Mg-deficient rats showed multifocal vacuoles in the retinal pigment epithelial (RPE) cells and irregular arrangement of the photoreceptor outer segments and pyknosis of the photoreceptor nuclei.

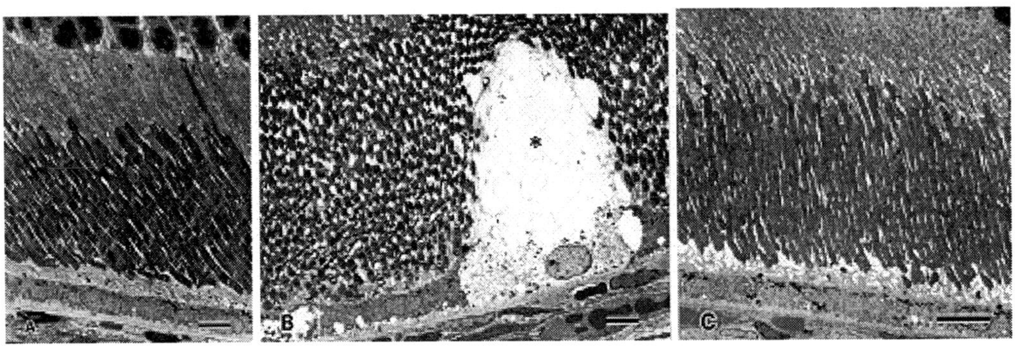

Figure 1.4.1. TEM micrographs of RPE and photoreceptor outer segments of control (A), Mg-deficient (B) and pair-fed control (C) rats. A shows the outer segment and RPE of a control rat retina. (B) shows a triangular defect (*) between the RPE and the outer segment layer. The RPE is necrotic. (C) shows the same view as (A). Bar: 5 μm(A),(B) and 10 μm (C).

Electron microscopic findings

In some places in the RPE layer, some RPE cells showed multifocal necrosis, breakdown of the nuclear membrane, sparse chromatin granules, breakdown of the cytoplasmic membrane, and destruction of intracytoplasmic organelles, such as mitochondria and lysosomes (Fig. 1.4.1). Photoreceptor cell outer segments facing such RPE cells were lost: the long-axis of photoreceptor cell outer segments was curved in contact with RPE cells to avoid adjacent necrotic cells (Fig. 1.4.2). Some RPE cells contained many lamellar bodies, probably outer segment discs. The RPE cells were much shorter than those of control rats. Many photoreceptor outer segment discs were seen as dense bodies between the tip of the outer segment and the microvilli of the RPE cells (Fig. 1.4.2). The outer segment discs showed neither vacuolation nor destruction.

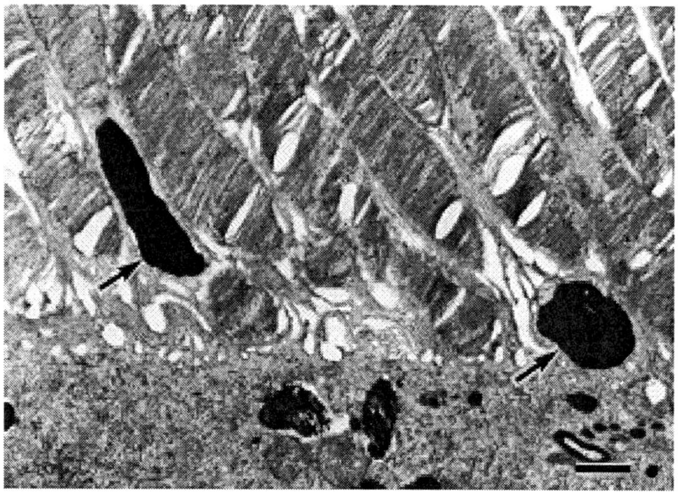

Figure 1.4.2. TEM micrograph of the retina of a rat fed a Mg-deficient diet for 6 weeks. The photoreceptor outer segment discs near the RPE show dark masses of abnormal shedding (arrows). There are many phagocytized lamellar structures in the RPE. Bar: 1μm.

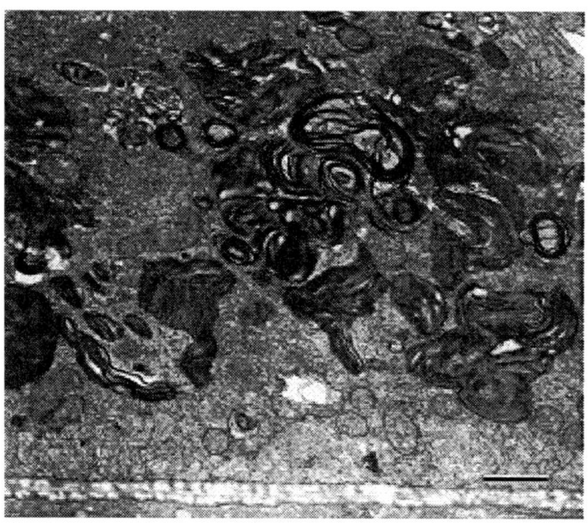

Figure 1.4.3. TEM micrograph of the RPE of a Mg-deficient rat showing many phagocytized lamellar structures. Bar: 1μm.

In many photoreceptor cell nuclei there were pyknotic apoptosis-like changes: crescent-shaped clumps of chromatin, abnormal distribution of clumped chromatin granules and shrinkage of the nucleus (Fig. 1.4.4). However, there were still eight to nine layers of photoreceptor cell nuclei.

Rats in control and pair-fed control groups showed no abnormalities in the retina.

In the heart ventricle muscle of Mg-deficient rats, myocardial necrosis was seen: blood capillary occlusion, destruction of sarcoplasmic organelles, interuption of myofibrils and extracellulary scattered debris of cells (Fig. 1.4.5). The control and pair-fed rats showed no abnormalities in the heart.

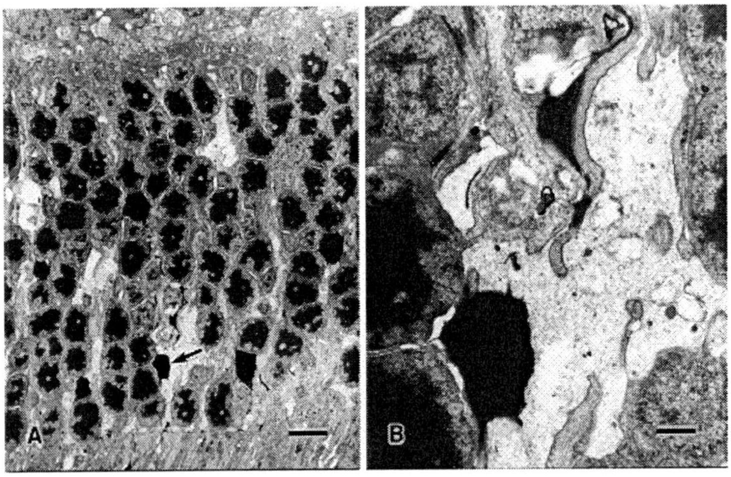

Figure 1.4.4. TEM micrographs of the retina of a rat fed a Mg-deficient diet for 6 weeks. (A) The chromatin in photoreceptor cell nuclei is clumped and condensed, suggesting pyknotic apoptosis-like changes (arrows). (B) is an enlargement of the pyknotic area. Bar: 5μm (A), 1μm (B).

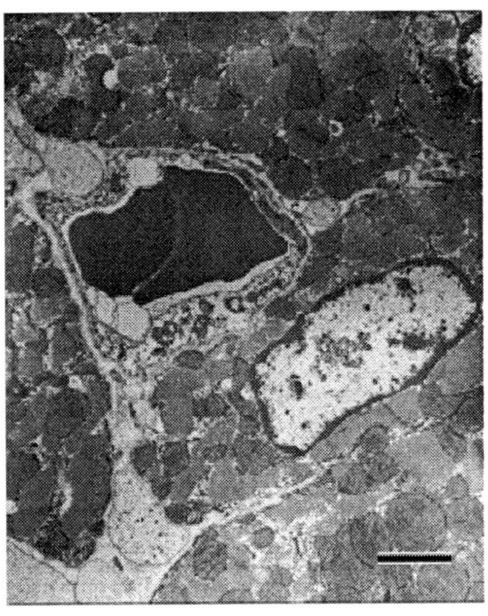

Figure 1.4.5. TEM micrograph of the heart ventricle muscle of a rat fed a Mg-deficient diet for 6 weeks. The myocardium shows emboli in capillaries and destruction of intrasarcoplasmic organelles, cell debris and abnormal deposition. Bar: 2μm.

Secondary ion mass spectrometry (SIMS)

SIMS images show a lower Mg and higher Ca concentration in the whole retina of the Mg-deficient rats than that in the controls (Table 1.4.1). The ratio of Ca to Mg concentration in the retina of the Mg-deficient rats is significantly higher than in the control rats ($p<0.0001$)(Table 1.4.1). This means decreased Mg and increased Ca in the retina.

Table 1.4.1. The ratio of calcium to magnesium concentration in retina (Ca: Mg).

Groups	Counts per sec		Ratio (Ca: Mg)	Number of the ratio counted
	Ca	Mg		
6 week old Mg-deficient rat	1711±708	1158±552	1.24±0.09*	9
Equivalent-age control rat	5672±794	9528±790	0.84±0.05	10

*P<0.0001 (Student test).

SIMS sequential analysis in the retina. Because of multifocal necrosis in the pigment epithelial cells, the whole amount of trace elements in the Mg-deficient rat is lower than that in controls, but the ratio of Ca to Mg concentration in the retina of Mg-deficient rats is significantly higher than in controls. It indicates that in the Mg-deficient rat retina, Mg is decreased and Ca is increased.

Discussion

Mg is essential for protein synthesis and mediates synaptic transmission in the retina (Kaneko and Shimazaki, 1975; Langdon, Manis, Freeman et al, 1988; Shils, 1997). Mg is involved in the activities of various enzymes. It has been proved Mg is abundant in retinal rod outer and inner segments (Somlyo and Walz, 1985), the retinal photoreceptor membranes might be influenced by changes in the concentration of Mg in the medium in vitro experiments (Van and Bazan, 1986 a, b), and a decreased concentration of Mg might cause retinal degeneration (Farber and Lolley, 1976), but all these studies are in vitro. In the retina Mg modulates glutamate receptors (Schmidt, 1999) and protects against ischemia (Szabo, Droy, Doly et al, 1992; Maynard, Quinones, Ogilvy et al, 1998). It also reduces N-methyl-D-asparate neurotoxicity in the retina (Gilson and Reif, 1985), influencing phospholipase D, phosphatidate phosphohydrolase and diacylglyceride lipase activities (Pasquare and Giusto, 1993; Salvador and Giasto, 1998) and retinal adhesiveness (Yao, Endo and Marmor, 1989; Yao, Hageman and Marmor et al, 1994).

Sudden death in patients with Mg deficiency has been considered to be due to myocardial focal necrosis (Elwood, Sweetman, Beasley et al, 1980). Electron microscopy of the heart muscle confirms that the rats fed a Mg-deficient diet in the current study are certainly deficient in Mg, and in the pair-fed control group the retina and heart show no histopathologic changes like those in the Mg-deficient rats. These results indicate that the changes in the photoreceptor nuclei and RPE are caused by Mg deficiency and show that Mg deficiency induces multifocal necrosis in RPE cells and pyknosis (apoptosis-like pyknosis) in photoreceptor cell nuclei. These retinal findings resemble the clinical features of acute posterior multifocal pigment epitheliopathy (Gass, 1968). The findings in the heart suggest that Mg deficiency might also cause focal necrosis in the retina. The similarity of retinal changes in Mg-deficient rats to the clinical features of acute posterior multifocal placoid pigment epitheliopathy (Gass, 1968) is characterized by a rapidly progressive bilateral loss of central vision caused by multifocal, yellowish-white lesions in the RPE (Gass, 1968). Multifocal lesions caused by Mg deficiency might be a secondary condition induced by drugs such as penicillin and sulfonamides which may chelate with Mg. Another cause of multifocal lesions of the RPE might be related to the higher Ca level associated with the low level of Mg (McCarron, 1983).

There are many Mg-containing enzymes involved in at least 300 reactions by which food constituents are metabolized and new products are formed (Shils, 1997). Mg^{2+} is involved in essentially all kinase reactions. Thus it is natural that the sensory retina and retinal pigment epithelium affected by many kinases are damaged by the disturbed enzyme activity due to low Mg in the serum and the retina. Mg deficiency is also related to increased serum phospholipids, triglycerides, variable total cholesterol, low free cholesterol, increased levels of oleic and linoleic acids, decreased levels of stearic and arachidonic acids and modifications of lipid and lipoprotein concentrations (Geuex, Mazur, Cardot et al, 1991). The photoreceptor cell has characteristic morphological structures consisting of a lipid-rich outer segment disc membrane, an inner segment with many mitochondria, and a nucleus. That is, the retina has increased susceptibility to free radical metabolism and pathology because of its high oxgen consumption and because its photoreceptor membranes have the highest concentration of readily oxidizable long chain polyunsaturated fatty acids of any tissue in the body (Castorina, Capisi, Di Giacomo et al, 1992). A sustained elevation of intracellular Ca^{2+} results in apoptotic cell death (Nicotera and Orsenius, 1998). Fox et al (1999) suggested that Ca^{2+} overload induced by alterations in cGMP phosphodiesterase activity may underline selective apoptotic rod cell death because Ca^{2+} enters the rod through the cGMP channel and then induces the opening of the mitochondrial permeability transition pore (PTP) by binding to the internal metal regulatory site of the mitochondrial PTP (He, Poblem, Medrano et al, 2000). In addition, Mg is related to CGMP hydrolysis in a rapid equilibrium random binding order of Mg^{2+} and cCMP to the rod phosphodiesterase (Srivastava, Fox and Hurwitz et al, 1995). Another possibility is that nitric oxide (NO) production induced by a high level of Ca might damage the RPE cells (Roth, 1997) and a higher level of Ca might cause apoptosis-like pyknosis of photoreceptor cell nuclei, because SIMS shows low Mg and high Ca levels in the retina of Mg-deficient rats. Elevated Ca^{2+} increases nitric oxide synthase in neurons and causes cytotoxicity (Nicotera and Orrenius, 1998). It has also been noted that in Mg-deficient cardiac tissue the activity of superoxide dismutase (SOD) is decreased (Kumar and Shivakumar, 1997), and in a low Mg medium SOD activity in retinal tissue is decreased (Szabo, Droy, Doly et al, 1992). Thus, disturbed metabolism and antioxidation may cause retinal damage due to Mg deficiency. A low Mg serum level is known to be accompanied by a high Ca serum level. However, it is assumed that the hypercalcemia in the Mg-deficient rat is secondary to an unknown factor (Shils, 1997).

V. The Optic Nerve

Results

Light microscopic findings

The diameter of the optic nerve of 6-week-old Mg-deficient rats was significantly shorter than that of control rats ($p<0.05$), but that of normal rats was not significantly different from that in the pair-fed control group (Table 1.5.1). The number of myelinated axons was obviously decreased only in the Mg-deficient rats (Fig. 1.5.1).

Table 1.5.1. Diameter of optic nerves.

Groups	Number of optic nerves counted	Diameter μm
Control	10	565±14
Mg-deficient	12	507±5.8
Pair-fed control	14	578±11

Diameter of optic nerves in control, pair-fed control and Mg-deficient rats measured in cross-sections taken about 3 mm behind the eyeball. There is a significant difference between the control and Mg-deficient groups ($p<0.05$). There is no significant difference between the control and pair-fed control groups ($p>0.25$).

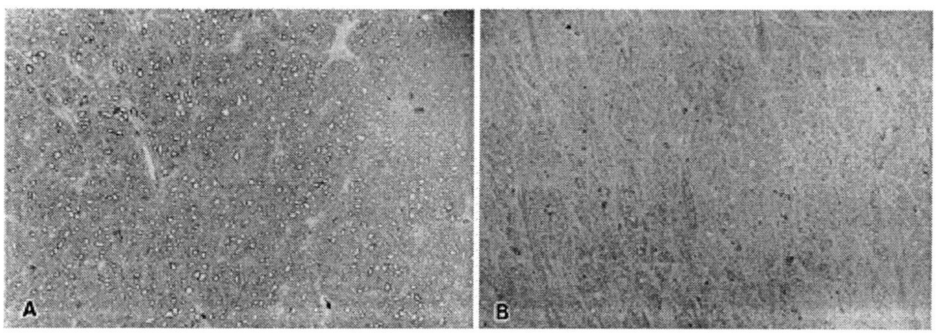

Figure 1.5.1. Light microgaphs of transverse sections of optic nerve 3 mm behind the globe stained with toluidine blue. In the control group (A), myelinated nerve fibers are round, compactly arranged and appear normal. In the Mg-deficient group (B), myelinated nerve fibers are irregular and loosely arranged and decreased. × 200 (A,B).

TEM findings

Electron microscopy of the control optic nerves showed compactly arranged myelinated nerve fibers (Fig. 1.5.2A). The myelin sheaths were thick and composed of an average of 12 layers. Axons contained neurotubules.

In the optic nerves of Mg-deficient rats, myelinated nerve fibers were prominently decreased ($p<0.001$; Table 1.5.2), and glial cells were increased (Fig. 1.5.2B). The diameters of the myelinated nerve fibers were significantly shorter ($p<0.0001$, Table 1.5.3). Small foci of necrosis were seen in the cluster of axons (Fig. 1.5.3). The myelin sheaths were thinner and the number of lamellae in myelin sheaths was much smaller than control ($p<0.0001$, Table 1.5.4) (Fig. 1.5.4). The axons were degenerated, and their myelin sheaths were deformed, destroyed and clumped (Fig. 1.5.4). There was scattered extracellular debris from the axoplasm and degenerated myelin lamellae (Fig. 1.5.5).

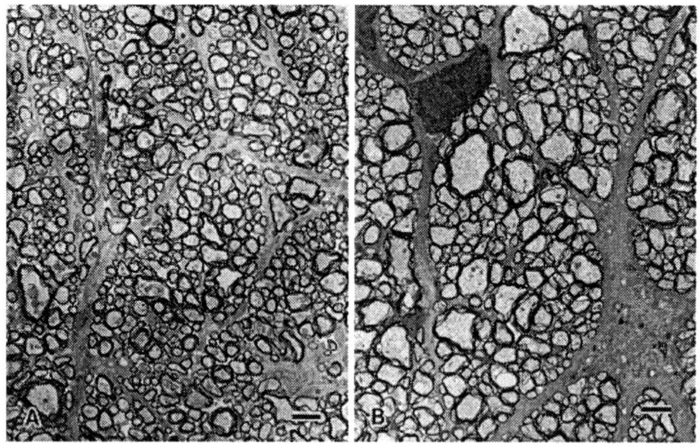

Figure 1.5.2. TEM micrographs of transverse sections of the optic nerves of control and Mg-deficient rats. (A) Myelinated nerve fibers are round and compactly arranged. Myelin sheaths are thick, and the arrangement of myelin lamellae is regular. (B) The optic nerve of a pair-fed control rat shows almost the same as that of a control rat. Bar: 2μm (A, B).

Table 1.5.2. Number of myelinated axons in optic nerves (600μm^2).

Groups	Number of optic nerves examined	Number of fields examined	Number of myelinated axons
Control	6	205	157±43
Mg-deficient	6	275	116±34
Pair-fed control	6	195	149±38

The number of myelinated axons is significantly higher in the normal control and pair-fed control groups than in the Mg-deficient group ($p<0.01$); the difference between the control and pair-fed control group is not significant ($p>0.05$).

Table 1.5.3. Diameter of myelinated nerve fibers.

Groups	Myelinated fibers counted/ optic nerves examined	Mean diameter μm
Control	228/6	0.89±0.23
Mg-deficient	276/6	0.54±0.30
Pair-fed control	176/6	0.76±0.35

The diameter of myelinated nerve fibers is significantly larger in the control and pair-fed control groups than in the Mg-deficient group ($p<0.0001$); the difference between the control and pair-fed control groups is not significant ($p>0.05$).

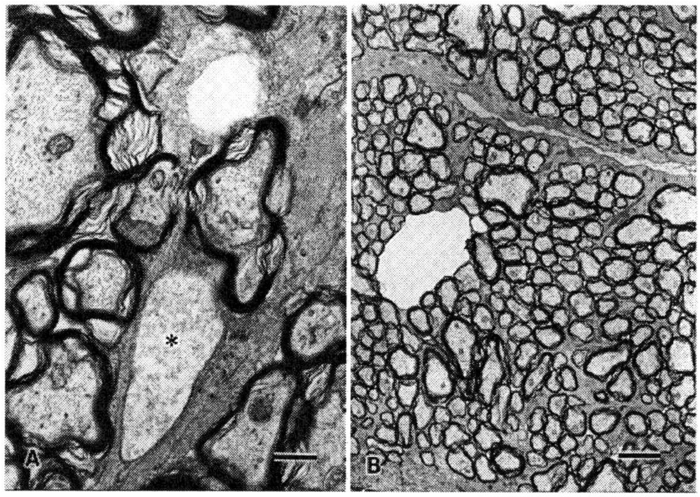

Figure 1.5.3. TEM micrograph of the optic nerve of a rat fed a Mg-deficient diet for 6 weeks. (A) Focal necrosis (*) begins at an astrocyte. (B) Focal necroses are seen in the astrocyte. Amorphous materials containing space (*) is clearly demarcated by a membrane. Myelin lamellae show irregular arrangement (A). (B) There is a completely vacant space which is surrounded by relatively normal-looking myelinated nerve fibers. Bar: 500nm (A), 2μm (B).

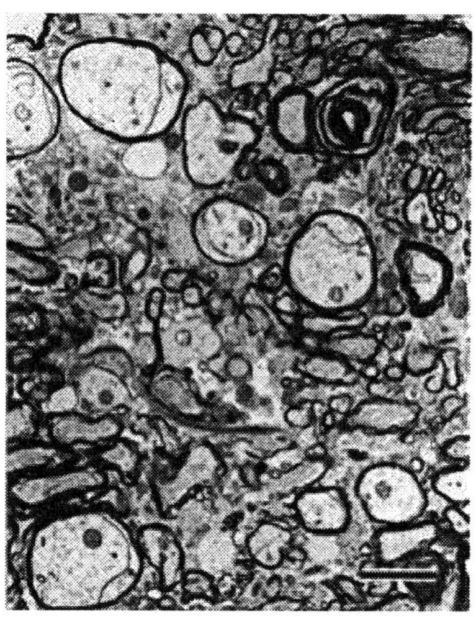

Figure 1.5.4. TEM micrograph of a transverse section of a optic nerve of a Mg-deficient rat. Myelinated nerve fibers are decreased, and myelinated axons show degeneration. Myelin sheaths are thin and destructed. Bar: 2μm.

The optic nerves of the pair-fed control rats had numerous myelinated nerve fibers densely arranged (149±38 at $600\mu m^2$) with diameters of 578±11μm. The number of myelin lamellae looked normal (Table 1.5.4). The number of myelinated nerve fibers and of myelin lamellae and the diameters of the myelinated nerve fibers were not significantly different between the controls and the pair-fed controls (Tables 1.5.1, 2, 4).

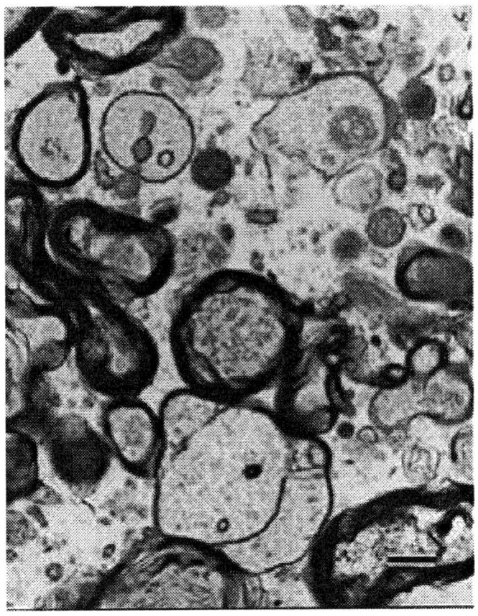

Figure 1.5.5. TEM micrograph of a transverse section of a optic nerve of a rat fed a Mg-deficient diet, showing thin myelin sheath and degenerated cytoplasmic components scattered after glial cell destruction. Bar: 500nm.

Table 1.5.4. Lamellar layers of myelinated fibers in optic nerves.

Groups	Myelinated fibers counted/ optic nerves examined	Number of layers
Control	256/6	12.8±3.4
Mg-deficient	272/6	6.7±3.7
Pair-fed control	255/6	11.8±4.2

The number of myelinated nerve fiber layers is significantly larger in the control and pair-fed control groups than in the Mg-deficient group ($p<0.0001$). The difference between the control and pair-fed control groups is not significant ($p>0.05$).

Discussion

Pair-fed control rats showed severe weight loss but no abnormal changes in the optic nerve. Thus, the changes in Mg-deficient rats must be due to Mg deficiency, not to starvation or severe weight loss. Furthermore, poor weight gain due to decreased dietary intake does not affect the early stage of ultrastructural development in the optic nerve if all nutrients are adequate.

Most intracellular Mg is associated with organic compounds and particularly with ATP (Di Polo and Beauge, 1984). Thus, a relatively small change in the percentage of bound Mg may lead to major changes in the amount of Mg^{2+} (Lester, Doll, Brumfeld et al, 1990).

Mg deficiency is also related to increased serum phospholipids, triglycerides, variable total cholesterol, low free cholesterol, increased levels of oleic and linoleic acids, decreased levels of stearic and arachidonic acids and modifications of lipid and lipoprotein concentrations (Altura, Brust, Bloom et al, 1990; Inagaki and Fujita, 1991; Kumar and Shivakumar, 1997). The activity of superoxide dismutase is also decreased in Mg-deficient cardiac tissue (Szabo, Droy, Doly et al, 1992) and in retinal tissue in vitro (Hamada, 1967). That is, Mg acts to stabilize cell membranes and cell walls. Since myelin lamellae are composed of lipids, disturbed metabolism and oxidation due to Mg deficiency may induce maldevelopment and destruction of myelin lamellae. In addition, Mg is contained in many enzymes as a cofactor and involved in essentially all kinase reactions (Shils, 1997). For instance, one of the Mg^{2+}-dependent reactions includes those catalized by thiamine pyrophosphotransferase (thiamine pyrophosphate), a key coenzyme in oxidative decarboxylation (Shils, 1997). The optic nerve requires much thiamine (Ascherio, 1997; Rayssiguier, Gueux, Bussiere et al, 1993), and the disturbance of the thiamine metabolism caused by Mg deficiency might lead to optic nerve damage.

Table 1.5.5. Optic nerve changes in deficiencies of trace elements.

	Optic nerve changes	Specificity
Mg deficiency	diameter of optic nerve: short; myelinated axons: decreased number, short diameter, decreased lamellae, thin lamellae	Multifocal lesion
Cu deficiency	myelin formation: delayed, thin myelin sheath, vacuolation, detached lamellae; nonmyelinated axons: increased number; astrocytes: increased number neurons: swollen, few neurotubules, few neurofilaments, vacuolation	
Zn deficiency	diameter of optic nerve: shorter myelinated axons: decreased, detached lamellae, vacuoles in the axons nonmyelinated axons: increased number; astrocytes: increased neurons: swollen, vacuolated, few neurofilaments	
Mn deficiency	diameter of optic nerve: shorter. myelinated axons: decreased, shorter diameter of axon, decreased number of lamellar layers, thin myelin sheath, vacuolated mitochondria. unmyelinated axons: increased oligodendrocytes: increased	

The optic nerve changes in Mg-deficient rats are very similar to those in rats with Zn, Mn or Cu deficiency: reduction in the number and size of myelinated axons, proliferation of astrocytes and oligodendrocytes and thinned and decreased myelin lamellae (Table 1.5.5) (Dake and Amemiya, 1991; Mishima Dake, Amemiya et al, 1996; Gong and Amemiya 1999; Gong and Amemiya, 2001). The optic nerve has a relatively simple structure: almost entirely myelinated axons and neurons. Deficiencies of Zn, Cu and Mn in superoxide dismutases seem to induce oxidation of lipid-rich myelin. Thus the common oxidative injury to myelin membranes in Zn, Cu, Mn and Mg deficiencies may induce very similar changes in the optic nerve although the lipid peroxidation process in Mg deficiency appears to be different from that seen in deficiencies of other trace elements through lipid peroxidation products (Nicotera and Orrenius, 1998). However, Mg deficiency shows a specific finding: mulifocal lesions in the optic nerve. Mg deficiency tends to induce multifocal cellular necrosis in the myocardium and RPE (Gong and Amemiya, 2001). Such foci of necrosis were even seen in the optic nerve in the current study. Necrotic foci were not always found in every tissue slice. Some showed no necrotic foci. The high death rate and severe general disturbances due to Mg deficiency mean that Mg is an essential trace element for life and that Mg deficiency may affect not only the optic nerve and retina (Gong, Amemiya and Takaya et al, 2001) but also the central nervous system in general. The author assumes that a small focus of necrosis occurs first in the optic nerve (Fig. 1.5.3) then extends to the severe wide degenerative lesions seen in Figs 1.5.4 and 5. Although the exact reason for focal necrosis is not known, it might be due to the absence of certain Mg-associated enzymes in each cell and/or tissue.

Several studies of trace elements have shown that deficiencies of Zn, Cu and Mn cause demyelination or destruction of the optic nerve fibers as was found in our study of Mg deficiency (Dake and Amemiya, 1991; Mishima, Dake, Amemiya et al, 1996; Gong and Amemiya, 1999). It is assumed that myelin lamellae composed of lipid membranes are oxidized and destroyed by Zn, Cu or Mn deficiency because these trace elements are present in superoxide dismutase, which prevents oxidation of the lipid membrane. Acyl CoA synthetase involved in Mg^{2+}-dependent reactions is related to fatty acyl CoA, the first product in the ß-oxidation of fatty acid (Shils, 1997). Thus the decreased activity of this synthetase due to Mg deficiency may induce maldevelopment and degeneration of myelin. The high level of Ca in the current study might induce nitric oxide production and damage the myelin lamellae and axons because elevated Ca^{2+} causes nitric oxide synthetase in neurons and nitric cytotoxicity (Di Polo and Beauge, 1981).

There is a controversy as to how nerve cells manage to maintain an exceedingly low Ca^{2+} concentration against very large electrochemical Ca^{2+} gradients. Di Polo and Beauge (1981) showed Ca^{2+}-Mg^{2+}-ATPase activity and Ca^{2+}-Mg^{2+}-dependent phosphorylation from ATP in plasma membrane fragments from squid optic nerves, which might be the mechanism responsible for the maintenance of the low-level of ionized Ca concentration in the nerve. In Mg deficiency, the optic nerve might not maintain its normal ATP-derived uncoupled Ca^{2+} pump with the result that myelinated nerve axons would be damaged.

The degeneration of the optic nerve in Mg deficiency might occur through secondary retrograde degeneration following retinal degeneration. However, in the same experiment, the retinal changes due to Mg deficiency are multifocal necrosis in the RPE and slight apoptosis-like pyknosis without prominent destruction of whole photoreceptor cells. It is assumed that Mg-deficient rats die too early to show the extension of photoreceptor and pigment epithelial lesions to the ganglion cells. Thus, it is less probable that myelin loss is secondary to retrograde loss of axons initiated by the loss of retinal fibers.

In the current study, infant rats were raised under low-magnesium conditions from the early stage of ocular development. Thus, poor myelination of axons may be due to maldevelopment as well as to destruction of myelin lamellae.

REFERENCES

Altura BT, Brust M, Bloom S, Barbour RL, Stempak JG, Altura BM. Magnesium dietary intake modulates blood lipid levels and atherogenesis. *Proc Natl Acad Sci USA.* 1990;87:1840-1844.

Ascherio A. Antimetabolites and an optic neuropathy epidemic in Cuba. *Am J Clin Nutr.* 1997;65:1092-1093.

Bachman WG, Wilson G. Essential ions for maintenance of the corneal epithelial surface. *Invest Ophthalmol Vis Sci.* 1985;26:1484-1488.

Black CB, Cowan JA. Magnesium dependent enzymes in general metabolism. In Cowan AJ, ed. *The Biologic Chemistry of Magnesium.* UK:VCH Publishers; 1995: 159-183.

Bunce GE, Saacke RG, Mulins J. The morphology and pathogenesis of magnesium deficiency-induced nephrocalcinosis. *Exp Mol Pathol.* 1980;33:203-210.

Caddell JL. Magnesium therapy in premature neonates with apnea neonatorum. *J Am Coll Nutr.* 1988;7:5-16.

Caddell JL. Hypothesis: The possible role of magnesium and copper deficiency in retinopathy of prematurity. *Magnes Res.* 1995;8:261-270.

Castorina C, Capisi A, Di Giacomo C, Sorrenti B, Russo A, Vanella A. Lipid peroxidation and antioxidant enzymatic systems in rat retina as a function of age. *Neurochem Res.* 1992;17:599-604.

Covacci V, Bruzzese N, Sgambato A, Janapathi R, Cittadini A, Wolf F. Effect of extra-cellular magnesium on topoisomerase II activity and expression in human leukemia HL-60 cells. *J Cell Biochem.* 2000;78:325-333.

Cowan JA. Introduction to the biologic chemistry of magnesium ion. In Cowan JA, ed. *The Biologic Chemistry of Magnesium.* UK:VCH Publishers;1995:1-23.

Dake Y, Amemiya T. Electron microscopic study of the optic nerve in copper deficient rats. *Exp Eye Res.* 1991;52:277-281.

DiPolo R, Beauge L. The effects of vanadate on calcium transport in dialyzed squid axons: Sidedness of vanadate-cation interactions. *Biochim Biophys Acta.* 1981;645:229-236.

DiPolo R, Beauge L. Interactions of physiological ligands with the Ca pump and Na/Ca exchange in squid axons. *J Gen Physiol.* 1984;84:895-914.

Elwood PC, Sweetnam PM, Beasley WH, Jones D, France R. Magnesium and calcium in the myocardium: cause of death and area differences. *Lancet.* 1980;2:720-722.

Farber DB, Lolley RN. Calcium and magnesium content of rodent photoreceptor cells as inferred from studies of retinal degeneration. *Exp Eye Res.* 1976;22:219-228.

Fox DA, Poblenz AT, He L. Calcium overload triggers rod photoreceptor apoptotic cell death in chemical-induced and inherited retinal degenerations. *Ann NY Acad Sci.* 1999;893:282-285.

Galle J, Mohr W, Lossnitzer K, Haferkamp O. Development of necrosis and its sequelae in the myocardium of polymyopathic hamsters (BIO 8262): An electron microscopic study. *Virchows Arch B Cell Pathol Incl Mol Pathol.* 1981;36:87-100.

Gass JD. Acute posterior multifocal placoid pigment epitheliopathy. Arch Ophthalmol. 1968;80:177-185.

Geuex E, Mazur A, Cardot P, Rayssiguier Y. Magnesium deficiency affects plasma lipoproteins in rats. *J Nutr.* 1991;121:1222-1227.

Gibson BL, Reife LL. Mg^{2+} reduces N-methyl-D-asparate neurotoxicity in embryonic chick neural retina in vitro. *Neurosci Lett.* 1985;57:13-18.

Gong H, Amemiya T. Optic nerve changes in magnesium-deficient rats. *Exp Eye Res.* 1999;68:313-320.

Gong H, Amemiya T, Takaya K. Retinal changes in magnesium deficient rats. *Exp Eye Res.* 2001;72:23-32.

Gong H, Amemiya T. Optic nerve changes in zinc-deficient rat. *Exp Eye Res.* 2001;72:363-369.

Gong H, Takami Y, Amemiya T, Tozu M, Ohashi Y. Ocular surface in Zn-deficient rats. *Ophthalmic Res.* 2004;36:129-138.

Hamada S. Experimental studies on influences of elevation of the intra-ocular pressure on thiamine contents in the ocular tissue. II. Concentrations of thiamine in the retina and the optic nerve of white rabbits with elevated intra-ocular pressure. *Nippon Ganka Gakkai Zasshi.* 1967;71:493-501.

He L, Poblenz AT, Medrano CJ, Fox DA. Lead and calcium produce rod photoreceptor cell apoptosis by opening the mitochondrial permeability transition pore. *J Biol Chem.* 2000;275:12175-12184.

Herse P, Adams L. Effect of hyperglycemia duration on rabbit corneal thichness and endothelial ATPase activity. *Acta Ophthalmol Scand.* 1995;73:158-161.

Inagaki O, Fujita Y. Long term effect of magnesium on lipid metabolism in uraemic rats. *Magnes Res.* 1991;4:191-195.

Ito M, Toda T, Kummerow FA, Nishimori I. Effect of magnesium deficiency on ultra-structural changes in coronary arteries of swine. *Acta Pathol Jpn.* 1986,36:225-234.

Kaneko A, Shimazaki H. Effects of external ions on the synaptic transmission from photoreceptors to horizontal cells in the carp retina. *J Psychol.* 1975;252:509-522.

Kumar BP, Shivakumar K. Depressed antioxidant defense in rat heart in experimental magnesium deficiency: Implications for the pathogenesis of myocardinal lesions. *Biol Trace Element Res.* 1997;60:139-144.

Langdon RB, Manis PB, Freeman JA. Goldfish retinotectal transmission in vitro: Component current sink-source pairs isolated by varying calcium and magnesium levels. *Brain Res.* 1988;441:299-308.

Lester DS, Doll I, Brumfeld V, Miller IR. Lipid dependence of surface conformation of protein kinase C. *Biochim Biophys Acta.* 1990;1039:33-41.

Maynard KI, Quinones HA, Ogilvy CS. Magnesium plus mexiletine inhibit energy usage and protect retinas against ischemia. *NeuroReport.* 1998;9:4141-4144

McCarron DA. Calcium and magnesium nutrition in human hypertension. *Ann. Internal Med.* 1983;98:800-805.

Mishima K, Dake Y, Amemiya T, Nishimura M. Electron microscopic study of optic nerves of macular mice. *Eye Eye Res.* 1996;63;85-90.

Nicotera P, Orrenius S. The role of calcium in apoptosis. *Cell Calcium.* 1998;23:173-180.

Ottlecz A,. Garcia CA, Eichberg J, Fox DA. Alteration in retinal Na^{+}, K^{+} ATPase in diabetes: streptozotocin-induced and zucker diabetic fatty rats. *Curr Eye Res.* 1993;12:111-121.

Pasquare SJ, Giusto NM. Differential properties of phosphatidate phosphohydrolase and diacylglyceride lipase activities in retinal subcellular fractions and rod outer segments. *Comp Biochem Physiol B Biochem*. 1993;104:141-148.

Rayssiguier Y, Gueux E, Bussiere L, Durlach J, Mazur A. Dietary magnesium affects susceptibility of lipoproteins and tissues to peroxidation in rats. *J Am Coll Nutr*. 1993;12:113-117.

Reinach P, Holmberg N. Calcium stimulated Mg dependent ATPase activity in a plasma membrane enriched fraction of bovine corneal epithelium. *Curr Eye Res*. 1987;6:399-405.

Riley MV. The role of the epithelium in control of corneal hydration. *Exp Eye Res*. 1971;12:128-137.

Roth S. Role of nitric oxide in retinal cell death. *Clin Neurosci*. 1997;4:216-223.

Salvador GA, Giusto NM. Characterization of phospholipase D activity in bovine photoreceptor membranes. *Lipids*. 1998;33:853-860.

Schmidt KF. Divalent cations modulate glutamate receptors in retinal horizontal cells of the perch (Perca fluviatilis). *Neurosci Lett*. 1999;262:109-112.

Shils ME. Magnesium. In O'Dell BL, Sunde RA, ed. *Handbook of Nutritionally Essential Mineral Elements*. New York: Marcel Dekker;1997:117-152.

Somlyo AP, Walz B. Elemental distribution in Rana pipiens retinal rods: quantitative electron probe analysis. *J Psychol*. 985;358:183-195.

Srivastava P, Fox DA, Hurwitz RL. Effects of manganese on cyclic GMP hydrolysis by the bovine retinal rod cyclic GMP phosphodiesterase. *Biochem J*. 1995;308:653-658.

Szabo ME, Droy LM, Doly M, Braquet P. Ischaemia — and reperfusion-induced Na^+, K^+, Ca^{2+} and Mg^{2+} shifts in rat retina: Effects of two free radical scavengers, SOD and EGB 761. *Exp Eye Res*. 1992;55:39-45.

Van RL, Bazan NG. Cationic amphiphilic drugs perturb the metabolism of inosititides and phosphatidic acid in photoreceptor membranes. *Biochem Biophys Res*. 1986a;134:378-385.

Van RL, Bazan NG. The inositide cycle in bovine photoreceptor membranes. *Life Sci*. 1986b;38:1685-1693.

Whikehart DR, Montaomery B, Wells JD. Age as a function of ATPase activity in cultured corneal endothelial cells. *Invest Ophthalmol Vis Sci*. 1989;30:335-338.

Whikehart DR, Montaomery B, Angelos P, Sorna D. Alteration of ATPase activity and duplex DNA in corneal cells grown in high glucose media. *Cornea*. 1993;12:295-298.

Yao XY, Endo EG, Marmor MF. Reversibility of retinal adhesion in the rabbit. *Invest Ophthalmol Vis Sci*. 1989;30:220-224.

Yao XY, Hageman GS, Marmor MF. Retinal adhesiveness in the monkey. *Invest Ophthalmol Vis Sci*. 1994;35:744-748.

Chapter 2

ZINC

I. SIGNIFICANCE

According to King and Keen (1999), zinc (Zn) essentiality was shown in animals in 1934 and Zn-deficiency syndrome in humans was demonstrated in 1956. Prasad et al (1963) indicated that the endemic hypogonadism and dwarfism in rural Iran is derived from Zn deficiency. Zn prevails in all organs, tissues, fluids, and secretions of the body and exists in cells as an intracellular ion with well over 95% of total-body Zn. Although Zn is associated with all organelles of the cell, about 60 to 80% of the cellular Zn is contained in the cytosol. Disposition of Zn within the cell is diverse. In the cell Zn may be used by the cell for Zn-dependent processes, become bound firmly to metallothionein and held within the cell, or pass through the cell. Zn, a metalloenzyme, has a catalytic, structural, or regulatory role. Over 200 Zn enzymes have been found in biologic systems.

Signs and symptoms of Zn deficiency in experimental animals are anorexia, cyclic feeding, growth retardation, dermatitis, abnormal bone growth and maturation. Many malformations due to Zn deficiency have been reported including eye defects.

Clinical manifestations of human Zn deficiency are growth retardation, delayed sexual maturation and impotence, hypooadism and hypospermia, alopecia, acroorificial skin lesions, other epithelial lesions including glossitis, alopecia, and nail dystrophy, immune deficiencies, night blindness, impaired taste, delayed healing of wounds, burns, and decubitus ulcers, impaired appetite and food intake and ocular symptoms such as photophobia and impaired dark adaptation.

Ocular tissues in humans contain high concentrations of Zn (Tauber and Krause, 1943; Galin, Nano and Hall, 1962; Yolton, 1981; Karcioglu, 1982). The descending order of Zn concentration in intraocular tissues is the retina, choroid, ciliary body, iris, optic nerve, sclera, cornea and lens (Tauber and Krause, 1943; Hirayama, 1990). Zn deficiency has been encountered sporadically when patients have been maintained on total parenteral nutrition with highly purified solutions lacking adequate Zn (Hamit, David and Stevens, 1980; Ortega, Cuchaza, Tovar et al, 1985; Sandstead, 1989). Zn deficient conditions occur in chronic alcoholism, (Prasad, 1985; Akar and Arcasoy, 1990; Vannucchi, Favaro, Cunha et al, 1995), liver cirrhosis (Scholmerich, Lohle, Kottgen et al, 1983; Ozsoylú, Kocak and Akgun, 1991), Crohn's disease (Heimburger, Tamura and Marks, 1990; Myung, Yang, Jung et al, 1998) and acrodermatitis enteropathia (Sturtevant, 1980; Chesters, 1997; Muga and Grider, 1999) and the administration of drugs such as ethambutol (Yolton, 1981), disulfiram and penicillamine (Klingberg, Prasad and Oberleas, 1976; Weismann, 1986).

II. Zn-Deficiency Experiment

Material and Methods

Twenty-one-day old male Wistar Kyoto rats weighing 40-50g were divided randomly into Zn-deficient and control groups. All rats were fed a commercially prepared Zn-deficient powdered diet obtained from Clea Japan Inc., Tokyo. This diet contained 0.007mg Zn per 100g and was complete in all other nutrients. Zn-deficient and control groups received the diet ad libitum. Distilled and deionized water was given freely to the Zn-deficient group, and the same water supplemented with 3mg Zn per 100g water to the control group. Recovery experiments were as follows. Rats fed a Zn-deficient diet for 7 weeks were freely given the Zn-deficient diet, but deionized water with 3mg Zn per 100g. The animals were killed 5 weeks later.

The Pair-fed control experiment: To confirm that the changes in Zn-deficient rats are due to Zn deficiency, not to starvation or severe weight loss, pair-fed control experiment was done as follows; in the pair-fed control group, infant rats were suckled by their mother rats fed a Zn-deficient diet and water supplemented with 3 mg Zn/100ml for 3 weeks, then for 7 weeks, they were given the Zn-containing water and the same amount of the diet that the Zn-deficient rats had taken on the previous day, then killed under anesthesia.

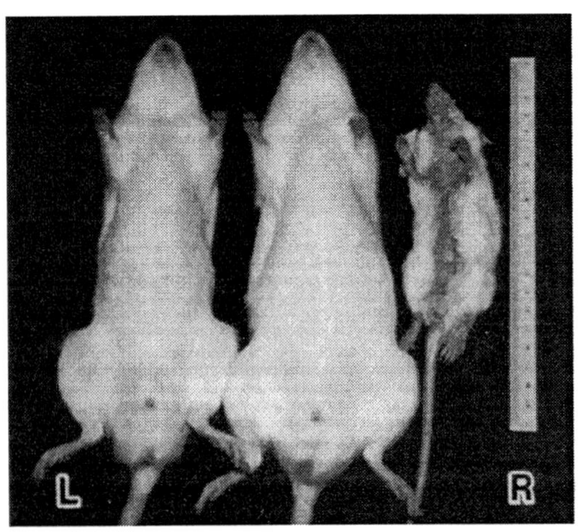

Figure 2.2.1. R: Gross appearance of a rat fed a Zn-deficient diet for 7 weeks; in the middle is an age-equivalent control rat; L, A rat given Zn-supplemented water for 5 weeks after 7 weeks on a Zn-deficient diet. The Zn-deficient rat exhibits extreme emaciation, marked hair loss and a small body, while the recovery rat is almost normal in appearance. The middle is a normal control rat.

Table 2.2.1. The body weight and the serum Zn concentration of control, Zn-deficient, recovery and pair-fed control rats (mean±SD).

Groups	Body Weight (g)	Age (week)	Serum Zn levels (μg/dl)	Age (week)
Control	194.3±39 * (N=8)	10-week-old	182.4±7 † (N=8)	10-week-old
Normal	410±30 (N=8)	18-week-old	177±12 † (N=6)	18-week-old
Zn-deficient	77.14±7 *, ** (N=7)	10-week-old	81.7±33 †, †† (N=7)	10-week-old
Recovery	390±15 * (N=9)	18-week-old	165.6±11 †, †† (N=9)	18-week-old
Pair-fed	104±7 *, ** (N=7)	10-week-old	131.9±9 †, †† (N=7)	10-week-old

Both the normal and the recovery rats are significantly heavier than the Zn deficient and pair-fed control rats (* $p<0.0001$); even the weights of the Zn-deficient and the pair-fed control rats are significantly different (** $p=0.03$).
The serum Zn level of the normal rats are significantly higher than those of the Zn-deficient, recovery and pair-fed control rats († $p<0.001$), and those of the recovery and pair-fed control rats are also significantly higher than those of the Zn-deficient rats (†† $p<0.001$).

Clinical Features of the Zn-Deficient Animal

In comparison with the values in the control group, serum Zn levels and body weight of Zn-deficient groups were obviously decreased at 4 and 7 weeks; the difference in Zn levels between the experimental and control groups was statistically significant at $p<0.001$ at 4 and $p<0.002$ at 7 weeks (Table 2.2.1). Growth retardation was already noted in the Zn-deficient rats by the end of the first week of the experiment. After the first week most of the Zn-deficient rats showed hair loss around the eyes and on the extremities. After 4 weeks on the diet, the Zn-deficient rats were much smaller than the controls (Fig. 2.2.1) and most of them died by the 7th week. The body weight of the Zn-deficient rats was significantly lower than that of the control rats (Table 2.2.2). In the recovery group, the serum levels of Zn reached almost the normal level and all symptoms disappeared.

Table 2.2.2. Body weight of the experimental rat (g)

Groups	Weeks after start of experiment		Weeks of recovery experiment
	4	7	5
Control	235.0±17.3 *(n=5)	342.5±91.0 *(n=5)	380.0±18.4 (n=5)
Zn-deficient	51.7±8.6 (n=8)	105.0±19.0 (n=5)	-
Recovery	-	-	250.0(n=1)

* $p<0.0001$ (Fisher's Protected Least Significant Difference). n=number of animals examined.

III. THE CONJUNCTIVA AND CORNEA

Scanning Electron Microscopic(SEM) Findings

The conjunctiva: The control conjunctiva showed a majority of clear cells with well-developed microvilli in the most superficial layer of the epithelium (Fig. 2.3.1). Goblet cells were frequently seen and have well-developed and expanded secretory granules (Fig. 2.3.1). In the Zn-deficient rats, on the other hand, microvilli of the most superficial layer of the epithelium were prominently reduced while the dark cells were prominently increased (Fig. 2.3.2). Goblet cells were also decreased in number (Fig. 2.3.2) (Table 2.3.1: $P<0.001$). The goblet cells of the Zn-deficient rats showed shrinkage, were small and irregular in shape and had poorly developed secretory granules which looked empty (Fig. 2.3.2).

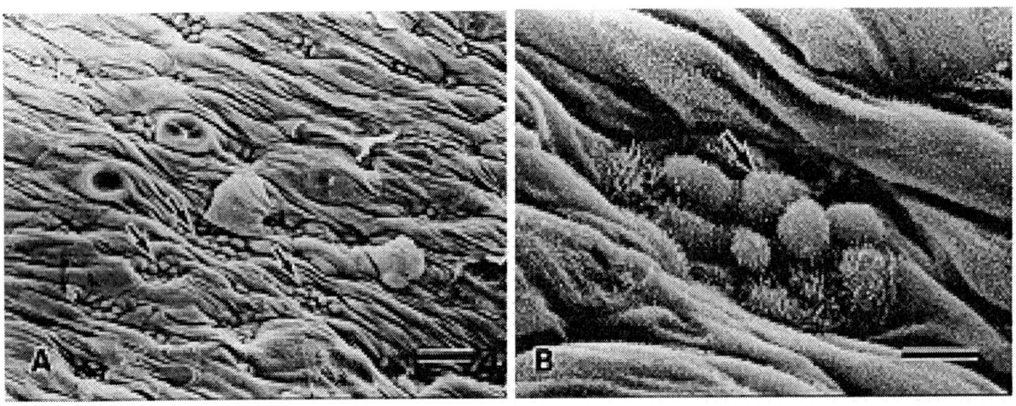

Figure 2.3.1. SEM micrographs of the conjunctival epithelium of control rats. A. A control rat shows many goblet cells with well-developed granules (arrows). B. Magnified view of the conjunctival surface and goblet cell of a control rat. The conjunctival epithelium shows numerous fine microvilli. A goblet cell with well-developed granules (arrow) is seen. Bar: A: 20μm; B: 5μm.

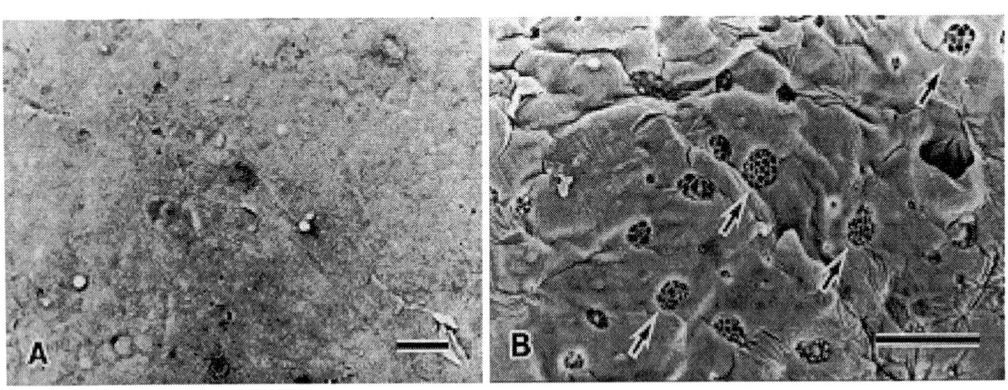

Figure 2.3.2. SEM micrographs of the conjunctival epithelium of Zn-deficient rats. A: The most superficial layer of the epithelium has lost microvilli, and no goblet cells are seen in this area. B: The conjunctival surface with goblet cells shows no microvilli. Goblet cells are irregular in shape and contain poorly developed secretory granules which look empty (arrows). Bar: A: 20μm; B: 50μn.

The cornea: The control corneas showed numerous microvilli and microplicae in the most superficial layer of the epithelium and a majority of clear cells. There were round holes in the epithelium (Fig. 2.3.3). On the other hand, the most superficial layer of the epithelium of the Zn-deficient rats had lost most of the microvilli and microplicae and had a majority of dark cells (Fig. 2.3.4).

In the rats recovered from Zn deficiency, the conjunctiva and cornea showed well-developed microvilli and microplicae in the epithelial cells and many goblet cells with well-developed secretory granules (Fig. 2.3.5).

Table 2.3.1. Numbers of goblet cells in conjunctiva.

Groups	Number of Fields Examined	Number of goblet cells / 300×200μm^2
Control	40	13.9±1.1*, ‡
Zn-deficient	56	9.2±3.4*,**, ***
Recovery	47	17.42±0.8**
Pair-fed control	42	12.8±2.2***, ‡

There are significantly more goblet cells in the conjunctiva of the control, pair-fed control and recovery groups than in that of the Zn-deficient group ($p<0.001$, $p<0.005$), but not between the control and pair-fed control groups ($p>0.05$). *, *** $p<0.001$; ** $p<0.05$; ‡ $p<0.05$.

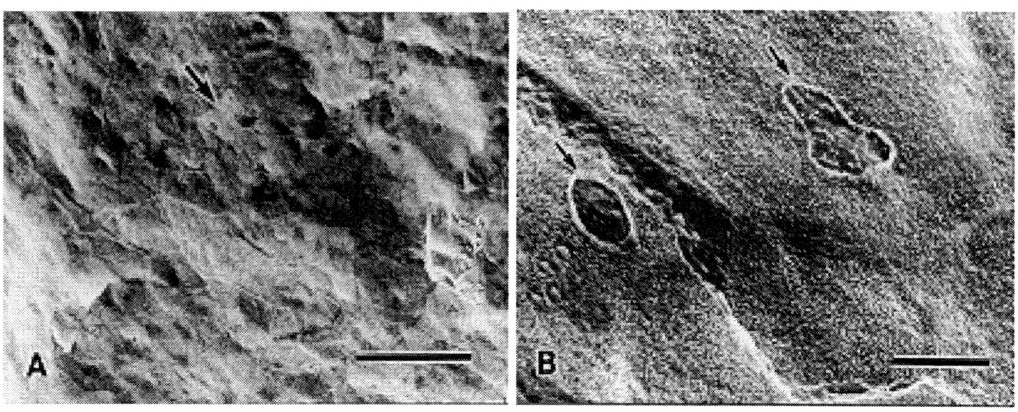

Figure 2.3.3. SEM micrographs of corneal epithelium of control rats. A: A low magnification of the epithelial surface shows many light cells with a high density of microvilli and microplicae. B: A higher magnification of most superficial corneal epithelium at the site of the arrow in Fig.2.3.3A shows numerous microvilli and microplicae and two epithelial holes (arrows). Bar: A: 50μm; B: 5μm.

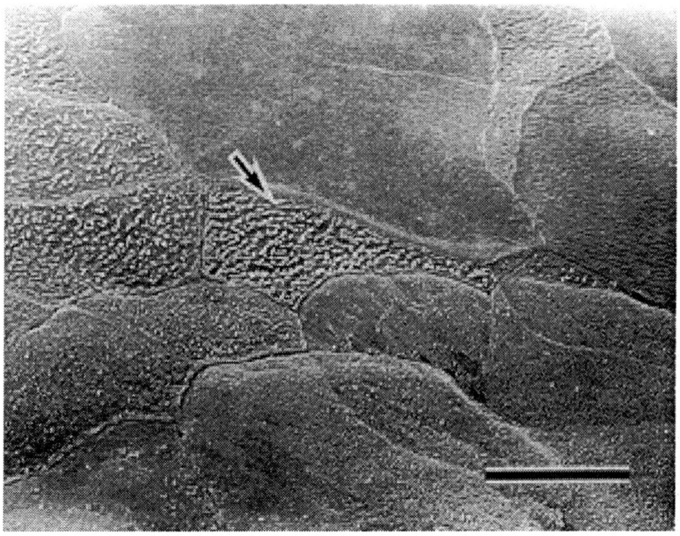

Figure 2.3.4. SEM micrograph of corneal epithelium of Zn-deficient rats. There are many dark cells with scarce microvilli in the most superficial epithelium. In light cells (arrow) microvilli remain but are not well-developed and are scattered. Bar: 10μm.

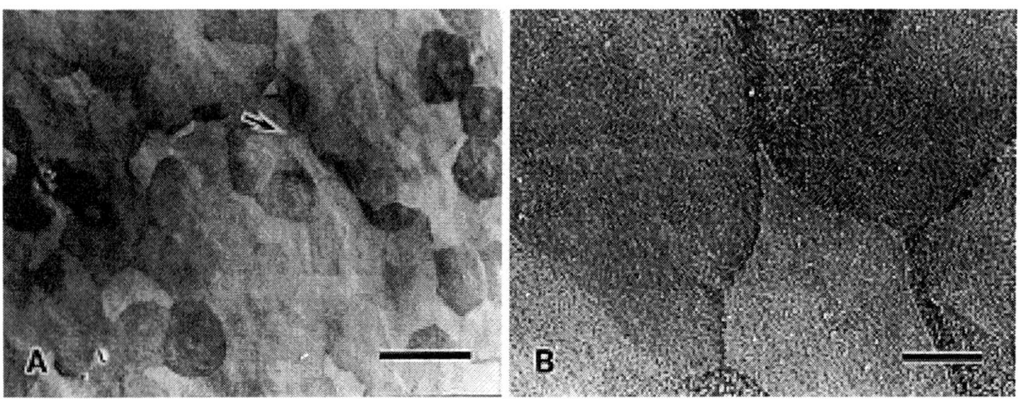

Figure 2.3.5. SEM micrographs of the corneal epithelium of rats recovered from Zn deficiency. There are many light cells (A) with numerous microvilli and microplicae (B). An arrow indicates a magnified site of Fig.2.3.5A. Bar: A: 50μm; B: 5μm.

TEM Findings

The conjunctiva: In the control rats the goblet cells showed well-developed secretory granules expansively filling the cytoplasm and compressing the nuclear to the basal portion (Fig. 2.3.6A). In the Zn-deficient rats, however, the remaining goblet cells showed a shrinkage pattern: small in size, with decreased and shrunken secretory granules, and a closed secretory orifice (Fig. 2.3.6B).

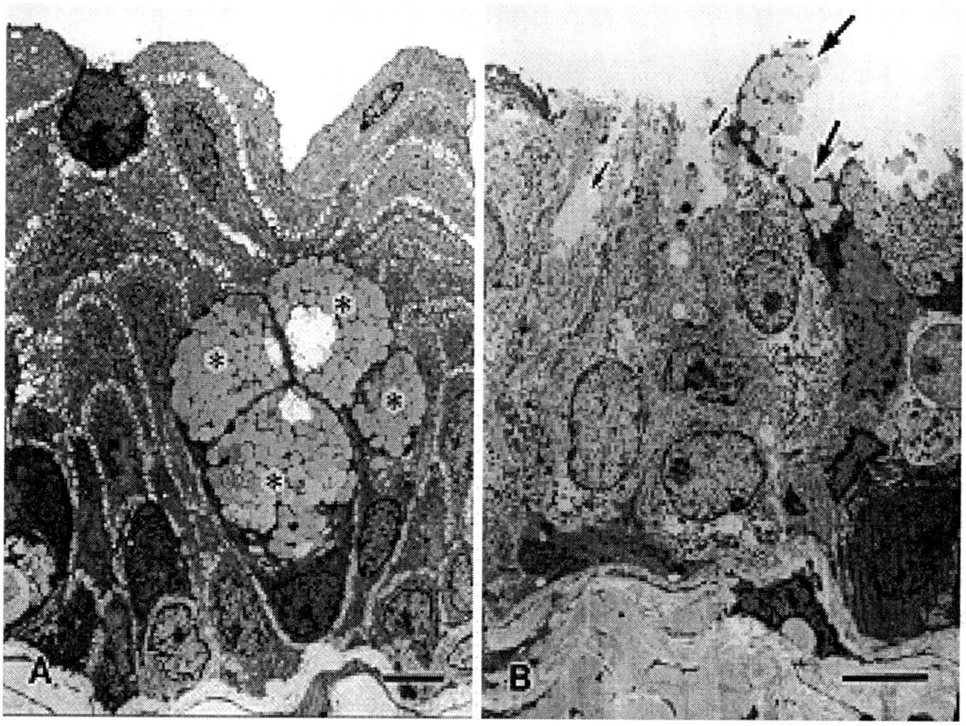

Figure 2.3.6. TEM micrographs of conjunctival epithelium of control and Zn-deficient rats. A: A control rat shows fine microvilli and goblet cells with well-developed granules (asterisks). B: In a Zn-deficient rat, some goblet cells (thin arrows) have no granules, while other (thick arrows) keep a few granules. Bar: A: 5μm; B: 5μm.

The cornea: In the control rats the most superficial epithelial cells had many microvilli, and epithelial cells contained many fibrils and tonofibrils, many desmosome-like intercellular junctions and nuclei with diffusely distributed chromatin granules (Fig. 2.3.7A, B). In the Zn-deficient rats, however, microvilli and microplicae in the most superficial epithelial cells were poorly developed (Fig. 2.3.7C, D). The epithelial cell cytoplasm had decreased fibrils and tonofibrils and desmosome-like attachments with scarce fibrils. The nucleus had clumped chromatin granules (Fig. 2.3.7C, D).

The rats recovered from Zn deficiency had many microvilli, fibrils and desmosome-like intercellular attachments in the epithelial cells of the conjunctiva (Fig. 2.3.8A) and cornea (Fig. 2.3.8B). The goblet cells contained well-developed secretory granules (Fig. 2.3.8A).

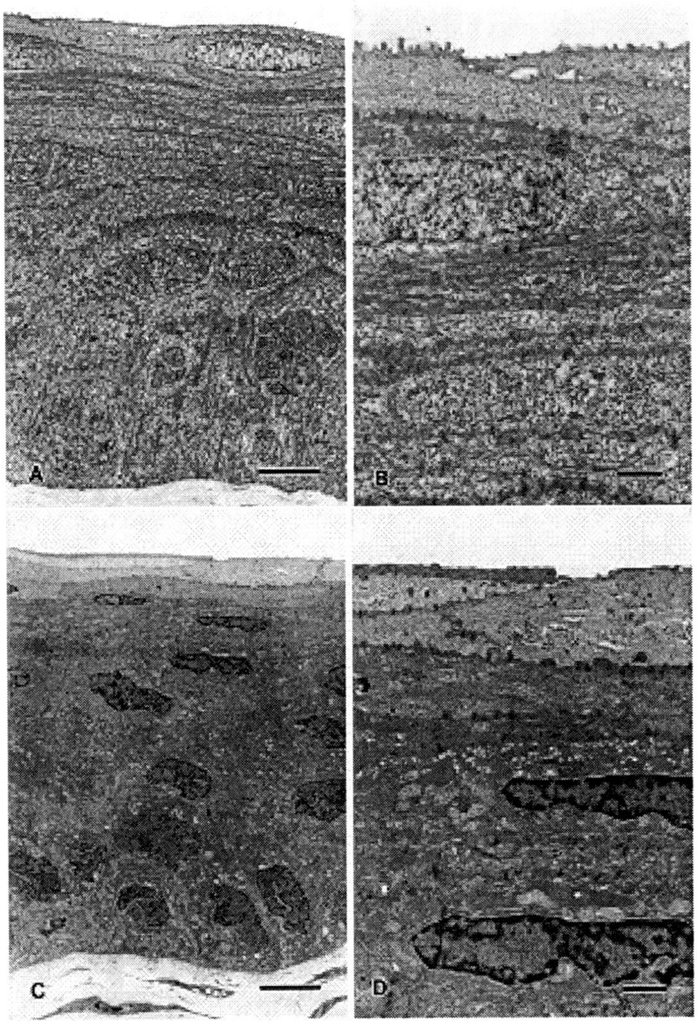

Figure 2.3.7. TEM micrographs of corneal epithelium of control and Zn-deficient rats. A: A low magnification of whole epithelial layers of a control rat shows compactly arranged epithelial cells. The most superficial epithelial cell has microvilli and epithelial cell nuclei have widely distributed chromatin granules and epithelial cytoplasm contains many ribosomes and fibrils. B: Magnified view of epithelium of the control rat cornea shows prominent microvilli in the most superficial epithelium, many desmosome-like intercellular junctions and ribosomes and fibrils in the cytoplasm. C: In the corneal epithelium of a Zn-deficient rat the nucleus is irregular in contour and has dense chromatin granules at the nuclear margin. There are many dark cells. D: In the corneal epithelium of a Zn-deficient rat microvilli are scarce in the most superficial epithelium and many dark cells are seen. Bar: A: 5μm; B: 1μm; C:5μm; D:1μm.

Element Analysis

In the conjunctiva, TOF-SIMS could detect the elements Zn, Na, Mg, K, Ca, and Fe with a primary positive Ga^+ ion source and S, P, Cl with a primary negative Ga^+ ion source. Tables 2.3.2 and 2.3.3 show statistically significant differences in the counts of each ion between the control and Zn-deficient groups. In the Zn-deficient group, Zn, Ca, Al and S counts were significantly lower than in the control group. On the other hand, K, Fe and Cl counts in the Zn-deficient group were significantly higher than in the control group. The counts of the other elements were not significantly different between the two groups. Although vitamins A and E could be detected, no significant difference was found between the control and Zn-deficient groups.

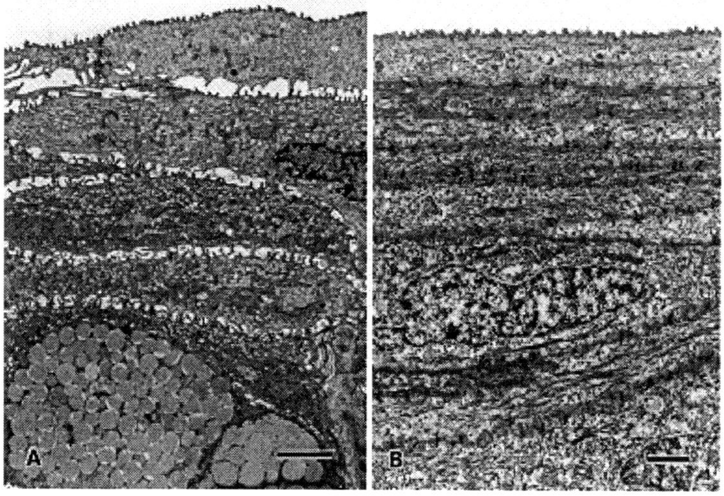

Figure 2.3.8. TEM micrographs of the conjunctival and corneal epithelia of rats recovered from Zn-deficiency. A: The epithelium of the conjunctiva of a recovered rat has well-developed microvilli in the most superficial epithelium and goblet cells filled with well-developed granules. B: The corneal epithelium of a recovered rat has well-developed microvilli in the most superficial epithelium; many desmosome-like intercellular junctions are seen, and fibrils are well-developed in the epithelial cytoplasm. Bar: A: 2μm; B: 1μm.

Table 2.3.2. Distributions of trace elements examined with TOF-SIMS by positive primary ion.

Conjunctiva	K	Ca	Fe	Al	Zn
Control	0.03±9.7E-3 n=6	6.6E-5±1.5E-5 n=6	1.3E-4±1.9E-5 n=6	3.3E-5±9.1E-6 n=6	7.9E-5±3.9E-5 n=6
Zn-deficient	0.06±0.02E-3 ↑ n=9	2.4E-5±1.8E-5 ↓ n=9	7.2E-5±1.4E-5 ↑ n=9	1.1E-5±3.2E-6 ↓ n=9	1.6E-5±1.2E-5 n=9
p value	<0.0105	<0.0002	<0.0001	<0.0001	<0.0003
Cornea		Ca			
Control	---	1.8E-5±8.0E-6 n=4	---	---	---
Zn-deficient	---	8.4E-6±1.2E-6 ↓ n=5	---	---	---
p value		<0.0188			

Table 2.3.3. Distributions of trace elements examined with TOF-SIMS by negative primary ion.

Conjunctiva	S	Cl	Vit. C
Control	7.6E-4±7.2E-5 *	2.0E-3±2.8E-5 †	5.2E-5±1.1E-5 #
	n=3	n=3	n=6
Zn-deficient	1.1E-3±1.4E-4 *, ** ↑	3.5E-3±9.2E-4 †, ‡↑	3.9E-5±5.8E-6 # ↓
	n=5	n=6	n=9
Recovery	8.3E-4±6.3E-5 **	2.1E-3±1.7E-4 ‡	---
	n=3	n=3	
p value	*<0.006	†<0.0002	#<0.0164
	**<0.002	‡<0.0002	
Cornea		**Ca**	**Vit. C**
Control	---	6.9E-3±1.9E-3 §	4.4E-5±8.6E-6 ¶
		n=4	n=4
Zn-deficient	---	0.014±7.1E-5 § ↑	2.8E-5±2.1E-6 ¶ ↓
		n=2	n=5
p value	---	§<0.0301	¶<0.038

In the cornea, authors detected the following elements with a primary positive Ga^+ ion source: Zn, Na, Mg, K, Ca, and Fe; and with a primary negative Ga^+ ion source S, P, Cl. Tables 2.3.2 and 2.3.3 show statistically significant differences in the ion counts of the elements between the control and Zn-deficient groups; the Cl and S count is significantly higher in the Zn-deficient than in the control group, while Ca is significantly less in the Zn-deficient group. The other elements showed no significant difference between the control and Zn-deficient groups. Although vitamins A and E could be detected, no significant difference was found between the control and Zn-deficient groups. However, the vitamin C level in the Zn-deficient group was significantly lower than in the control group ($P<0.0164$).

In pair-fed control rats, the conjunctiva and cornea showed no abnormalities.

Discussion

The ocular surface symptoms such as foreign body sensation and tearing, in Zn deficiency in humans (Karcioglu, 1982) can be explained by the changes in the conjunctiva and cornea noted in authors' study (Gong, Takami, Amemiya, 2004): atrophy and decreased numbers of goblet cells in the conjunctiva and loss of microvilli and microplicae in the most superficial epithelial cells. That is, reduced production of mucin by atrophic goblet cells and poorly developed microvilli and microplicae in the conjunctiva and cornea may lead to undeveloped glycocalix layers in the conjunctiva and deficient tear film in the cornea. This may result in serious damage to the defense mechanism against infection on the ocular surface and explain the reduced immunity of the cornea in Zn deficiency. However, it is not known why Zn deficiency causes those morphological changes in the conjunctiva and cornea.

Zn is active in many metabolic functions such as protein (Kirchgessner, Moser and Roth, 1996), nucleic acid (Satre, Jessen, Clegg et al, 2001) and collagen synthesis (Agren, 1991) through Zn-containing enzymes. The decrease of ribosomes in the epithelial cells in Zn deficiency may be due to the reduced activity of RNA-polymerase which contains Zn (Roth and Kirchgessner, 1980). Myosin-like substance, actin filaments and tonofibrils are important structural components of microplicae and microvilli in the epithelium. Maldevelopment of these structural components in Zn deficiency may be related to disturbances of Zn-containing enzyme activities in protein and collagen synthesis.

Despite the relatively modest effects of Zn deficiency on Cu·Zn SOD activity, Zn-deficient animals often show evidence of oxidative damage to membranes, which has been attributed, in part, to the loss of the stabilizing role of Zn (Virgili, Canali, Figus et al, 1999). In addition, the absence of Zn in the membrane increases the odds that redox active metals, such as iron and copper, will bind to membranes where they can facilitate the production of hydroxy radicals (Zidenberg-Cherr, Keen, Lönndal et al, 1983; Zidenberg-Cherr, Har, Dubick et al, 1991; Bray and Bettger, 1990). Some of the increased oxidative damage observed in Zn-deficient animals may be secondary to an inadequate ability to clear hydroxy radicals (Cao and Chen, 1991).

Since inorganic and organic substances have rarely been studied histologically, it is very difficult to discuss the significance of the present results showing up and down changes of elements and vitamins. The common phenomena in the conjunctiva and cornea in Zn deficiency were decreased Ca and increased Cl. Changes of the elements and vitamins in Zn deficiency were more prominent in the conjunctiva than in the cornea and are mainly decreased amounts of S, Ca, Al, Zn and vitamin C in the conjunctiva. Thus these changes following Zn deficiency should be understood as phenomena to be explained in the future. The decrease of S in the conjunctiva might be related to the decrease of goblet cells and scarcity of secretory granules, because mucin is composed of many S-containing substances. In the same way the decrease in the amount of many elements might be due to the scarcity of goblet cells and their secretory granules.

Although the level of Zn in the serum was low, it was not significantly low in the cornea, but it was significantly low in the conjunctiva. This discrepancy remains to be explained. Basnuclin, a Zn-finger protein, is present in various stratified squamous epithelial cells and is related to cellular proliferative ability (Tseng, 1998). K154 (formerly GKLF), a Zn-finger transcription factor, plays an important role in cell proliferation and/or differentiation and in goblet cell-specific differentiation in the colon (Katz, Perreault, Goldstein et al, 2002). Similarly low levels of Zn in the serum and tissues might cause poorly developed stratification of the conjunctiva and corneal epithelium.

IV. THE RETINA

Analysis of Zn in the Retina with the TOF-SIMS

The percentage of the ratio of spattered Zn ion count to the total counts of all ions spattered is shown in Table 2.4.1. The Zn level in the retina was significantly lower in the Zn-deficient group than in the control (P<0.014) and recovered (P<0.0125) groups, but there was no significant difference in Zn level between the control and recovered groups (P>0.5250).

Table 2.4.1. Ratio of the count of zinc and vitamin A ions to total ion count in control, Zn-deficient and recovery rat retinas (mean±SD).

Groups	Zn	Vit. A (184 amu)	Vit. A (224)
Control	2.671E-5±2.153E-5 * (N=42)	2.016E-4±1.313E-4 (N=42)	2.258E-5±1.114E-5 (N=42)
Zn-deficient	7.190E-6±2.649E-6 *, ** (N=14)	2.103E-4±4.745E-5 (N=14)	1.986E-5±3.464E-6 (N=14)
Recovery	3.272E-5±1.608E-5 ** (N=15)	2.464E-4±2.621E-4 (N=15)	1.862E-5±9.676E-6 (N=15)

The ratio of the Zn ion count to the total ion count is significantly higher in normal control and recovery rat retinas than in Zn-deficient retinas (* p<0.014, ** p<0.0125), but there is no significant difference in vitamin A in the retinas of the three groups (p<0.05).

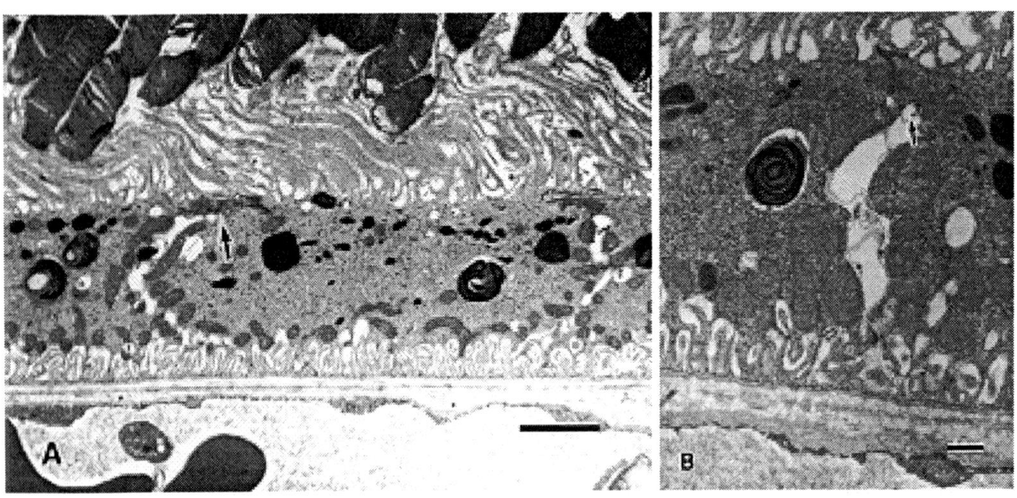

Figure 2.4.1. TEM micrographs of the RPE and outer segment (OS) of a Zn-deficient rat. (A) shows a low magnification of the OS and RPE. The tip of OS discs are separated as masses. A wide space (arrow) is present between lateral cell walls of the RPE in a Zn-deficient rat. Electron densities in the OS discs vary from place to place. (B) is a high magnification of part of intercellular dehiscence. It contains intercellular debris. The terminal bar (arrow) looks tight. Bar: 3μm (A): 500 nm (B).

TEM Findings

In rats fed the Zn-deficient diet for 7 weeks, the tip of photoreceptor outer segment discs was separated as masses near the apical portion of the retinal pigment epithelium (RPE) (Fig. 2.4.1). The distance between outer segment discs was significantly wider in Zn-deficient rats than in the controls (P<0.0001) (Table 2.4.2) (Fig. 2.4.2) and the number of outer segment discs in the axial length of 500 nm was also significantly less in Zn-deficient rats than in the controls (P<0.0001) (Table 2.4.3) (Fig. 2.4.2). On the other hand, photoreceptor inner segments and nuclei looked intact (Fig. 2.4.3).

Table 2.4.2. Distance between outer segment discs in control, Zn-deficient, recovery and pair-fed control rat retinas.

Groups	Number of Fields Examined	Number of Outer Segment Discs Examined	Distance Between Outer Segment Discs (nm)
Control	96	1205	34±5.4 *
Zn-deficient	120	1475	39±7.1 *, **, ***
Recovery	82	1020	33±5.0 **
Pair-fed	90	1100	35±3.6 ***

The distance between the outer segment discs is significantly greater in the Zn-deficient rat retina than in normal, recovery and pair-fed groups (*, ** and *** p<0.0001).

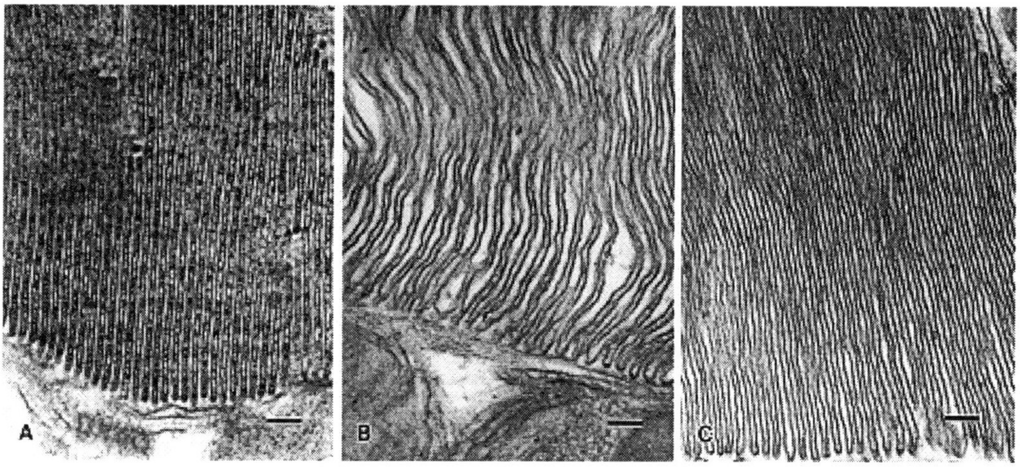

Figure 2.4.2. TEM micrographs of high magnification of OS discs in an axial length of 500nm in a control (A), a Zn-deficient (B) and a recovered rat (C). (A) shows the OS discs arranged regularly and compactly. (B) shows the OS discs arranged irregularly and loosely. The distance between the two discs is wider in B. The distance between OS discs is almost the same in A and C. Bar: 100nm (A—C).

Table 2.4.3. Number of outer segment discs in normal, Zn-deficient, recovery, pair-fed control rat retinas.

Groups	Number of Fields examined	Number of Outer Segment Discs (500nm length) Examined
Control	76	11.4±1.1 *
Zn-deficient	82	9.7±0.9 *, **, ***
Recovery	61	11.6±1.1 **
Pair-fed	55	11.1±1.8 ***

The number of outer segments in an axial length of 500 nm of Zn-deficinet rat retinas is significantly lower than that in control, recovery and pair-fed control groups (* and ** p<0.0001, *** P<0.001).

The RPE seemed to contain large vacuoles and spaces similar to artifacts (Fig. 2.4.1). However, they were found to be intercellular spaces caused by intercellular dehiscence. This dehiscence stopped at the terminal bar (Fig. 2.4.1), and contained cellular debris. The cytoplasm of the RPE contained mitochondria, lysosomes, ribosomes, smooth-surfaced endoplasmic reticulum and rough-surfaced endoplasmic reticulum which looked normal (Fig. 2.4.1). However, many lamellar structures were present in the RPE of Zn-deficient rats even when the retina was removed 6h after the beginning of light exposure. On the other hand, the RPE of control and pair-fed control rats contained very few lamellar structures (Fig. 2.4.3). There was a statistically significant difference in the number of lamellar structures 6h after the beginning of light exposure between the control and pair-fed control rats and Zn-deficient rats (Table 2.4.4).

In control and pair-fed control rats, the photoreceptor cells and RPE showed no abnormal findings.

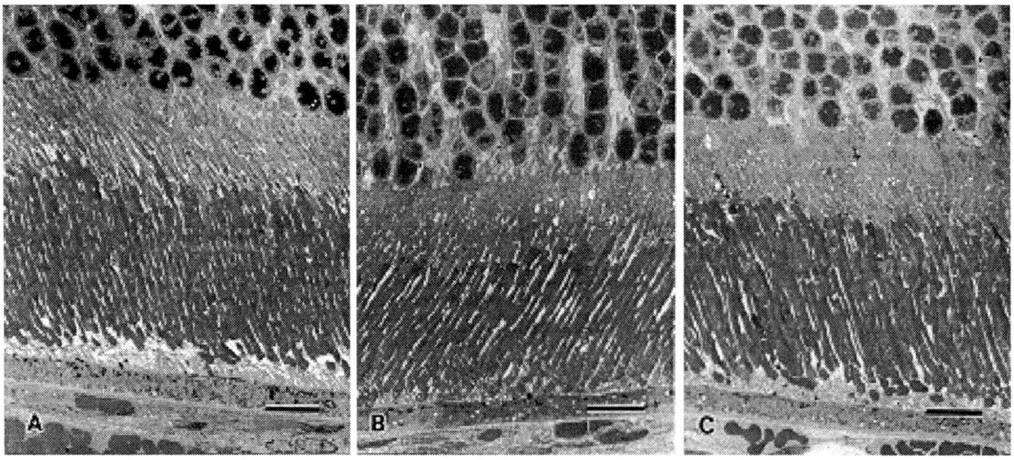

Figure 2.4.3. TEM micrographs of the RPE, OS, inner segments and photoreceptor cell nuclei (PRN) of normal control (A) and pair-fed control (B) and recovery rats (C). In (A), (B) and (C) the OS discs and PRN are arranged regularly and compactly. In recovery rats the RPE shows regular arrays of OS disc membranes and no dehiscence of lateral walls. Bar: 10μm (A—C).

Table 2.4.4. Changes in number of lamellar structures phagocytized by retinal pigment epithelium in control, Zn-deficient, recovery and pair-fed control rats.

Groups	Number of Fields Examined	Number of Lamellated Structures (20μm length)
Control	32	0.344±0.602 *
Zn-deficient	35	2.314±2.055 *, **, ***
Recovery	37	0.622±0.681 **
Pair-fed	43	0.413±0.638 ***

In retinas removed 6h after the beginning of light exposure, the number of lamellar structures phagocytized by RPE in 20μm baseline of retinal tissue is significantly more in Zn-deficient rats than in control rat (* $p<0.0001$), recovery (** $p<0.0001$) or pair-fed control rats (*** $p<0.0001$). However, there is no significant difference among the control, recovery and pair-fed control rats ($p>0.05$).

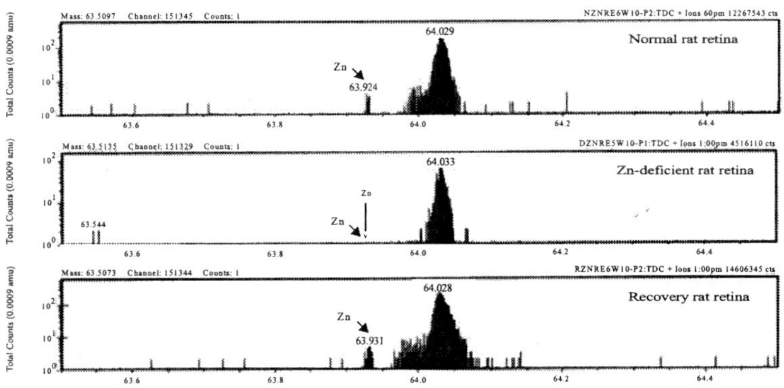

A

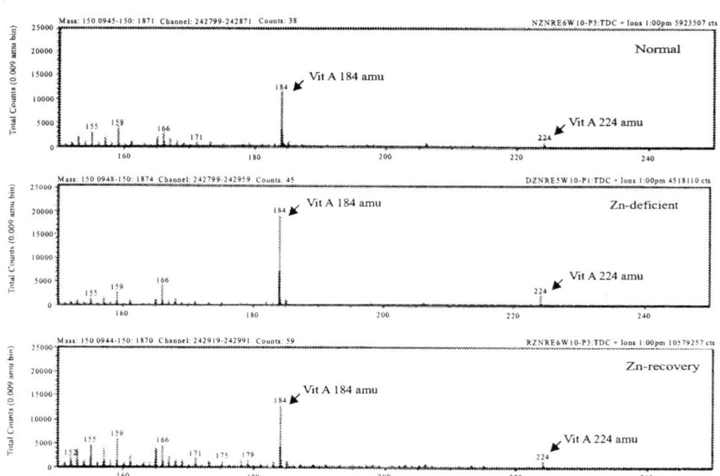

B

Figure 2.4.4. (A) Spectrums of Zn detected with TOF-SIMS in whole retina of normal control, Zn-deficient and Zn recovery rats. The total Zn ion count is significantly lower in Zn-deficient rats than in normal control and Zn recovery rats. (B) Spectrums of vitamin A detected with TOF-SIMS in whole retina of normal control, Zn-deficient and Zn recovery rats. (B) shows the total ion counts of vitamin A 154 amu and 224 amu in normal control, Zn-deficient, and Zn recovery rats: the differences are not significant.

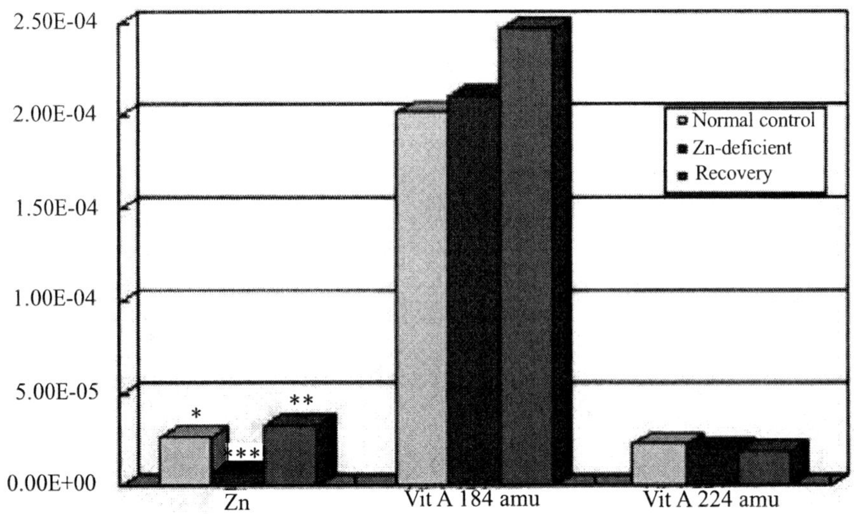

Figure 2.4.5. Ratios of counts of vitamin A 184 amu and, 224 amu and Zn to total count of ions spattered in the whole retina detected with TOF-SIMS. There is no significant difference in the distributions of vitamin A 184 amu and 224 amu among the 3 groups. However, there is a significant difference in the amount of Zn between the normal control and Zn-deficient groups (*P=0.0196) and between the recovery and Zn-deficient groups (**P=0.0326).

Discussion

There is a theory that a major interaction exists between Zn and vitamin A (Solomons and Russell, 1980). Zn deficiency may interfere with vitamin A metabolism by decreasing retinal-binding protein (RBP) production and/or release from the liver (Solomons and Russell, 1980; Smith, McDaniel, Fan et al, 1973; Smith, Brown and Smith 1974; Smith, Brown, McDaniel et al, 1976). RBP, the carrier protein for vitamin A is a rapid turnover protein with a half life of 12h. Zn deficiency in man leads to a decrease in the serum level of rapid turnover protein such as prealbumin and transferrin, and Zn supplementation increases or normalizes these levels (Bates and McClain, 1981).

Zn is also an integral part of alcohol dehydrogenase, the metalloenzyme that catalyzes the interconversion of vitamin A alcohol (retinal). Huber and Gershoff (1975) have demonstrated altered vitamin A metabolism in the eyes of Zn-deficient rats manifested by a decreased activity of alcohol dehydrogenase and decreased conversion of retinol to retinal. They also reported that alcohol dehydrogenase in the retina was much more sensitive than hepatic alcohol dehydrogenase to effects of Zn deficiency (Raskin, Sligar and Steinberg, 1973). Pyrazole (an inhibitor of alcohol dehydrogenase) administered rats decreased the retinolaldehyde level in the retina and altered the function of the retina as assessed by electroretinography (Leure-duPree and McClain, 1982). Thus, Zn deficiency may induce retinal changes very similar to those in vitamin A deficiency: vesiculation of the outer segment discs, loss of the outer segment and loss of lamellar structures in the RPE (Amemiya, 1968; Dowling and Gibbons, 1961). The retinal changes in the current study scarcely resemble those seen in the initial stage of vitamin A deficiency. Actually TOF-SIMS reveals that the vitamin A levels (amus 184 and 224) are not lower in the Zn-deficient rats than in the controls, although authors don't know why vitamin A defracts into two amuses. Thus vitamin A may be less available when the Zn level is low. The phagocytosis of outer segment discs follows a circadian rhythm and is maximal 2h after exposure to light and minimal or almost zero after 6h of light exposure (LaVail and Ward, 1978). However, the RPE of Zn-deficient rats contains lamellar structures 6h after the beginning of light exposure, indicating a continuation of light phagocytosis. This accelerated phagocytosis of the RPE may be due to degeneration of the discs following acute Zn deficiency. The number of outer segment discs is certainly decreased in the Zn-deficient rats. According to Dowling and Gibbons (1961), the most characteristic finding in vitamin A-deficient rats is the absence of lamellar structures in the RPE. In the current study, no such phenomenon occurs because Zn-deficient rats never survive long enough for all discs to degenerate and disappear.

The damaging effect on membranes might also be augmented in Zn deficiency. Zn plays a vital role in membrane stability (Bettger and O'Dell, 1981). One of the biochemical functions of Zn is its role in metalloenzymes such as Cu·Zn superoxide dismutase (Cu·Zn SOD) which is thought to protect cells from the deleterious effects of free radicals (Kondo, 1997). Since outer segment disc membranes are composed of lipid, vitamin A and long chain polyunsaturated fatty acids (Castorina, Campisi, Di Geacomo et al, 1992), the lower activity of Cu·Zn SOD due to Zn deficiency may lead to degeneration of the disc membrane following peroxidation of lipid membrane, Zn deficiency enhances lipid peroxidation and damage to lipid membranes, and thus the combination of retinyl esters and Zn deficiency might have a synergistic deleterious effect on the retina (Sullivan, Jetton, Hahn et al, 1980; Prasad and Oberleas, 1974).

Cadherin and integrin $ß_4$, cell adhesive molecules, have been reported to be present in the cornea where they are related to Zn and vitamin A (Shams, Hanninen, Chaves et al, 1993). Shams et al (1993) demonstrated that laminin, bullous pemphigoid antigen and a component of adhesion complex are decreased in the corneal basal epithelial cells of vitamin A deficient rats. In the RPE cell adhesion molecules have not been seen, but RPE cells are tightly attached by terminal bars. Since RPE cells in the Zn-deficient experiment are tightly attached to each other and terminal bars look morphologically intact, some adhesion abnormality in the lateral walls might be present in Zn deficiency. Because Zn is related to vitamin A metabolism through alcohol dehydrogenase, Zn-containing enzyme activity's disturbance caused by Zn deficiency might lead to lowered vitamin A activity, resulting in weak cell to cell adhesion of RPE if it has any cell adhesion molecules related to vitamin A as in corneal epithelial cells. Another possibility is that Zn deficiency itself causes cell to cell adhesion to be weak because some cell adhesion molecules contain Zn, which plays a role in expression (Nakamoto, Yamagata, Sakai et al, 2000). Further study of cell adhesion molecules in RPE is needed.

Leure-duPree (1981) reported the frequent appearance of osmiophilic inclusion bodies in the RPE of Zn-deficient rats and that of rats given Zn chelator, dithizone and 1.10-phenanthroline. However, there are no such inclusion bodies in the current long and patient examinations of a large number of Zn-deficient rats. No one knows the reason, but it might be because of the differences between Spraugue-Dawley and Wistar Kyoto rats.

V. The optic nerve

Results

The serum zinc levels and body weights of control and Zn-deficient rats are shown in Tables 2.5.1 and 2.5.2

Table 2.5.1. Serum zinc levels (μg dl^{-1}).

Groups	Weeks after start of experiment		Weeks of recovery experiment
	4	7	5
Control	175.7±10.3 * (n=3)	189±8.7 ** (n=4)	184.6±10.2 (n=4)
Zinc-deficient	46.3±27.0 (n=3)	105±9.0 (n=3)	
Recovery	---	---	162 (n=1)

*p<0.001, ** p<0.002 (Fisher's Protected Least Significant Difference). n=number of animals examined.

Table 2.5.2. Body weight of the experimental rat (g).

Groups	Weeks after start of experiment		Weeks of recovery experiment
	4	7	5
Control	235.0±17.3 * (n=5)	342.5±91.0 ** (n=5)	380±18.4 (n=5)
Zinc-deficient	51.7±8.6 (n=8)	10.5±19.0 (n=5)	
Recovery	---	---	250 (n=1)

*, ** p<0.0001 (Fisher's Protected Least Significant Difference). n=number of animals examined.

Table 2.5.3. Diameter of the optic nerves (μm).

Groups	Number of optic nerves counted	Diameter
Control	9	659±86
Zinc-deficient	10	466±42
Recovery	---	---

Diameter of optic nerves calculated in control rats and Zn-deficient rats fed on a Zn-deficient diet for 7 weeks in cross sections taken about 3mm behind the eyeball. There is significant difference between the control and Zn-deficient groups (p<0.0001).

Table 2.5.4. Number of myelinated axons in the optic nerve (100μm²).

Groups	Weeks after start of experiment		Weeks of recovery experiment
	4	7	5
Control	48.0±7.5 * (n=120)	37.4±10.8 ** (n=100)	40.0±6.5 * (n=72)
Zinc-deficient	26.8±7.4 (n=120)	20.3±6.7 (n=100)	
Recovery	---	---	9.3±4.7 (n=119)

* p<0.0001, ** p<0.0125 (Fisher's Protected Least Significant Difference), n=number of animals examined.

The diameter of the optic nerves in rats fed a Zn-deficient diet for 7 weeks was significantly shorter than that of control rats ($p<0.0001$) (Table 2.5.3). The number of myelinated axons and thickness of myelin sheaths in 4- and 7-week deficient rats are shown in Table 2.5.4 and 2.5.5, respectively. The difference between the deficient and control groups at both 4 and 7 weeks was statistically significant, and the difference between the recovery and control groups was also statistically significant.

Table 2.5.5. Thickness of the myelin sheath in the optic nerve (nm).

Groups	Weeks after start of experiment		Weeks of recovery experiment
	4	7	5
Control	112.5±17.5 * (n=120)	135.6±29.5 ** (n=140)	148.6±37.2 *** (n=142)
Zinc-deficient	85.6±19.5 (n=120)	72.6±11.5 (n=150)	
Recovery	---	---	56.6±11.5 (n=179)

* $p<0.005$, ** $p<0.001$, *** $p<0.0002$ (Fisher's Protected Least Significant Difference). n=number of myelin sheaths counted.

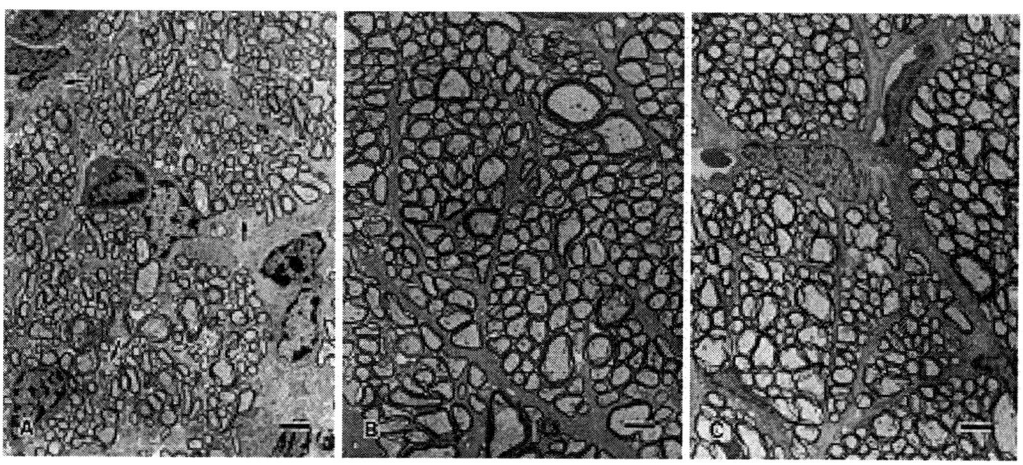

Figure 2.5.1. TEM micrographs of transverse sections of the optic nerves. In a rat fed Zn-deficient diet for 4 weeks (A), myelinated axons are decreased and unmyelinated axons are more numerous than in the control (B) and age-equivalent control rats (C). Destruction of myelin (arrows) and proliferation of glial cells are seen in the Zn-deficient rat (A). Bar: 5µm (A, B, C).

TEM Findings

Electron microscopy demonstrated that in the postlaminar part of the optic nerve of rats on the Zn-deficient diet for 4 or 7 weeks, unmyelinated axons were more numerous (Fig. 2.5.1A) than in the controls (Fig. 2.5.1B). In the initial stage of deficiency destruction of myelin and proliferation of glial cells were local changes but were not diffuse in the optic nerve. However, this tendency became more prominent with time. The optic nerve in the 4 and 7 week deficient rats had few axons, many glial cells, mainly astrocytes, and their well-developed processes occupied the space between axons. In comparison with the control group, the myelin in the Zn-deficient rats was thinner and its lamellae were detached (Fig.

2.5.2). Vacuoles in the axonal cytoplasm were seen in the Zn-deficient group. Swollen neurons contained few neurofilaments and many vacuoles (Fig. 2.5.2). Most of the Zn-deficient rats die by the end of the 7th week and only one rat in the recovery experiment remained alive. This rat showed a further decrease of myelinated nerve fibers (Fig. 2.5.3). In the control group there were no abnormal findings.

In the pair-fed control experiment, the optic nerve showed no abnormalities.

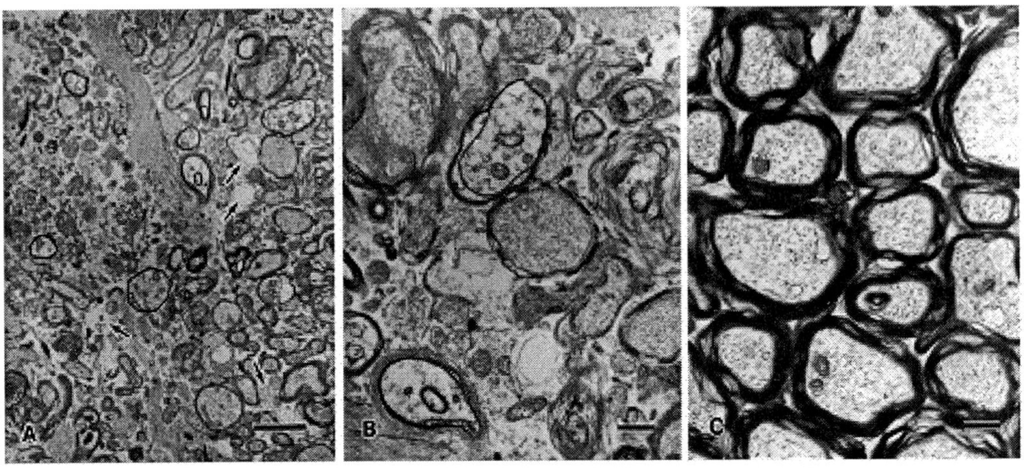

Figure 2.5.2. TEM micrographs of transverse sections of optic nerves. In a rat fed a Zn-deficient diet for 7 weeks (A and B), there are many vacuoles (arrows) among the myelinated axons: swollen neurons contain few neurofilaments. The lamellae of myelin are detached from the cytoplasmic membrane and myelin layer is very thin. Myelinated nerve fibers are scarce and in irregular arrangement. (B) is a high magnification of (A). (C) is an optic nerve of an age-equivalent control rat. Bar: 5μm (A), 1μm (.B, C).

Discussion

The optic nerves of Zn-deficient rats showed a decrease in the number of myelinated nerve fibers. Even when Zn-deficient rats were fed a Zn-sufficient diet, their optic nerves did not recover: the number of myelinated axons is lower in the recovery group than in the Zn-deficient group. The same findings were noted in the Mn-deficient and recovery rats (Gong and Amemiya, 1999) and in the Mg-deficient and recovery rats (Gong, Amemiya and Takami, 2001). It appears that axons continue to degenerate after resumption of a normal diet. This means that when CNS degeneration occurs, there is never a recovery. Thus the loss of myelin may be secondary to axon degeneration caused by Zn deficiency. Another possibility is that the myelin loss is secondary to retrograde loss of axons initiated by the loss of retinal fibers. These changes are also induced by vitamin deficiency such as vitamins A (Chapter 13), B_2 (Takami, Gong and Amemiya, 2004), B_{12} (Amemiya, Kawata and Maekawa, 1987; Agamanolis, Chester, Victor et al, 1976), C (Tsuda, 2002) and E (Chapter 13). It is interesting that the synergistic interaction exists between Zn and vitamin A and between vitamins A and E (Kanazawa, Kitaoka, Ueda et al, 2002; Fujikawa, Gong and Amemiya, 2003; Chapter 13).

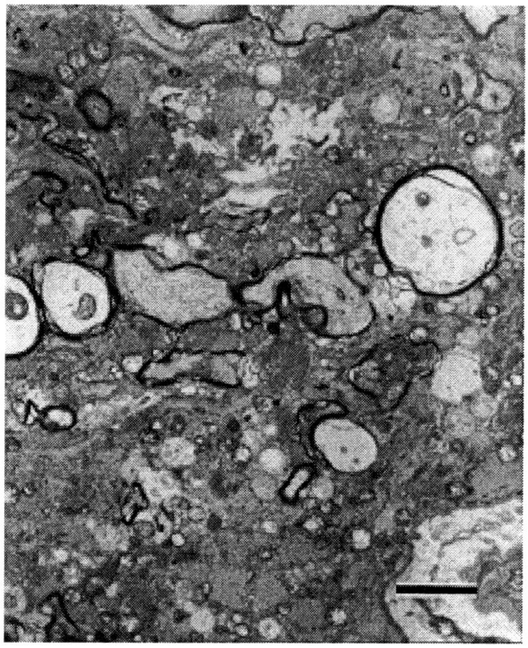

Figure 2.5.3. TEM micrograph of transverse section of a rat in the 5 week recovery experiment. There are fewer myelinated axons than in the optic nerve of Zn-deficient rats. Debris of myelin lamellae, mitochondria and processes of glial cells are scattered between degenerated axons. Bar: 2μm.

In patients whose serum levels of Zn fall due to the administration of drugs such as ethambutol, disulfiram, oxyquinoline, penicillamine, soniazed, etc., optic neuritis, optic atrophy and optic neuropathy have been reported (Klingberg, Prasad and Oberleas, 1976; Yolton, 1981; Weismann, 1986). These conditions are thought to be toxic neuropathies. However, no histopathological study of the optic nerve has been reported. The decreased number of myelinated axons and demyelination induced by Zn deficiency are similar to those seen in the optic nerve fibers of rhesus monkeys treated with ethambutol (Sandstead, Vo-khactu and Solomons, 1976). Although demyelination of optic fibers due to ethambutol administration has been thought to be a toxic effect of ethambutol, these optic nerve changes may be a secondary effect of the low Zn condition following ethambutol toxicity. One of the biochemical findings of Zn is its role in metalloenzmes such as Cu-Zn superoxide dismutase (Cu·Zn SOD) (Coleman, 1992; Vallee and Falchuk, 1993), which is thought to protect cells from the deleterious effects of superoxide free radicals (Kraus, Roth and Kirchgessner, 1997). It has been suggested that the changes in myelin lamellae produced by Zn-deficiency are related to the role of Cu·Zn SOD in lipid membrane stability. (Bettger and O'Dell, 1981). That is, decreased activity of this enzyme due to Zn deficiency may lead to an increase of lipid peroxidation in biomembranes. This hypothesis is the third possibility to account for the loss of myelin. Deficiencies of copper and manganese cause a decrease of myelinated axons and demyelination (Dake and Amemiya, 1991; Mishima, Dake, Amemiya et al, 1996; Gong and Amemiya, 1999). These elements are contained in SOD. Thus decreased activity of SODs may be common to demyelination due to increased lipid peroxidation in the myelin sheath, although details of optic nerve abnormalities are different in deficiencies of Zn, Cu, and Mn.

Part II. Contribution of Zinc to Corneal Epithelial Wound Healing

I. Significance

In the cornea, the effect of Zn on stromal wound healing has been studied, but two opposite conclusions remain. There are reports that wound healing is delayed in Zn deficiency (Sandstead and Shephard, 1968; Oberleas, Seymour, Lenaghan et al, 1971; Rahmat, Norman and Smith et al, 1974; Senapati and Thompson, 1985), but it is reported not to be prolonged under the normal condition (Norman, Rahmat and Smith et al, 1975; Senapati and Thompson, 1985). The purpose of the current study is to clarify whether wound healing is promoted by Zn supplementation under a normal condition. In this study, the injury is in the corneal epithelium, not the stroma.

II. Experiment

Materials and Methods

Animal

We used 21-day-old Wistar Kyoto rats weighing 40 to 50g and divided them randomly into 4 groups: Group 1 (controls) was fed a usual diet with distilled and deionized water. Group 2 (Zn-deficient group) was fed a Zn-deficient diet with distilled and deionized water. Group 3 (recovery group). Zn-deficient rats were fed a usual diet and distilled and deionized water supplemented with 3.0mg Zn/100g water starting immediately after corneal abrasion. Group 4 (Zn-supplemented group) was fed a usual diet with distilled and deionized water supplemented with 3.0mg Zn/100g water. Rats were housed in stainless steel wire bottom cages equipped with plastic bottles and maintained at a constant temperature of 21°C with 12h light and dark cycles at the Laboratory Animal Center for Biomedical Research, Nagasaki University.

Diet

The Zn-deficient diet containing 0.06mg Zn/100g is complete in all other nutrients. This diet is a commercially prepared Zn-deficient powdered diet obtained from Clea Japan Inc., Tokyo. The usual diet contains 4.7mg Zn/100g with all other nutrients. All the animals received the diet ad libitum. Water was given freely to all animals.

Corneal Epithelial Abrasion

Under a stereomicroscope the epithelium in all the rats was completely abraded with a razor blade from limbus to limbus 6 weeks after birth under Nembutal anesthesia and surface anesthesia. The completeness of the abrasion was confirmed with fluorescent test paper.

The rats were killed under Nembutal anesthesia 12h, 1, 3, 5 days, and 1 and 2 weeks after epithelial abrasion and the corneas were examined. At least 5 rats in each group were killed on each day mentioned above. Ultrathin sections for electron microscopy were cut from the central part of the corneas.

Immunohistochemical Study

Immunohistochemical examination was performed on paraffin sections fixed in 4% paraformaldehyde in 0.1M phosphate buffer (pH 7.4) at 4°C overnight to examine the relationship of integrin β_4, integrin β_5, cadherin and laminin to corneal wound healing. We used mouse anti-human integrin β_5 monoclonal IgG1 (Upstate Biotechnology, Inc), mouse anti-human integrin β_4 monoclonal antibody (Chemicon International, Inc), mouse anti-Pan cadherin monoclonal antibody (SIGMA, MO, USA) and rabbit anti-laminin affinity isolated antibody (SIGMA, MO, USA). We also used ED-1 monoclonal antibody (Serotec, Oxford, UK, macrophage/monocyte marker) for the labeling of rat macrophages. The sections were incubated overnight at 4°C with anti-β_4 integrin antibody, anti-β_5 integrin antibody, anti-laminin antibody and anti-cadherin antibody or ED-1 antibody diluted with KPBS containing 1% BSA. The optimal antibody dilution which gave distinct staining at antigen sites with negligible background staining was 1:600 for anti-β_4 integrin antibody, 1:50 for anti-β_5 integrin antibody, 1: 20 for anti-laminin antibody, 1:200 for cadherin antibody and 1:100 for ED-1 antibody. Nonimmunized mouse or rabbit serum with 1% BSAA was used as a negative control. These sections were examined by light microscopy.

Clinical Features

There was a statistically significant difference in body weight at 5 weeks of age between the normal and Zn-deficient groups (p<0.001). The Zn-deficient rats lost hair around the eyes and on the extremities. There was a statistically significant difference in the body weight 2 weeks after corneal abrasion between the Zn-deficient and the recovery groups (P<0.001). The serum Zn level in all groups is shown in Table. 2.7.1.

Table 2.7.1. Serum zinc levels (μg/dl).

Group	Time after corneal abrasion (Mean±SD)				
	12h	1 day	3 days	5 days	1 week
Control	96.5 ± 9.0* (n=3)	96.5 ± 9.0* (n=3)	96.5 ± 9.0* (n=3)	96.5 ± 9.0** (n=3)	96.5 ± 9.0** (n=3)
Control+ Zinc	77.3 ± 7.3 (n=3)	86.7 ±5.8 (n=3)	109.0 ± 3.2 (n=3)	111.5 ± 2.9 (n=3)	129.3 ± 2.7 (n=3)
Zinc deficient	67.0 ± 2.6* (n=3)	66.3 ± 3.3* (n=3)	62.0 ± 3.2*‡ (n=3)	52.0 ± 2.1**‡ (n=3)	47.7 ± 1.5**‡‡ (n=3)
Zinc-deficient recovery	70.7 ± 1.8 (n=3)	70.0 ± 1.2 (n=3)	74.7 ± 2.6‡ (n=3)	89.0 ± 4.0‡ (n=3)	91.3 ± 5.2‡‡ (n=3)

Control rats and zinc-deficient rats: * P<0.05, ** P<0.001

Zinc deficient rats and recovery rats: ‡P<0.05, ‡‡P<0.001

(Fisher's Protected Least Significant Difference), n=number of animals examined.

There were statistically significant differences in the serum Zn level 2 weeks after corneal abrasion between the control and Zn-supplemented group, the control and Zn-deficient groups and the Zn-deficient and recovery groups ($P<0.05$).

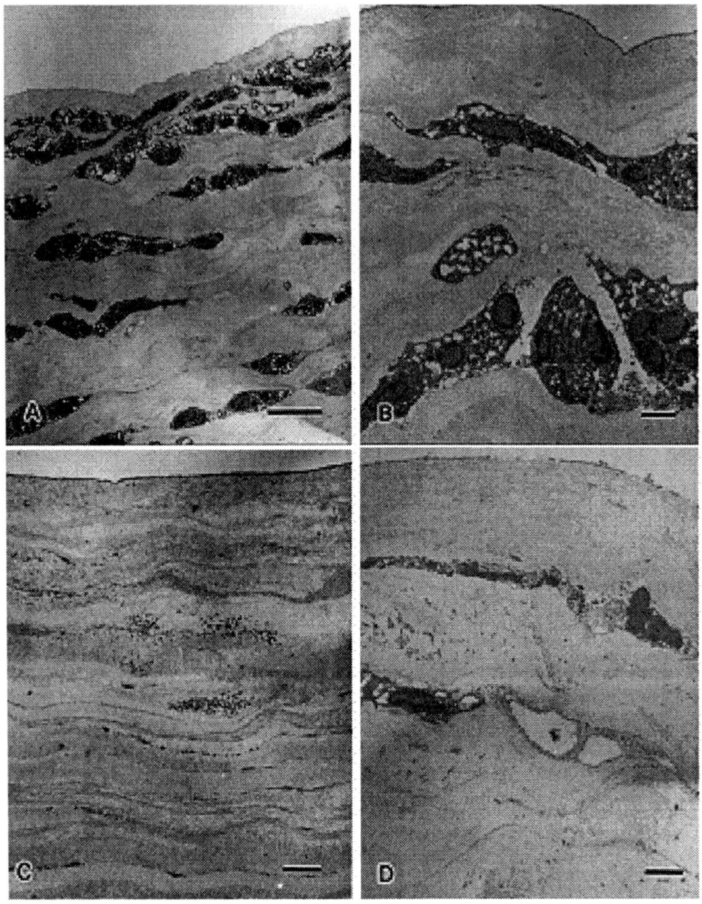

Figure 2.7.1. Electron micrographs of corneas 12h after epithelial abrasion. A: The cornea of a control rat shows no epithelial cells, but many polymorphic cells in the stroma. B: The cornea of a control rat with Zn supplementation shows no epithelial cells, but many polymorphic cells in the stroma. C: The cornea of a Zn-deficient rat shows neither epithelial cells nor polymorphic cells in the stroma. D: The cornea of a Zn-deficient rat treated with Zn supplementation has polymorphic cells, but fewer than those of a normal rat: no epithelial cells but some polymorphic cells in the stroma. Bar: 10μm (A), 2μm (C, D), 0.3μm (B).

III. Results

Electron Microscopic Findings

At 12h after corneal abrasion, no epithelial cells were seen in any of the corneas. However, the corneas of rats in the normal control, Zn-supplemented and recovery groups had many polymorphic cells in the stroma (Fig. 2.7.1). The immunohistochemical methods for macrophages failed to stain them. On the other hand, the corneas of Zn-deficient rats showed no polymorphic cells in the stroma. On the first day after corneal abrasion, epithelial cells appeared in the normal rats with Zn supplementation, but no epithelial cells appeared in the Zn-deficient, normal control and Zn-supplemented groups (Fig. 2.7.2). On the 3rd day after abrasion, epithelial cells were seen in all groups, and they had desmosomes, but there were only a few in the Zn-deficient group (Fig. 2.7.3). On the 5th day after corneal abrasion, the corneal epithelial cells formed 10 layers in the normal control, Zn-supplemented and recovery groups, but only 8 in the Zn-deficient group. In the recovery group, epithelial cells were compactly arranged, but they were loosely arranged in the control and Zn-deficient groups (Fig. 2.7.4). No polymorphic cells were found in the stroma in all 4 groups. In corneas 2 weeks after epithelial abrasion, epithelial cells were almost regularly and compactly arranged in the control, Zn-supplemented and recovery groups, but the epithelial cell layer was still less in number in the Zn-deficient group (Fig. 2.7.5).

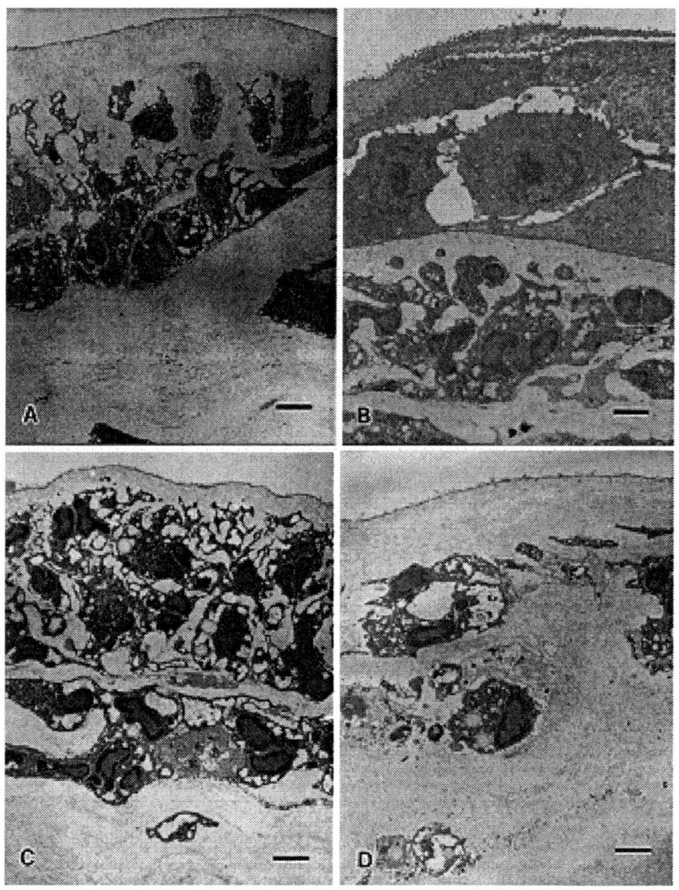

Figure 2.7.2. Electron micrographs of corneas 1 day after epithelial abrasion. A: The cornea of a control rat shows no epithelial cells but many polymorphic cells in the stroma. B: The cornea of a control rat with Zn supplementation shows 3 layers of epithelial cells and many polymorphic cells in the stroma. C: The cornea of a Zn-deficient rat shows no epithelial cells but many polymorphic cells in the stroma. D: The cornea of a Zn-deficient rat treated with Zn shows no epithelial cells but many polymorphic cells in the stroma. Bar: 2μm (A-D).

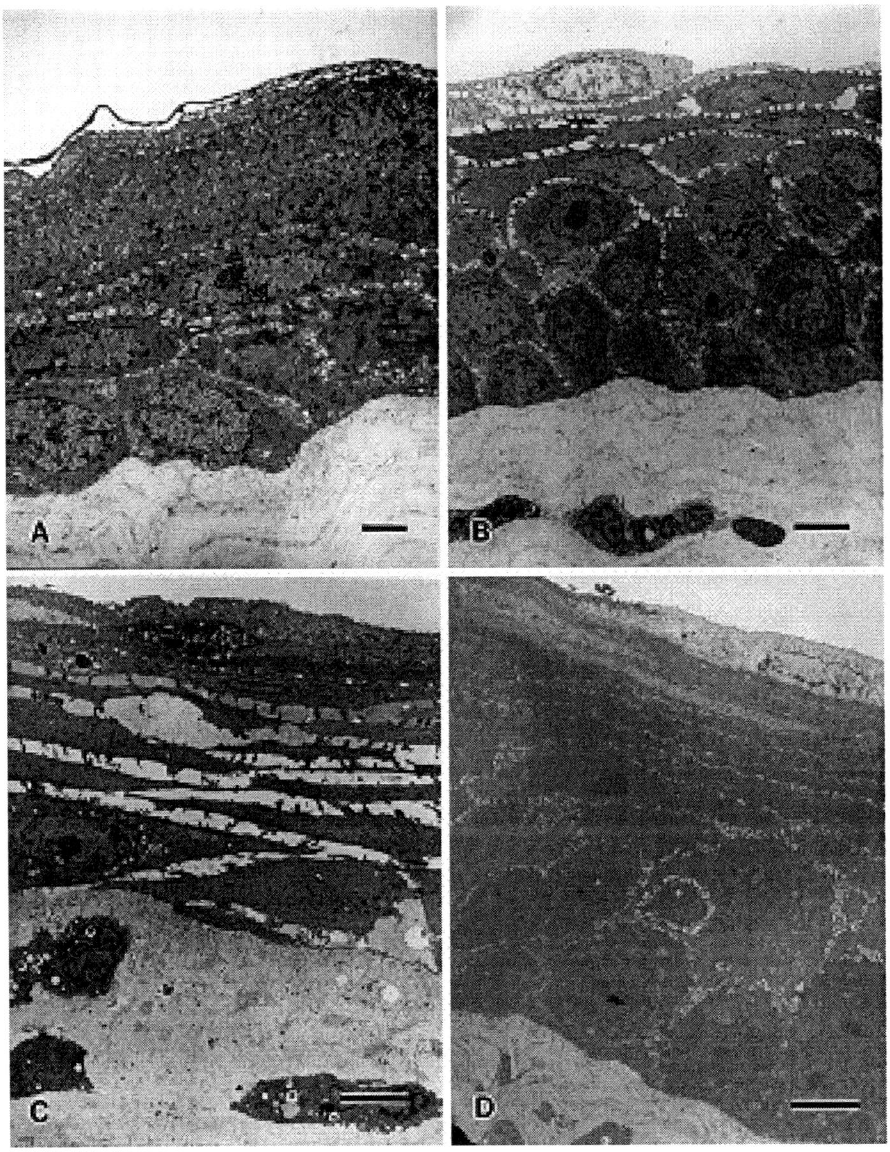

Figure 2.7.3. Electron micrographs of corneas 3 days after epithelial abrasion. A: In a control rat corneal epithelial cells form a few layers, and polymorphic cells are scarcely seen in the stroma. B: In a control rat treated with Zn corneal epithelial cells form several layers. C: A Zn-deficient rat cornea shows regeneration of epithelial cells, but dehiscence between cells is seen despite connections with desmosomes. Polymorphic cells still remain in the stroma. D: In the cornea of a Zn-deficient rat treated with Zn epithelial cells form several layers and are compactly arranged. Large fibroblast cells are seen in the stroma. Bar: 2μm (A), 5μm (B-D).

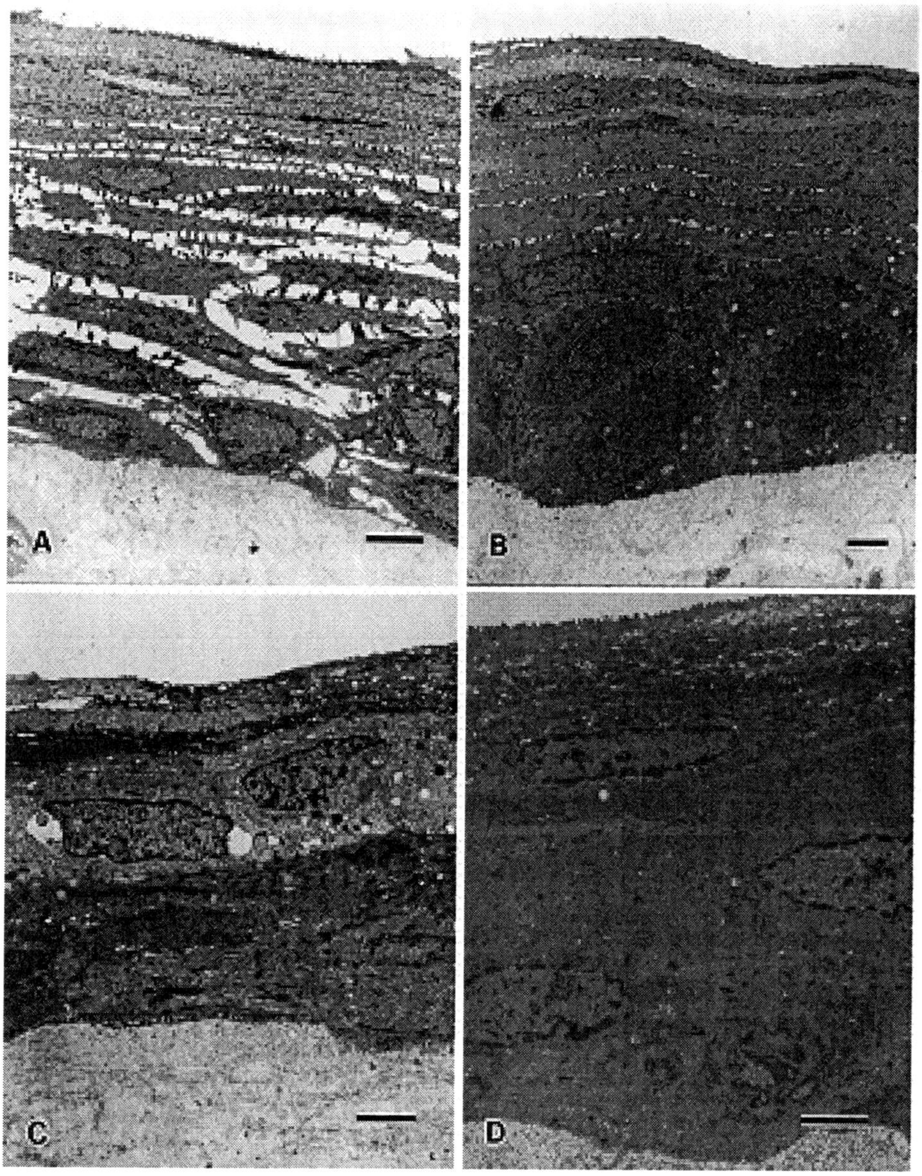

Figure 2.7.4. Electron micrographs of cornea 5 days after epithelial abrasion. A: In a control rat corneal epithelial cells form 11 layers and have many microvilli and desmosomes, but the intercellular spaces are large. B: In a control rat treated with Zn corneal epithelial cells form 11 layers and the intercellular spaces are compact. C: A Zn-deficient rat cornea shows regeneration of epithelial cells. D: In the cornea of a Zn-deficient rat treated with Zn epithelial cells form several layers and are compactly arranged. Bar: 5μm (A, C, D), 2μm (C).

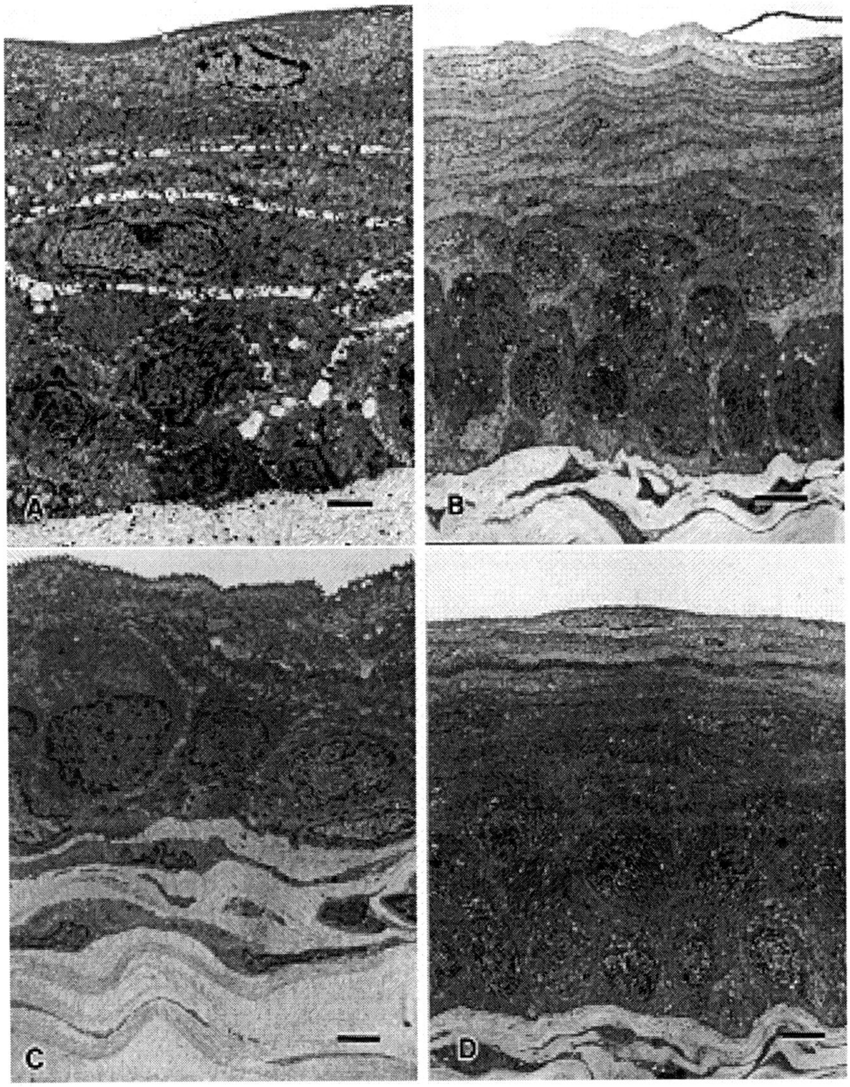

Figure 2.7.5. Electron micrographs of corneas 2 weeks after epithelial abrasion. A: In a control rat corneal epithelial cells form many layers. B: In a control rat treated with Zn corneal epithelial cells look almost normal. C: In a Zn-deficient rat corneal epithelial cells form several layers which are compactly arranged. D: In the cornea of a Zn-deficient rat treated with Zn epithelial cells form many layers which are compactly arranged. Bar: 2μm (A, C), 5μm (B, D).

Immunohistochemical Findings

Macrophage ED-1: No immunoreactivity of macrophage ED-1 was observed in the cornea after abrasion in all groups.

Integrin $ß_4$: The maximum immunoreactivity of integrin $ß_4$ in the corneal epithlium was observed on the 3rd day after abrasion in all 4 groups. The immunoreactivity of integrin $ß_4$ was observed not only around basal cells but also around superficial and wing cells in the control and recovery groups. These results are shown in Table 2.7.2. The intensity of expression of integrin $ß_4$ was strongest in the basal cells of the corneal epithelium in all 4 groups 3 days after abrasion (Fig. 2.7.6).

Table 2.7.2. Immunohistochemical results of integrin β_4 in corneal epithelium after corneal abrasion.

Rats	Epithelium	Time after abrasion					
		12h	1d	3d	5d	1w	2w
Control	superficial epithelial cell	-	-	+	+	+	-
	basal epithelial cell	-	-	+	++	+	++
	basement membrane	-	-	-	-	-	-
Control + Zn	superficial epithelial cell	-	-	-	+	-	-
	basal epithelial cell	-	-	++	+	+	+
	basement membrane	-	-	+	+	+	+
Zn-deficient	superficial epithelial cell	-	-	-	+	+	-
	basal epithelial cell	-	-	+	+	+	+
	basement membrane	-	-	-	-	+	+
Zn-deficient recovery	superficial epithelial cell	-	-	+	+	+	-
	basal epithelial cell	-	-	+	+	+	+
	basement membrane	-	-	+	+	+	+

Staining intensity: ++, strongly positive; +, weakly positive; ±, faintly positive; –, negative.

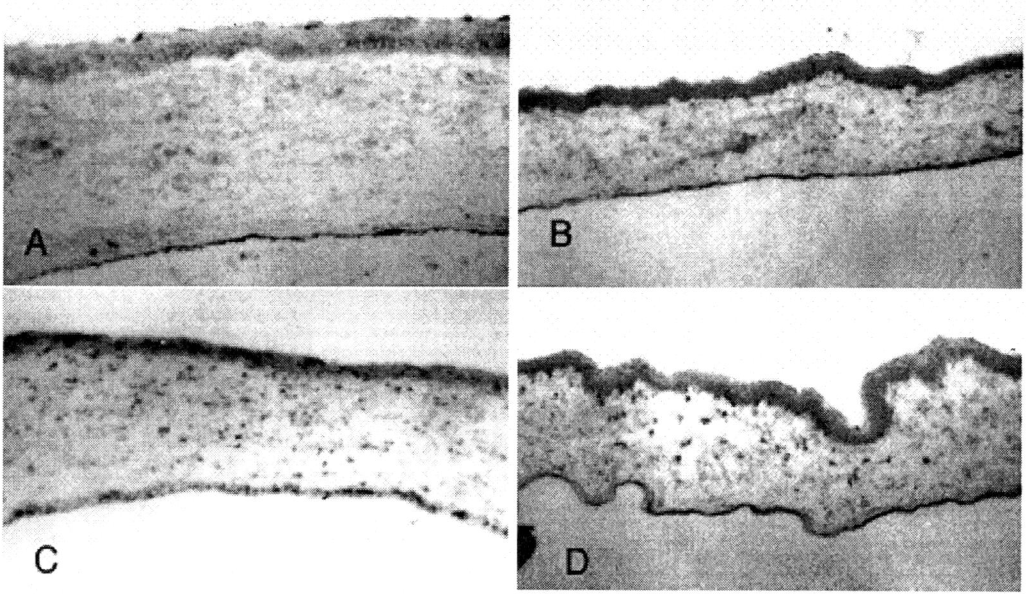

Figure 2.7.6. Immunohistochemical staining for integrin ß4 is seen in the superficial layer of the epithelium and the basal epithelium of the cornea 5 days after epithelial abrasion. It is stronger in a control (A) and a Zn-deficient (C) rat than in a control treated with Zn (B) and a Zn-deficient rat treated with Zn (D). × 200.

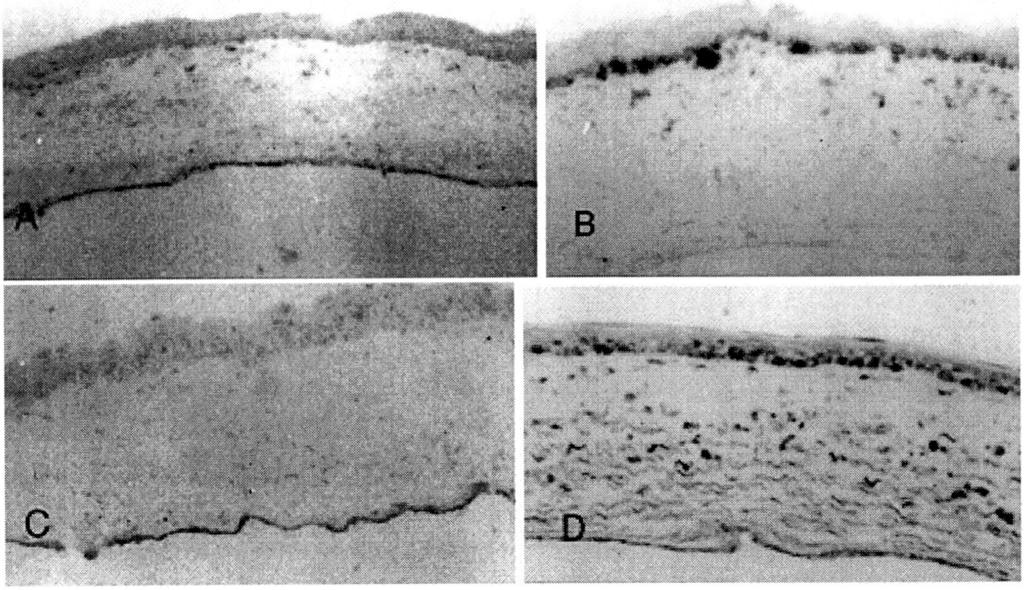

Figure 7.7. Immunohistochemical staining for integrin ß5 expression is present in the superficial layer of the epithelium and basal epithelium in the cornea 3 days after epithelial abrasion, but a control rat treated with Zn (B) and a Zn-deficient rat treated with Zn administration (D) show stronger expression than do a control (A) and a Zn-deficient (C) rat. × 200.

Table 2.7.3. Immunohistochemical results of integrin β_5 in corneal epithelium after corneal abrasion.

Rats	Epithelium	Time after abrasion					
		12h	1d	3d	5d	1w	2w
Control	superficial epithelial cell	-	-	+	-	+	-
	basal epithelial cell	-	-	+	+	+	+
	basement membrane	-	-	-	-	-	-
Control + Zn	superficial epithelial cell	-	-	+	-/+	-	-
	basal epithelial cell	-	-	++	+	+	+
	basement membrane	-	-	-	-	-	-
Zn-deficient	superficial epithelial cell	-	-	+	-	-	-
	basal epithelial cell	-	-	+	+	+	+/-
	basement membrane	-	-	-	-	-	-
Zn-deficient recovery	superficial epithelial cell	-	-	+	-	-	-
	basal epithelial cell	-	-	++	+	+	++
	basement membrane	-	-	-	-	-	-

Staining intensity: ++, strongly positive; +, weakly positive; ±, faintly positive; –, negative.

Integrin β_5 activity was strong in the basal epithelial cells on the 3rd day (Fig. 2.7.7) and returned to normal on the 7th day after abrasion in 3 groups, but in the Zn-deficient group, it was weaker than in the control and recovery groups (Fig. 2.7.7). On the 5th day after abrasion, integrin β_5 was more intense in the basal epithelial cells in the recovery group than in the control and Zn-deficient groups. In the Zn-supplemented group, the integrin β_5 level was high from the 3rd to the 7th day when it returned to normal; it appeared earlier in the Zn-supplemented group than in the control, Zn-deficient and recovery groups. These results are shown in Table 2.7.3.

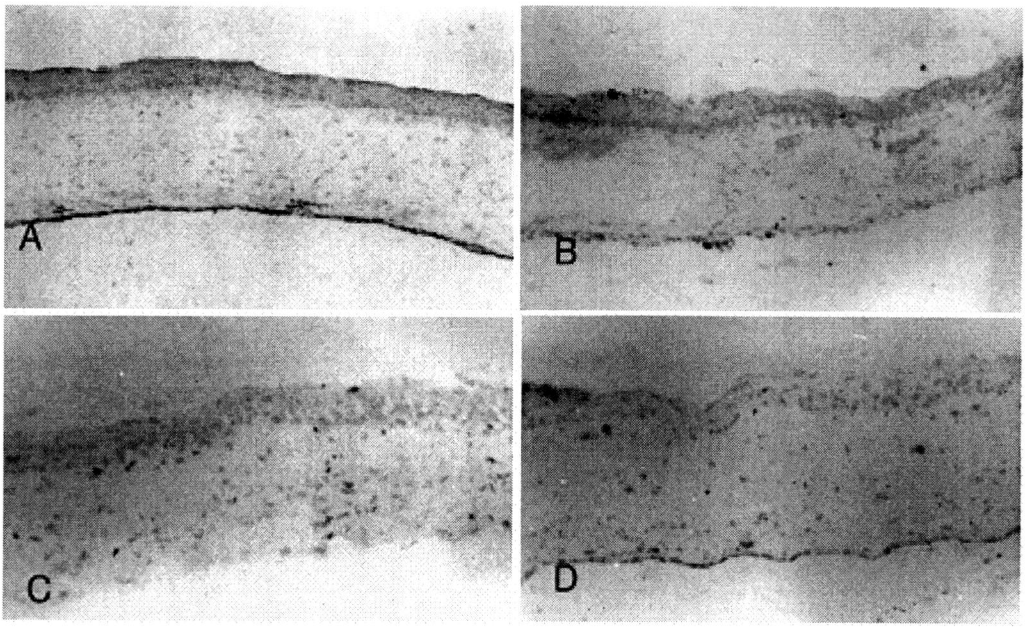

Figure 2.7.8. Immunohistochemical staining for cadherin is seen in the superficial layer of the epithelium, basal epithelium and basement membrane of the basal cell in the cornea 3 days after epithelial abrasion. (A) a control rat, (B) a control rat treated with Zn, (C) a Zn-deficient rat and (D) a Zn-deficient rat treated with Zn. × 200.

Table 2.7.4. Immunohistochemical study of cadherin in corneal epithelium after corneal abrasion.

Rats	Epithelium	Time after abrasion					
		12h	1d	3d	5d	1w	2w
Control	superficial epithelial cell	-	-	+	+	-	-
	basal epithelial cell	-	-	+	+	+	+
	basement membrane	-	-	+	+	-	-
Control + Zn	superficial epithelial cell	-	-	+	+	+	-
	basal epithelial cell	-	-	+	+	+	+
	basement membrane	-	-	+	+	+	+
Zn-deficient	superficial epithelial cell	-	-	+	+	+	+
	basal epithelial cell	-	-	+	+	+	+
	basement membrane	-	-	+	+	+	+
Zn-deficient recovery	superficial epithelial cell	-	-	+	+	+	-
	basal epithelial cell	-	-	+	+	+	++
	basement membrane	-	-	+	+	+	+

Staining intensity: ++, strongly positive; +, weakly positive; ±, faintly positive; –, negative.

Cadherin appeared on the 3rd day in the superficial epithelial cells, basal epithelial cells and basement membrane of the basal cells in all 4 groups (Fig. 2.7.8). These results are shown in Table 2.7.4.

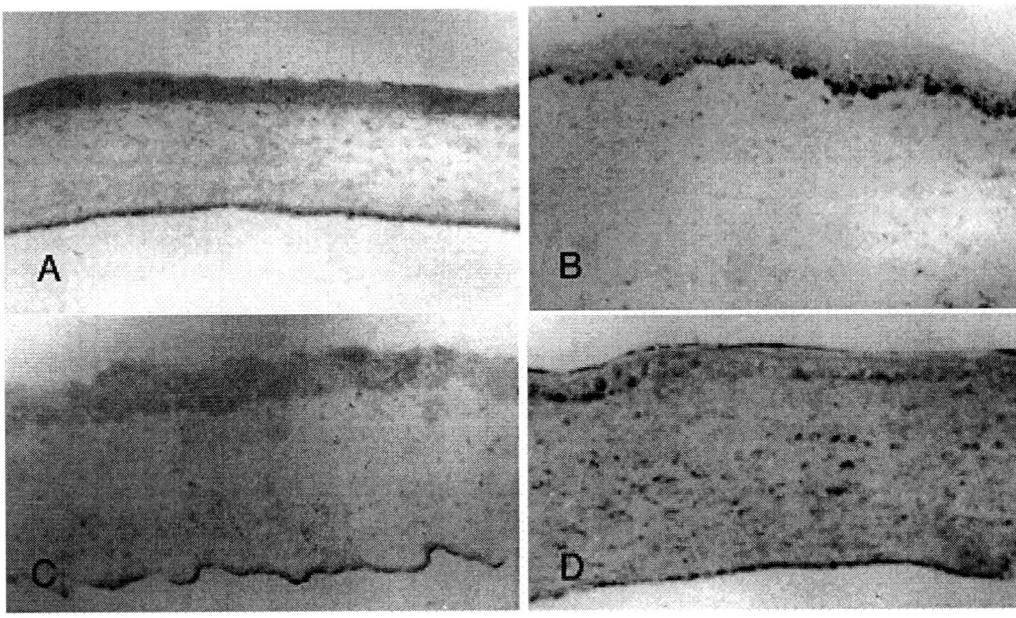

Figure 2.7.9. Immunohistochemical staining for laminin is positive in the superficial layer of the epithelium and basal epithelium of the cornea 3 days after epithelial abrasion, but a control rat treated with Zn (B) and a Zn-deficient rat treated with Zn (D) show stronger staining than a control rat (A) and a Zn-deficient rat (C). × 200.

Table 2.7.5. Immunohistochemical study of laminin in corneal epithelium after corneal abrasion.

Rats	Epithelium	Time after abrasion					
		12h	1d	3d	5d	1w	2w
Control	superficial epithelial cell	-	-	-	+	++	+
	basal epithelial cell	-	-	+	+	+	+
	basement membrane	-	-	+	+	+	+
Control + Zn	superficial epithelial cell	-	-	-	+	+	+
	basal epithelial cell	-	-	+	+	+	++
	basement membrane	-	-	++	+	+	++
Zn-deficient	superficial epithelial cell	-	-	-	-	-	-
	basal epithelial cell	-	-	+	+	+	+
	basement membrane	-	-	-	-/+	-	+
Zn-deficient recovery	superficial epithelial cell	-	-	+	+	+	+
	basal epithelial cell	-	-	+	+	+	+
	basement membrane	-	-	+	+	+	++

Staining intensity: ++, strongly positive; +, weakly positive; ±, faintly positive; –, negative

Laminin appeared on the 3rd day in all 4 groups, but its level was higher in basal cells and basement membrane of basal cells in the Zn-supplemented and recovery groups than in the normal control and Zn-deficient groups (Fig. 2.7.9). These results are shown in Table 2.7.5.

Discussion

Zn-containing plant extracts were used for wound repairs in ancient Egypt (Prasad, Miale, Farid et al, 1963) and many experiments on the wound healing ability of Zn have been reported (Hubbard, Herron, Andrews et al, 1969; Rahmat, Norman and Smith et al, 1974; Lee, Green, Long et al, 1976; Wacker, 1976; Williams, Meltzer, Brown et al, 1979), but its mechanism of action is still controversial. Zinc has a significant beneficial effect on wound healing in vascular tissues (Hubbard, Herron, Andrews et al, 1969; Leure-Dupree, 1986), first recognized by Strain and co-workers in the mid-1950's when they observed enhanced wound healing in animals fed diets supplemented with zinc (Strain, Dutton and Heyer, 1953).

In the current study, the rats fed a Zn-deficient diet certainly had Zn-deficiency confirmed by their low serum level of Zn, decreased weight gain, loss of hair and decrease of corneal epithelial microvilli. The effects of Zn administration were also confirmed by recovered or increased serum levels of Zn and recovery of hair in the recovery group.

The experimental results showed that the recovery of epithelial layers after corneal abrasion was delayed in Zn-deficiency and that Zn supplementation accelerated the regeneration of epithelium. It was confirmed that the addition of Zn to the normal diet definitely accelerated epithelial regeneration. Under normal and Zn-supplemented conditions, desmosomes between epithelial cells were proved to develop well, and intracytoplasmic components such as fibrils and ribosomes also did well. In the stroma, polymorphic cells with curled slender processes appeared by the first day after corneal abrasion and disappeared by the 5th day in rats on the normal diet, but Zn supplementation accelerated its appearance.

On the other hand, in immunohistochemical studies negative staining for macrophages with ED-1 antibody showed that curled slender cells were not macrophages.

In ocular tissues Zn is present in the cornea, especially in the corneal epithelial cells, and in the retina (Leiner and Leiner, 1942; Tauber and Krause, 1943; Eckhert, 1983; Grahn, Paterson, Gottschall-Pass et al, 2001). Zn deficiency induces loss of microvilli and a decrease of fibrils in epithelial cells (Mizoguchi and Amemiya, 1990: Gong and Amemiya, 2001). Since Zn is involved in collagenase (Berman, 1973; Berman, 1975; Francois, 1977; Burns, Paterson, Gray et al, 1990), collagen synthesis (Tengrup, Ahonen and Zederfeldt, 1980; Tengrup, Ahonen and Zederfeldt, 1981; Trujillo, 1993; Tumer, Kama, Tumer et al, 1999), protein synthesis (Prasad, 1985; Senapati and Thompson, 1985; Franzen and Ghassemifar, 1992; Prasad, 1995), and amino acid utilization (Vallee and Falchuk, 1993), corneal stromal wound healing is assumed to be delayed in Zn deficiency. However, it has actually been unclear whether Zn accelerates corneal stromal wound healing. The regeneration cycle of the corneal epithelial cell is 5-7 days. In addition, Zn-deficiency causes more damage in the corneal epithelium than in the stroma. Thus the effects of Zn on wound healing is more apparent in the epithelium than in the stroma.

Integrins, situated on the cell surface, play a role in cell to cell and in cell to extracellular matrix connections. The intergrins are formed by $\alpha\beta$ heterodimers, and combinations of them impart ligand specificity (Hynes, 1987; Ruoslahti, 1991). In the cornea, integrins have been reported to be located in the basal cells of the epithelium (Lauweryns, Van Den Ood, Volpes et al, 1991; Paallysaho and Williams, 1991; Tervo, Tervo, Van Setten et al, 1991; Trinkaus-Randall, Tong, Thomas et al, 1993). The current study showed integrin β_4 in the superficial cells, basal cells and basement membrane. In this study, integrin β_5 expression was observed in normal corneal superficial epithelial cells and basal epithelium. Integrin β_5 may act only in attachments between epithelial cells (Rayner, Gallop, George et al, 1998), while integrin β_4 may contribute not only to attachments between epithelial cells, but also to those between basement membranes and basal epithelial cells (Stepp, Spurr-Michaud and Gipson, 1993; Stepp, Zhu and Cranchill, 1996). (Tenaud et al. 2000) reported that Zn gluconate increases integrin subunit expression. Zn finger protein exists in promoters of several metalloproteinases (MMPs), which are Zn-dependent proteases that can digest various extracellular matrix proteins or cell surface proteins (Nakamoto, Yamagata, Sakai et al, 2000). These data show that Zn may play an important role in the production of integrin and in wound healing.

Laminin is related to cell adhesion, movement, differentiation and proliferation (Fukuda, Chikama, Nakamura et al, 1999). Thus, laminin in the epithelial cells may play a role in the movement of cells from the limbal portion to the central portion, from the deep layer to the superficial layer and from the normal part to the defective part with proliferation and differentiation. Laminin may also play a role in cell to cell adhesion in regular arrangements, relaxation of intercellular junctions in cell removal and loss of cellular connections in desquamation. In the current study, these roles were proved by immunohistochemical evidence showing the weak expression of laminin in the corneal epithelium in Zn deficiency and strong expression under normal conditions. Zn is found to be most effective at enhancing laminin-entactin and laminin-collagen type IV binding (Ancsin and Kisilevsky, 1996). Thus, the current results suggest that Zn contributes to wound healing partially through laminin.

Cadherin expression was observed in corneal superficial epithelial cells and basal epithelial cells in the current study. Cadherin is a calcium dependent cell adhesion molecule (Mohan, Lee and Panjwani et al, 1995). It functions in the formation and maintenance of the epithelium, is located in the adherent junction and plays an important role in cell to cell interactions that influence cell migration and morphogenesis (Mohan, Lee and Panjwani et al, 1995). It may act at the desmosome-like intercellular junctions in the epithelium (Danjo and Gipson, 1998). Thus, the determination of the location of cadherin in the current study should be correct. Zn-finger transcription acts as an important candidate mediator of E-cadherin downregulation (Comijn, Berx, Vermassen et al, 2001). This activity may contribute to the repair of epithelial wounds through cadherin in the presence of Zn.

Considering the previously reported role of Zn in stromal wound healing, scarring must be hastened by elevated collagen production activated by excessive Zn since collagenase is a Zn-containing enzyme related to collagen production. Zn is also contained in some enzymes related to protein synthesis. Such enzymes may also induce well-developed fibrils and the appearance of many ribosomes. On the other hand, the corneal epithelial wound healing described in the present study is different from stromal wound healing and is associated not only with many mechanisms involving Zn-containing enzymes, but also with some cell adhesion molecules. Zn may regulate the activity of integrin ß4, integrin ß5, laminin and cadherin by the Zn-finger protein. Therefore, it is assumed that corneal wound healing is regulated by Zn and cell to cell matrix adhesion similar to integrin ß4, integrin ß5, laminin and cadherin.

REFERENCES

Agamanolis DP, Chester EM, Victor M, Kark JA, Hiness JD, Harris JW. Neuropathology of experimental vitamin B_{12} deficiency in monkeys. *Neurology*. 1976;26:905-914.

Agren MS. Collagen synthesis in connective tissue of wounded rat mesentery: effect of dietary zinc deficiency. *Eur J Surg*. 1991;157:453-455

Akar N, Arcasoy A. Alcohol and zinc deficiency: contribution to villous atrophy. *J Intern Med*. 1990;228:412-413.

Amemiya T. Cytochemical and electron microscopic examination of the retina of rats with hypovitaminosis A. *Acta Soc Ophthalmol Jpn*. 1968;72:1074-1099.

Amemiya T, Kawata T, Maekawa A. Ocular pathology of vitamin B_{12}-deficient rats. In Takaku F, Uchino H, ed. *Kyoto symposium on Methyl B_{12}*. Tokyo: Kyodo Tsushin;1987:80-85.

Ancsin JB, Kisilevsky R. Laminin interactions important for basement membrane assembly are promoted by zinc and implicate laminin zinc finger-like sequences. *J Biol Chem*. 1996;271:6845-6851.

Bates J, McClain CJ. The effect of severe zinc deficiency on serum levels of albumin, transferrin, and prealbumin in man. *Am J Clin Nutr*. 1981;34:1655-1660.

Berman MB, Manabe R. Corneal collagenases. Evidence for zinc metallo-enzymes. *Ann Ophthalmol*. 1973;5:1193-1209.

Berman BM. Collagenase inhibitors: rationale for their use in treating corneal ulceration. *Int Ophthalmol Clin*. 1975;15:49-66.

Bettger WJ, O'Dell BL. A critical physiological role of zinc in the structure and function of biomembranes. *Life Sci*. 1981;28:1425-1438.

Bray TM, Bettger WJ. The physiological role of zinc as an antioxidant. *Free Radic Biol Med*. 1990;8:281-291.

Burns FR, Paterson CA, Gray RD, Wells JT. Inhibition of pseudomonas are aeruginosa elastase and pseudomonas keratitis using a thiol-based peptide. Antimicrob. *Agents Chemother*. 1990;34:2065-2069.

Cao GH, Chen JD. Effects of dietary zinc on free radical generation, lipid peroxidation, and superoxide dismutase in trained mice. *Arch Biochem Biophys*. 1991;291:147-153.

Castorina C, Campisi A, DiGiacomo C, Sorrenti V, Russo A, Vanella A. Lipid peroxidation and antioxidant enzymatic systems in rat retina as a function of age. *Neurochem Res*. 1992;17:599-604.

Chesters JK. Zinc. In O'Dell BL, Sunde RA ed. *Handbook of Nutritionally Essential Mineral Elements*. New York, Basel, Hong Kong:Marcel Dekker Inc;1997:185-230.

Coleman JE. Zinc proteins—enzymes, storage proteins, transcription factors, and replication proteins. *Annu Rev Biochem*. 1992;61:897-946.

Comijn J, Berx G, Vermassen P, Verschueren K, van Grunsven L, Bruyneel E, Mareel M, Huylebroeck D, van Roy F. The two handed E box binding zink finger protein SIP 1 downregulates E-cadherin and induces invasion. *Mol Cell*. 2001;7:1267-1278.

Dake Y, Amemiya T. Electron microscopic study of the optic nerve in copper deficient rats. *Exp Eye Res*. 1991;52:277-281.

Danjo Y, Gipson IK. Actin 'purse string' filaments are anchored by E-cadherin-mediated adherens junctions at the leading edge of the epithelial wound, providing coordinated cell movement. *J Cell Sci*. 1998;111:3323-3332.

Dowling JE, Gibbons IR. The effect of vitamin A deficiency on the fine structure of the retina. In:Smelser GK, ed. *The Structure of the Eye*. New York: Academic Press Inc;1961:85-99.

Eckhert CD. Elemental concentrations in ocular tissues of various species. *Exp Eye Res*. 1983;37:639-647.

Francois J. The Seventh Frederick H. Verhoeff Lecture. Collagenase and collagenase inhibitors. *Trans Am Ophthalmol Soc*. 1977;75:285-315.

Franzen LE, Ghassemifar MR. Connective tissue repair in zinc deficiency. An ultrastructural morphometric study in perforated mesentery in rats. *Eur J Surg*. 1992;158:333-337.

Fujikawa A, Gong H, Amemiya T. Vitamin E prevents changes in the cornea and conjunctiva due to vitamin A deficiency. *Graefes Arch Clin Exp Ophthalmol*. 2003;241:287-297.

Fukuda K, Chikama T, Nakamura M, Nishida T. Differential distribution of subchains of the basement membrane components type IV collagen and laminin among the amniotic membrane, cornea, and conjunctiva. *Cornea*. 1999;18:73-79.

Galin MA, Nano HD, Hall T. Ocular zinc concentration. *Invest Ophthalmol Vis Sci*. 1962;1:142-148.

Gong H, Amemiya T. Optic nerve changes in manganese-deficient rats. *Exp Eye Res*. 1999;68:313-320.

Gong H, Amemiya T, Takaya K. Retinal changes in magnesium-deficient rats. *Exp Eye Res*. 2001;72:23-32.

Gong H, Amemiya T. Optic nerve changes in Zn-deficient rats. *Exp Eye Res*. 2001;72:363-369.

Gong H, Takami Y, Amemiya T, Tozu M, Ohashi Y. Ocular surface in Zn-deficient rats. *Ophthalmic Res*. 2004;36:129-138.

Grahn BH, Paterson PG, Gottschall-Pass KT, Zhang Z. Zinc and the eye. *J Am Coll. Nutr*. 2001;20:106-118.

Hamit HF, David HE, Stevens JC. Dermatitis due to zinc deficiency associated with prolonged malnutrition and total parenteral nutrition. *World J Surg*. 1980;4:693-698.

Heimburger DC, Tamura T, Marks RD. Rapid improvement in dermatitis after zinc supplementation in a patient with Crohn's disease. Am J Med. 1990;88:71-73.

Hirayama Y. Histochemical localization of zinc and copper in rat ocular tissues. *Acta Histochem*. 1990;89:107-111.

Hubbard GB, Herron BE, Andrews JS, Elliott JH. Influence of topical and oral zinc upon corneal wound healing. *Br J Ophthalmol*. 1969;53:407-411.

Huber AM, Gershoff SN. Effect of zinc deficiency on the oxidation of retinol and ethanol in rats. *J Nutr.* 1975;105:1486-1490.

Hynes RO. Integrins: a family of cell surface receptors. *Cell.* 1987;48:549-554.

Jern NA, Van Beber AD, Gorman MA, Weber CG, Liepa GU, Cochran CC. The effects of zinc supplementation on serum zinc concentration and protein catabolic rate in hemodialysis patients. *J Renal Nutr.* 2000;10:148-153.

Kanazawa S, Kitaoka T, Ueda Y, Gong H, Amemiya T. Interaction of zinc and vitamin A on the ocular surface. *Graefes Arch Clin Exp Ophthalmol* 2002;240:1011-1021.

Karcioglu ZA. Zinc in the eye. *Surv Ophthalmol.* 1982;27:114-122.

Katz JP, Perreault N, Goldstein BG, Lee CS, Labosky PA, Yang VW, Kaestner KH. The zinc-finger transcription factor klf4 is required for terminal differentiation of goblet cells in the colon. *Development* 2002;129:2619-2628.

King JC , Keen C. Zinc, In: Shils ME, Olson JA, Shike M, Ross C, ed. *Modern Nutrition in Health and Disorder.* 9th ed. Philadelphia: Lippincott Williams & Wilkins; 1999: 223-239.

Kirchgessner M, Moser C, Roth HP. Activity and subcellular distribution of protein kinase C(PKC) in muscle and brain of force-fed zinc-deficient rats. *Biol Trace Element Res.* 1996;52:273-280.

Klingberg WG, Prasad AG, Oberleas D. Zinc deficiency following penicillamine therapy. In: Prasad AS, ed. *Trace Elements in Human Health and Diseases. Zinc and Copper.* Vol. 1. New York, NY:Academic Press Inc;1976:51-65.

Kondo T, Sharp FR, Honkaniemi J, Mikawa S, Epstein CT, Chan PH. DNA fragmentation and prolonged expression of c-fos, c-jun, and hsp 70 in kainic acid-induced neuronal cell death in transgenic mice overexpressing human CuZn-superoxide dismutase. *J Cereb Blood Flow Metab.* 1997;17:241-256.

Kraus A, Roth HP, Kirchgessner M. Influence of vitamin C, vitamin E and beta-carotene on the osmotic fragility and the primary antioxidant system of erythrocytes in zinc-deficient rats. *Arch Tierernahl.* 1997;50:257-269.

Lauweryns B, Van Den Oord JJ, Volpes R, Foets B, Missotten L. Distribution of very late activation integrins in the human cornea. An immunohistochemical study using monoclonal antibodies. *Invest Ophthalmol Vis Sci.* 1991;32:2079-2085.

LaVail MM, Ward PA. Studies on the hormonal control of circadian outer segment disc shedding in the rat retina. *Invest Ophthalmol Vis Sci.* 1978;17:1189-1193.

Lee PW, Green MA, Long WB, 3rd, Gill W. Zinc and wound healing. *Surg Gynecol Obestet.* 1976;143:549-554.

Leiner M, Leiner G. Der Zinkgehalt in den Augen von Knochenfischen. *Biol Zentralbl.* 1942;62:119-132.

Leure-duPree AE. Electron-opaque inclusions in the rat retinal pigment epithelium after treatment with chelators of zinc. *Invest Ophthalmol Vis Sci.* 1981;21(1 pt1):1-9.

Leure-duPree AE, McClain CJ. The effect of severe zinc deficiency on the morphology of the rat pigment epithelium. *Invest Ophthalmol Vis Sci.*.1982;23:425-434.

Leure-duPree AE. Vascularization of the rat cornea after prolonged zinc deficiency. *Anat Rec.* 1986;216:27-32.

Leure-duPree AE, Connor MJ. The effect of deferoxamine, an iron chelator, on the morphology of the retina. *Prog Clin Biol Res*. 1987;247:517-529.

McClain CJ, Su LC, Gilbert H, Cameron D. Zn deficiency –induced retinal dysfunction in Crohn's disease. *Dig Dis Sci*. 1983;28:85-87.

Mizoguchi T, Amemiya T. Ultrastructural study of corneal epithelium in zinc-deficient rats — deficiency and recovery. *Trace element Med*. 1992;9:84-89.

Mishima K, Dake Y, Amemiya T, Nishimura M. Electron microscopic study of optic nerves of macular mice. *Exp Eye Res*. 1996;63:85-90.

Mohan R, Lee B, Panjwani N. Molecular cloning of the E-cadherin cDNAs from rabbit corneal epithelium. *Curr Eye Res*. 1995;14:1136-1145.

Muga SJ, Grider A. Partial characterization of a human zinc-deficiency syndrome by differential display. *Biol Trace Element Res*. 1999;68:1-12.

Myung SJ, Yang SK, Jung HY, Jung SA, Kang CH, Ha HK. Hong WS, Min YI. Zinc deficiency manifested by dermatitis and visual dysfunction in a patient with Crohn's disease. *J Gastroenterol*. 1998;33:876-879.

Nakamoto T, Yamagata T, Sakai R, Ogawa S, Honda H, Ueno H, Hirano N, Yazaki Y, Hirai H. CIZ, a zinc finger protein that interacts with p/30(cas) and activates the expression of matrix metalloproteinases. *Mol Cell Biol*. 2000;20:1649-1658.

Norman JN, Rahmat A, Smith G. Effects of supplements of zinc salts on the healing of granulating wounds in the rat and guinea pig. *J Nutr*. 1975;105:815-821.

Oberleas D, Seymour JK, Lenaghan R, Hovanesian J, Wilson RF, Prasad AS. Effect of zinc deficiency on wound-healing in rats. *Am J Surg*. 1971;121:566-568.

Ortega SS, Cachaza JA, Tovar IV, Feijoo MF. Zinc deficiency dermatitis in parenteral nutrition : an EM study. *Dermatologica* 1985;171:163-169.

Ozsoylu S, Kocak N, Akgun N. Zinc deficiency in cirrhosis. *Gut* 1991;32:458.

Paallysaho T, Williams DS. Epithelial cell-substrate adhesion in the cornea: localization of actin, talin, integrin, and fibronectin. *Exp Eye Res*. 1991;52:261-267.

Prasad AS, Miale AJ, Farid Z, Sandstead HH, Darby WJ. Biochemical studies on dwarfism, hypogonadism, and anemia. *Arch Int Med*. 1963;111:407.

Prasad AS, Oberleas D. Thymidine kinase activity and incorporation of thymidine into DNA in zinc-deficient tissue. *J Lab Clin Med*. 1974;83:634-639.

Prasad AS. Clinical manifestations of zinc deficiency. Annu Rev Nutr. 1985;5:341-363.

Prasad AS. Zinc: an overview. *Nutrition*. 1995;11:93-99.

Rahmat A, Norman JN, Smith G. The effect of zinc deficiency on wound healing. *Br J Surg*. 1974;61:271-273.

Raskin NH, Sligar KP, Steinberg RH. Dark adaptation slowed by inhibitors of alcohol dehydrogenase in the albino rat. *Brain Res*. 1973;50:496-500.

Rayner SA, Gallop JL, George AJ, Larkin OF. Distribution of intergins alpha v beta 5, alpha v beta 3 and alpha v in normal human cornea: possible implications in clinical and therapeutic adenoviral infection. *Eye*. 1998;12:273-277.

Roth HP, Kirchgessner M. Zn metalloenzyme activities. Changes and biochemical aspects in Zn deficiency. *World Rev Nutr Diet*. 1980;3:144-160.

Ruoslahti E. Integrins. *J Clin Invest*. 1991;87:1-5.

Sandstead HH, Vo-khactu KP, Solomons N. Conditioned Zn deficiencies. In Prasad AS, ed. *Trace Elements in Human Health and Diseases*. Zinc and Copper. Vol. l. New York, NY: Academic Press Inc; 1976:33-49.

Sandstead HH. Discovery of zinc deficiency in patients receiving total parenteral alimentation, clinical correlations. *Nutrition*. 1989;5:21-22.

Satre MA, Jessen KA, Clegg MS, Keen CL. Retinal binding protein expression is induced in HepG2 cells by zinc deficiency. *FEBS Lett*. 2001;491:266-271.

Scholmerich J, Lohle E, Kottgen E, Gerok W. Zinc and vitamin A deficiency in liver cirrhosis. *Hepatogastroenterology*. 1983;30:119-125.

Senapati A, Thompson RP. Zinc deficiency and the prolonged accumulation of zinc in wounds. *Br J Surg*. 1985;72:583-584.

Shams NB, Hanninen LA, Chaves HV, Frangieh G, Reddy CV, Azar DT, Kenyon KR. Effect of vitamin A deficiency on the adhesion of rat corneal epithelium and the basement membrane complex. *Invest Ophthalmol Vis Sci*. 1993;34:2646-2654.

Smith JC Jr, McDaniel EG, Fan FF, Halsted JA. Zinc: a trace element essential in vitamin A metabolism. *Science*. 1973;181:954-955.

Smith JE, Brown ED, Smith JC Jr. The effect of zinc deficiency on the metabolism of retinol-binding protein in the rat. *J Lab Clin Med*. 1974;84:692-697.

Smith JC Jr, Brown ED, McDaniel EG, Chan W. Alterations in vitamin A metabolism during zinc deficiency and food and growth restriction. *J Nutr*. 1976;106:569-574.

Solomons NW, Russell RM. The interaction of vitamin A and zinc: implications for human nutrition. *Am J Clin Nutr*. 1980;33:2031-2040.

Stepp MA, Spurr-Michaud S, Gipson IK. Integrin in the wounded and unwounded stratified squamous epithelium of the cornea. *Invest Ophthalmol Vis Sci*. 1993;34:1829-1844.

Stepp MA, Zhu L, Cranfill R. Changes in beta 4 integrin expression and localization in vivo in response to corneal epithelial injury. *Invest Ophthalmol Vis Sci*. 1996;37:1593-1601.

Strain WH, Dutton AM, Heyer HB. *Experimental studies on the acceleration of burn and wound healing*. University of Rochester Reports. New York:University of Rochester;1953:

Sturtevant EM. Zinc deficiency, acrodermatitis enteropathica, optic atrophy, subacute myelo-optic neuropathy, and 5,7-dihalo-8-quinolinols. *Pediatrics*. 1980;65:610-613.

Sullivan JF, Jetton MM, Hahn HK, Burch RE. Enhanced lipid peroxidation in liver microsomes of zinc-deficient rats. *Am J Clin Nutr*. 1980;33:51-56.

Takami Y, Gong H, Amemiya T. Riboflavin deficiency induces ocular surface damage. *Ophthalmic Res*. 2004;36:156-165.

Tauber RW, Klause AC. The role of iron, copper, zinc and manganese in the metabolism of the ocular tissue with special reference to the lens. *Am J Ophthalmol*. 1943;26:260-266.

Tenaud I, Leroy S, Chebassier N, Dreno B. Zinc, copper and manganese enhanced keratinocyte migration through a functional modulation of keratinocyte integrins. *Exp Dermatol*. 2000;9:407-416.

Tengrup I, Ahonen J, Zederfeldt B. Granulation tissue formation in zinc-treated rats. *Acta Chir Scand*. 1980;146:1-4.

Tengrup I, Ahonen J, Zederfeldt B. Influence of zinc on synthesis and accumulation of collagen in early granulation tissue. *Surg Gynecol Obstet*. 1981;152:323-326.

Terril-Robb LA, Clemons DJ, Besch-Williford C, O'Brien DP, O'Dell BL. Morphophysiologic characterization of peripheral neuopathy in zinc-deficient guinea pigs. *Proc Soc Exp Biol Med.* 1996;213:50-58.

Tervo K, Tervo T, Van Setten G, Virtanen I. Integrins in human corneal epithelium. *Cornea.* 1991;10:461-465.

Trinkaus-Randall V, Tong M, Thomas P, Cornell-Bell A. Conforcal imaging of the alpha 6 and beta 4 integrin subunits in the human cornea with aging. *Invest Ophthalmol Vis Sci.* 1993;34:3103-3109.

Trujillo EB. Effects of nutritional status on wound healing. *J Vasc Nurs.* 1993;11:12-18.

Tseng H. Basonuclin, a zinc finger protein associated with epithelial expression and proliferation. *Front Biosci.* 1998;3:985-988.

Tsuda Y. Optic nerve changes in ascorbic acid-deficient rats. *Acta Med Nagasaki.* 2002;47:161-166.

Tumer AR, Kama NA, Tumer L, Reis E, Muftuoglu S. Effects of 5-fluorouracil and zinc on healing of colonic anastomoses in rabbits. *Eur J Surg.* 1999;165:369-377.

Vallee BL, Falchuk KH. Biochemical basis of zinc physiology. *Physiol Rev.* 1993;73:79-118.

Vannucchi H, Favaro RM, Cunha DF, Marchini JS. Assessment of zinc nutritional status of pellagra patients. *Alcohol.* 1995;30:297-302.

Virgili F, Canali R, Figus E, Vignolini F, Nobili F, Mengheri E. Intestinal damage induced by zinc deficiency is associated with enhanced Cu•Zn superoxide dismutase activity in rats: effects of dexamethasone or thyroxine treatment. *Free Radic Biol Med.* 1999;26:1194-1201.

Wacker ECW. Role of zinc in wound healing: A critical review. In Ananda SP, ed. *Trace elements in human health and disease.* New York:Academic Press Inc;1976:107-113.

Weisman K. Chelating drugs and zinc. *Dan Med Bull.* 1986;38:208-211.

Welsmann K, Kvist N, Kobayashi T. Bullous acrodermatitis due to zinc deficiency during total parenteral nutrition: an ultrastructural study of the epidermal changes. *Acta Derm Venereol.* 1983;63:143:146.

Williams KJ, Meltzer R, Brown RA, Tanaka Y, Chiu RC. The effect of topically applied zinc on the healing of open wounds. *J Surg Res.* 1979;27:62-67

Williams RB, Cheaters JK. The effect of early zinc deficiency on DNA and protein synthesis in rat. *Br J Nutr.* 1970;24:1053:-1054.

Yolton DP. Nutritional effects of zinc on ocular and systemic physiology. *J Am Optom Assoc.* 1981;52:409-414.

Zidenberg-Cherr S, Keen CL, Lönnerdal B, Hurley LS. Superoxide dismutase activity and lipid peroxidation in the rat: developmental correlations affected by manganese deficiency. *J Nutr.* 1983;113:2498-2504.

Zidenberg-Cherr S, Han B, Dubick MA, Keen CL. Influence of dietary-induced copper and manganese deficiency on ozone-induced changes in lung and liver antioxidant systems. *Toxicol* Lett. 1991;57:81-90.

Chapter 3

COPPER

PART I. COPPER DEFICIENCY

I. Significance

Copper is most frequently present in biologic systems as Cu^{2+}, including at least three types of bound Cu^{2+} which are found in copper-containing enzymes. Copper-containing enzymes include amine oxidases (monoamine oxidase, diamine oxidase etc.), ferroxidases (ceruloplasmin and ferroxidase II), cytochrome-c oxidase, dopamine β-hydroxylase, superoxide dismutase and tyrosinase. Albumin is also bound to copper, but not an enzyme.

Since copper is essential for cross-linking of collagen and elastin through lysyl oxidase, copper plays a role in bone formation, skeletal mineralization, and the integrity of the connective tissue in the heart and vascular system.

Copper is required for formation or maintenance of myelin, composed primarily of phospholipids. Cytochrome-oxidase activity is related to phospholipid synthesis. Thus, copper deficiency may lead to poor development of myelin, necrosis of nerve tissue, and neonatal ataxia. The role of cuproenzymes in catecholamine metabolism suggests a function in normal neurotransmission (Prohaska, 1990).

Copper is required for melanin synthesis in the pigmentation of skin, hair and eyes. Copper is known to be both prooxidant and antioxidant. The antioxidant enzymes such as ceruloplasmin and superoxide dismutase decrease in copper deficiency and induce impaired antioxidant conditions (Johnson and Fisher, 1992).

In humans, copper deficiency has been reported in patients treated with total parenteral nutrition, in premature infants fed milk formulas, in infants recovering from malnutrition usually due to chronic diarrhea, in infants undergoing chronic peritoneal dialysis and in severely handicapped patients. The clinical features are anemia, leukopenia, neutropenia, arthritis, arterial disease, loss of pigmentation, myocardial disease, and neurologic effects (Danks, 1988). Menkes' disease and Wilson disease are due to genetic defects in copper metabolism.

Copper deficiency has been induced experimentally and observed in areas with copper-deficient soil in rats, mice, guinea pigs, rabbits, chicken, pigs, dogs, cattle, goats and sheep.

Generally speaking, the deficiencies induced in animals are more severe than those in humans. Anemia, neutropenia, and osteoporosis are seen and other manifestations include skeletal abnormalities, fractures, spinal deformities, neonatal ataxia, depigmentation of hair, impaired keratinization of hair and fur, reproductive failure, cardiovascular disorders, rupture of blood vessels, and impaired immune function.

An adequate supply of copper is needed in the development of the nervous and cardiovascular systems in the neonatal period (Prohaska and Wells, 1974; Kitano, 1980). Some enzymes containing copper are related to lipid synthesis, collagen formation and neurotransmitters, etc (Gallager and Reeve, 1970; Morgan and O'Dell, 1977; Siegel, Pinnel and Martin, 1970). The depression of enzymatic activity caused by copper deficiency may result in various morphological biological alterations. For instance, cytochrome oxidase contains 1 mol each of cytochromes a and a_3, 2 mol Cu mol enzyme^{-1}, and activity of the complex in copper deficiency declines to 25% of control values (Prohaska and Wells, 1974). Carlton and Kelly (1967) demonstrated that reduction of cytochrome oxidase activity may be a biochemical lesion leading to the morphologic alterations induced by tissue hypoxia. Clinically, copper deficiency has been demonstrated in Menkes' disease and is considered to be due to impaired intracellular copper transport (Danks and Cartwright, 1973).

Dietary copper deficiency in neonates has been induced experimentally in pigs, mice and rats (Everson, Tsai and Wang, 1967; Prohaska and Wells, 1975; Prohaska, 1983). Focal necrotic and edematous neural tissues, impairment of myelin formation and swollen mitochondria have been observed morphologically in the cerebrum and cerebellum (Carlton and Kelly, 1967; Dipaodo, Kanfer and Newberne, 1974). However, the effect of copper deficiency on the ocular tissues has not been examined. Hirayama (1990) demonstrated that trace metal copper is located in the cornea, iris, ciliary body, retina and retinal pigment epithelial layer. But its role in ocular tissues also has not yet been fully examined.

II. Copper Deficient Experiment

Materials and Methods

Experiment I

Maturing female Wistar albino rats weighing 200g were mated with males fed commercial rat pellets. After mating all females were individually housed in plastic tubs for delivery, and divided into copper-deficient and control groups. During gestation and lactation, females were given deionized water and a purified diet low in copper prescribed by the American Institute of Nutrition (1977). The control group was given the same purified diet and supplemented copper in their drinking water as copper sulphate (Cu: 20ppm). All litters were reduced to 6-8 pups per mother within 7 days after birth. At 3 weeks of age, the pups were weaned to the same diet and water as their dams and transferred to suspended stainless steel cages.

After 3, 5 or 7 weeks on a copper-deficient diet, the eyes were enucleated under pentobarbital anesthesia and blood was drawn from the aorta for measurement of the plasma copper level. At least five rats were killed at each experimental week.

Experiment II

Since the C_3H mouse is a blind mouse with abnormal retinas, C_3H female heterozygote macular mice were mated with $C_{57}BL_6J$ male mice. Fourteen-day- and 1-month-old male hemizygote macular mice were used for the experiments and female heterozygotes and normal male littermates as controls. Seven-day-old hemizygotes under diethylether anesthesia were injected 50μg $CuCl_2$ per 0.1ml distilled into the abdomens.

Clinical features of copper deficient animals

Experiment I: Body weights were not significantly different between the two groups at the beginning of the experiment. In the deficient rats, however, weight gain became gradually depressed. Within 4 weeks, the copper-deficient rats exhibited body tremor, inactivity and progressive gait disturbance. Some copper-deficient rats developed complete paralysis of their hind limbs. In addition, seizures were observed in a severe case at 5 weeks of age and many copper deficient rats died suddenly after 11 weeks of age. However, spontaneous elevation of the tail and hypertension to noise were not observed.

The serum copper levels of the deficient group were obviously decreased at every experimental week than those of the control group; the difference between the two groups was statistically significant (Table 3.2.1).

Table 3. 2. 1. Serum copper level ($\mu g\ dl^{-1}$).

Groups	Weeks after start of experiment			
	3*	5*	7*	11*
Copper deficiency	12.4±2.4	10.2±0.25	17.1±3.5	20.3±7.6
	(n=5)	(n=12)	(n=18)	(n=3)
Control	58.2±9.9	89.9±8.1	76.3±11.9	102.3±17.2
	(n=5)	(n=12)	(n=18)	(n=3)
*p<0.01				

Experiment II: Hemizygote macular mice (Fig. 3.2.1) showed inadequate suckling on the 10th day, then gradually lost weight (Fig. 3.2.2). They died, on average, at 14 days of age (Fig. 3.2.2). Since hemizygote macular mice have a congenital disturbance of copper metabolism, they could be revived and their body weight increased by the administration of 50μg $CuCl_2$ per 0.1ml distilled water, but their growth was poorer than that of the controls (Fig. 3.2.3).

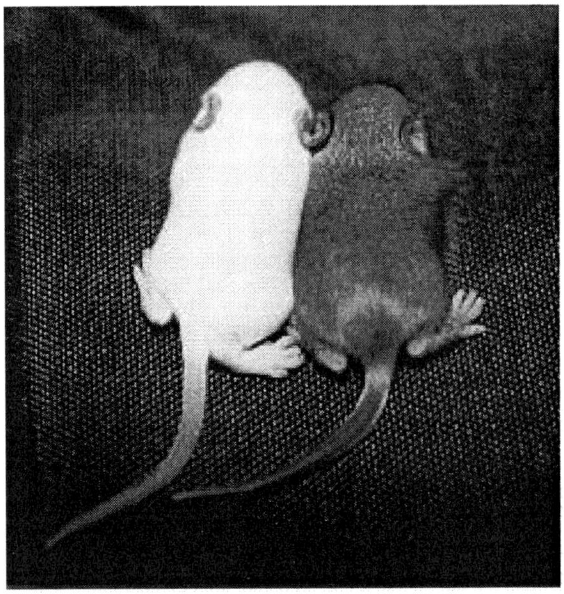

Figure 3.2.1. Left side, a control mouse and right side, hemizygote macular mouse.

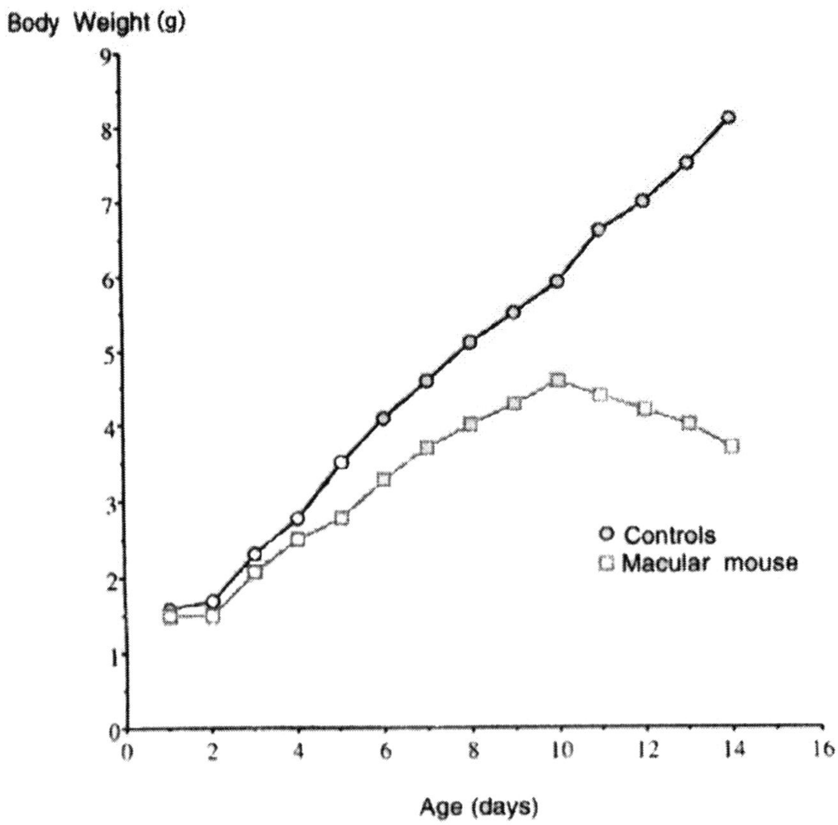

Figure 3.2.2. Body weight of male hemizygote and normal lettermates (controls).

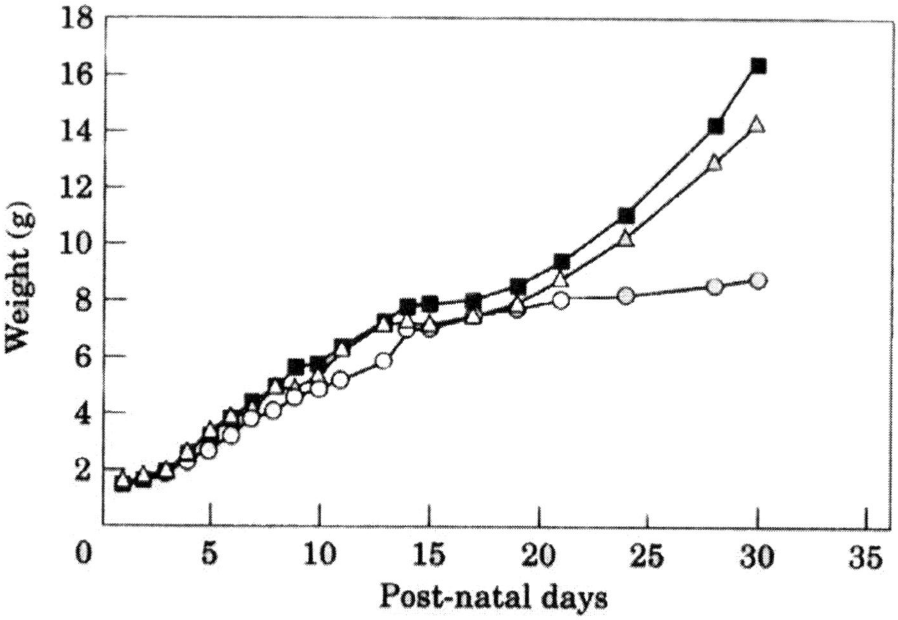

Figure 3.2.3. Body weights of hemizygote treated with $CuCl_2$ (▯), heterozygote (△), and normal littermate (■). *50μg $CuCl_2$ per 0.1ml distilled water injected into the abdominal cavity of hemizygote macular mouse on seven postnatal day.

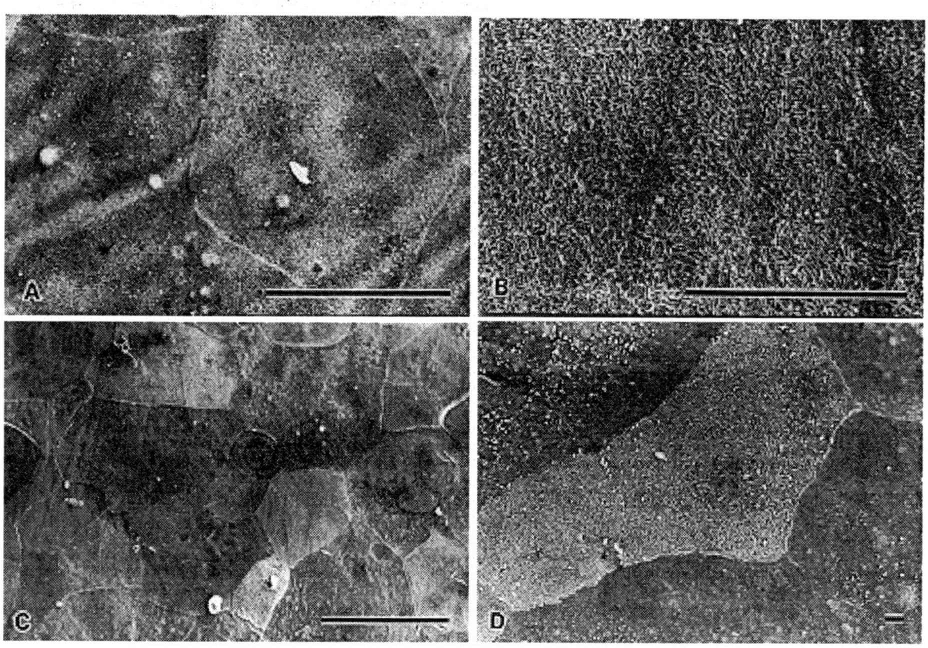

Figure 3.3.1. SEM micrographs showing the corneal surface of a 14-day-old control mouse (A, B) and of a 14-month-old hemizygote macular mouse (C, D). The surface seems to have a little bit more dark cells in a hemizygote macular mouse than in a control mouse. Dark cells have scarce microvilli (C, D). Bar: 20μm (A), 10μm (B), 50μm (C), 1μm (D).

III. The Cornea

Results

Experiment II

Scanning Electron Microscopic (SEM) Findings

In the copper deficient rat, dark cells were slightly increased in the most superficial epithelial cell layer as compared with those in the control rat, and they had fewer microvilli and microplicae (Fig. 3.3.1).

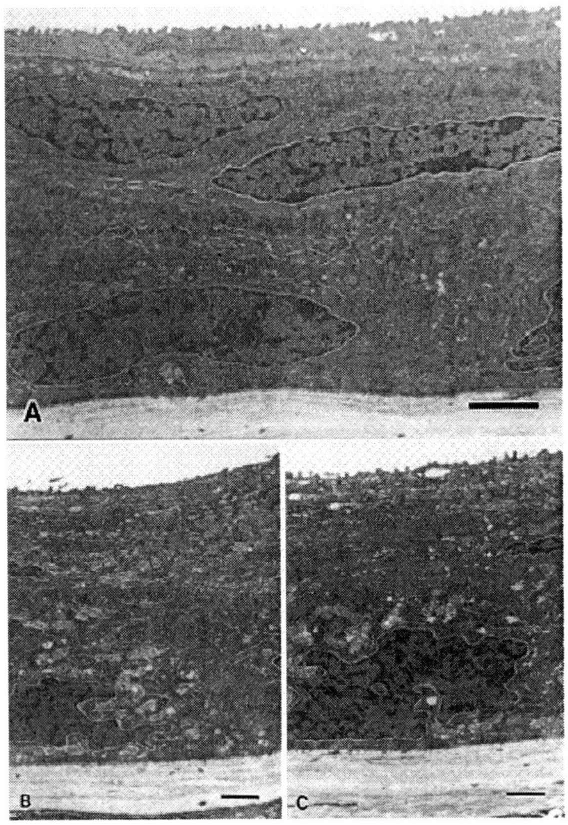

Figure 3.3.2. TEM micrographs of the corneal epithelium of macular and control mice. A control mouse shows prominent microvilli (A), but a macular mouse has scarce microvilli at some site (B) but many at some site (C). Bar: 2μm (A), 1μm (B, C).

Transmission Electron Microscopic Findings

In macular mice TEM showed that the epithelial microvilli and microplicae were decreased (Fig. 3.3.2), but showed no changes on the cytoplasmic organelles such as fibrils, intercellular junctions, mitochondria and ribosomes. In the endothelium macular mice showed wavy endothelium, i.e. normally thick at some sites and very thin at some sites (Fig. 3.3.3). At the normal thick endothelium, a large vacuole was seen containing amorphous materials.

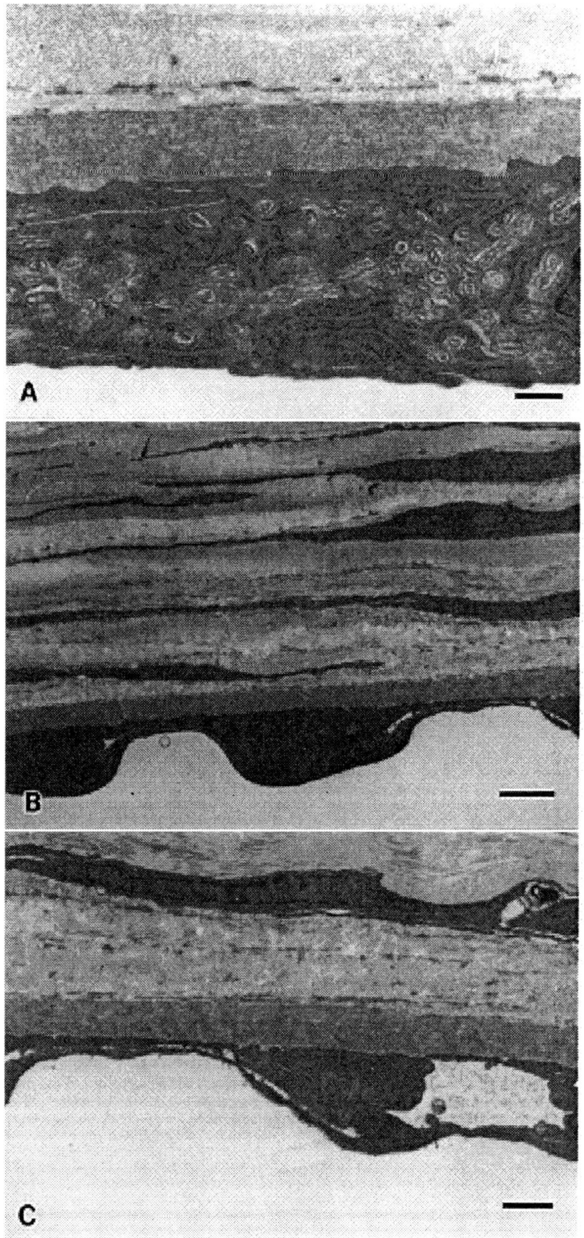

Figure 3.3.3. TEM micrographs of the endothelium of control and hemizygote macular mice. The endothelium of control mouse cornea is thick and contains many mitochondria and well-developed rough-surfaced endoplasmic reticulum (A). However, the endothelium of a macular mouse is a wavy figure, i.e. very thin at some site and almost normal thick at some site (B). At some site the endothelial cell contains a large vacuole with amorphous materials (C). Bar: 500nm (A), 2μm (B), 1μm (C).

Discussion

In chemical studies, copper has been shown to be present in high concentrations in the iris, corneal epithelium, retina, lens, optic nerve, choroid, sclera, and conjunctiva in ascending order (Bowness, Morton, Shakir et al, 1952; Eckert, 1983; Tauber and Krause,

1943). Hirayama (1990) demonstrated histochemically that trace metal copper is located in the cornea, iris, ciliary body, retina and pigment epithelium. In the cornea, he strongly showed histochemical localizations of Cu in the epithelium, but endothelium and Descemet membrane was observed weekly. Histochemistry failed to demonstrate Cu in the stroma, but chemical analysis showed highest Cu concentration in the epithelium which was about two times more than in the stroma (Tauber and Klause 1943).

Cytochrome oxidase, a Cu-containing enzyme, has been demonstrated histochemically in the retina (Kageyama and Wong-Riley, 1984; Lachica, Condo and Gasagrande, 1987; Kageyama and Meyer, 1988) and in the cornea (Tuberville, Wood and McLaughlin, 1986, 1987; Hayashi and Kenyon, 1988). Cu·Zn superoxide dismutase (Cu·Zn SOD), a Cu-containing enzyme, is also demonstrated in the epithelium and endothelium (Redmond, Duke, Coles et al, 1984).

In the cornea of macular mice, dark cells were slightly increased in the most superficial layer of the epithelium. Dark cells had scarce microvilli and microplicae. More severe epithelial damages due to Cu deficiency might be expected because Cu, cytochrome oxidase and Zn·Cu SOD coexist in the epithelium. However, epithelial damages due to Cu deficiency was slight: decreased microvilli and microplicae, but endothelial changes were prominent: wavy endothelium and large vacuoles. But what the wavy endothelium means is unclear. It is assumed that macular mice died without supplementation of Cu until 14 days after birth before epithelial damages appeared due to functional disturbance induced by Cu deficiency and reduced activities of Cu-containing enzymes such as cytochrome oxidase and Cu·Zn SOD.

IV. The Retina

Experiment I

Method for demonstration of cytochrome oxidase activity

After 11 weeks on a copper deficient diet, the eyes were enucleated under pentobarbital anesthesia. Specimens were cut into 80μm thick slices with a vibratome. According to the diaminobenzidine (DAB) method of Seligman et al (1968), slices were incubated for light and electron microscopy (Dake, 1992).

Reactive products resulted from oxidation of DAB deposit on the mitochondrial intermembrane-intracristal space and tended to grow into these spaces.

The area of mitochondrial intermembrane-intracristal space in electron micrographs at the magnification of 70,000 was measured with a computed image analyzer Zeiss IBAS by a point count method (Hirai, Ogawa, Wang et al, 1989). The area occupied by deposition of the reactive product under an adequate threshold was measured with the same method. Tangential sections of mitochondria were eliminated from the measurement. The percentage of the area occupied by the reaction product in each mitochondrion was calculated and statistically analyzed.

Results

Histochemical findings of cytochrome oxidase in the retina

The nerve fiber layer, ganglion cell layer, inner and outer plexiform layers, pigment epithelial layer and photoreceptor inner segment layer were stained dark brown in the control group. The photoreceptor inner segment layer showed an intensely positive reaction (Fig. 3.4.1A). On the other hand, the deficient group showed light yellow staining in each layer and less stainability. The reaction to cytochrome oxidase in the photoreceptor inner segments was apparently reduced (Fig. 3.4.1B). Negative controls incubated with the medium containing 0.1M NaN_3 showed no staining, indicating complete inhibition of reaction.

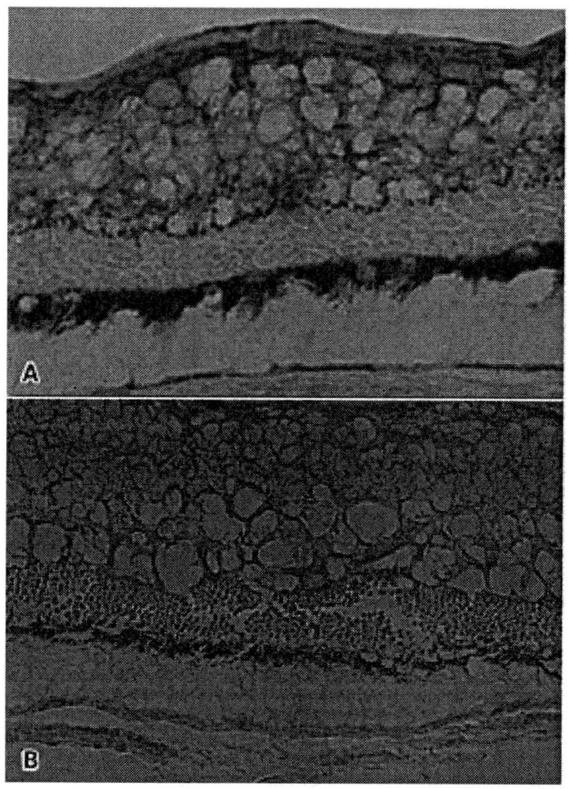

Figure 3.4.1. Cytochrome oxidase histochemical findings. A control rat: the nerve fiber layer, ganglion cell layer, inner and outer plexiform layers, pigment epithelial layer and photoreceptor inner segment layer are stained dark brown with DAB reaction products in a control rat. × 200. B. A copper deficient rat shows light yellow staining in each cell layer of the retina with DAB histochemistry. Photoreceptor inner segments of a copper deficient rat show less staining with DAB. × 100.

Electron microscopic and cytochemical findings

Although many copper deficient rats died after 11 weeks of age, the photoreceptor inner segment showed no morphological changes.

In the control rats, DAB-OsO_4 reaction products (osmium black) resulting from oxidation of DAB were identified as dense nondroplet depositions on the inner membranes and intracristal spaces of the mitochondria. The deposit of osmium black showed an intense, homogeneous staining pattern and grew into the intermembrane-intracristal space in mitochondria indicating high activity (Fig. 3.4.1). The intracristal spaces of the mitochondria were filled with osminum black (Fig. 3.4.2).

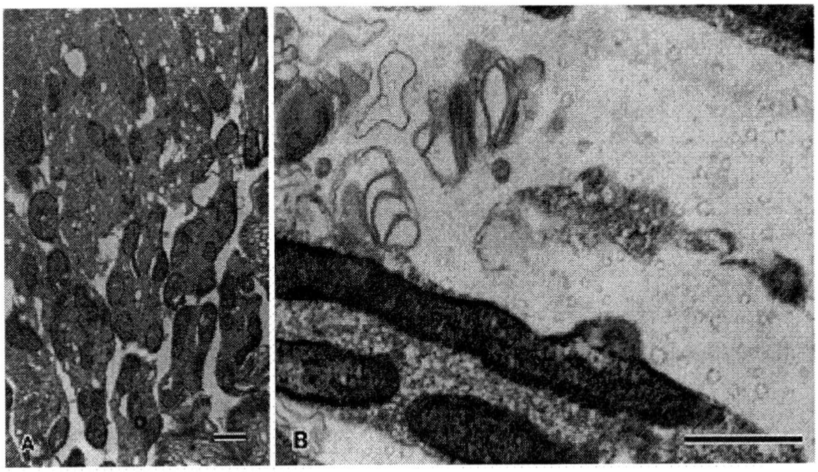

Figure 3.4.2. Electron micrograph of photoreceptor inner segments of a control rat. DAB-OsO_4 reaction products are seen as dense non-droplet depositions on the inner membranes and in the intracristal spaces of mitochondria (A, B). Bar: 1μm (A, B).

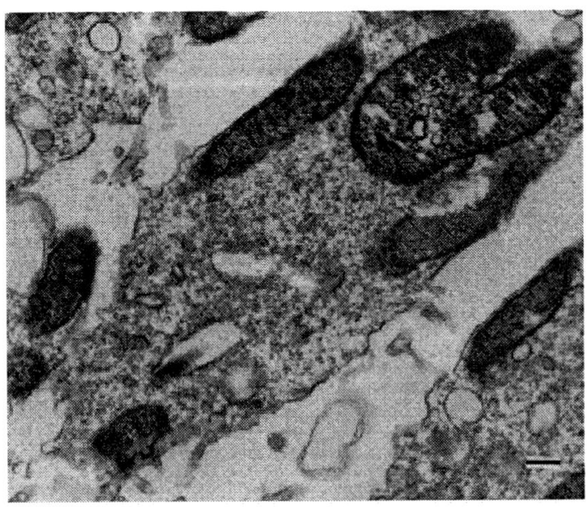

Figure 3.4.3. Electron micrograph of photoreceptor inner segments of a rat fed a copper deficient diet for 11 weeks. Reaction products are located on the inner membranes and narrow areas of the intracristal spaces of mitochondria. Bar: 0.5μm.

In copper deficient rats, depositions of osminum black were fewer than in the controls. DAB reaction products in the copper deficient group were insignificant and showed a localized staining pattern along the inner membrane and then occupied narrow areas of the intracristal spaces of the mitochondria (Fig. 3.4.3). The negative controls had no DAB-OsO_4 reaction products on the inner membranes or intracristal spaces of the mitochondria.

The area of reaction products resulting from oxidation of DAB was measured with the image analyzer. The results are shown in Table 3.4.1. Each value is a mean % area occupied by reaction products in the intermembrane-intracristal space. The paired t-test showed that cytochorome oxidase activity of the copper deficient group is significantly lower than that of the control group.

Table 3.4.1. Cytochorome oxidase activity (% area).

Control Group	65.2±8.9%* (n=30)
Copper-deficient group	38.0±18.0%* (n=30)
	* (p<0.01)

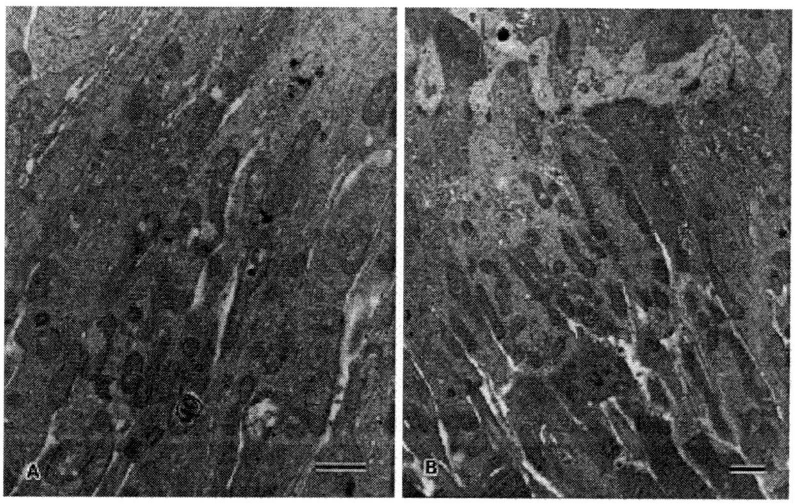

Figure 3.4.4. Electron micrograph showing the photoreceptor inner segment of a 12-day-old hemizygote macular mouse. Mitochondria contain swollen cristae and degeneration (B). A control littermate shows no abnormalities in mitochondria (A). Bar: 2μm (A, B).

Experiment II Results

Electron microscopic findings

Electron microscopy showed that the mitochondria in the photoreceptor inner segment of the hemizygote macular mouse retinas had a lower electron density in the matrix than did those in normal littermates and that they were swollen and contained swollen cristae and matrix (Figs 3.4.4). Swollen mitochondria were more numerous in the 14-day-old than in the 12-day-old macular mice. The development of the other parts of the retina, such as the inner limiting membrane, nerve fiber layer, ganglion cell layer, inner plexiform layer, inner nuclear layer, outer plexiform layer and outer nuclear layer, was almost the same as in normal littermates.

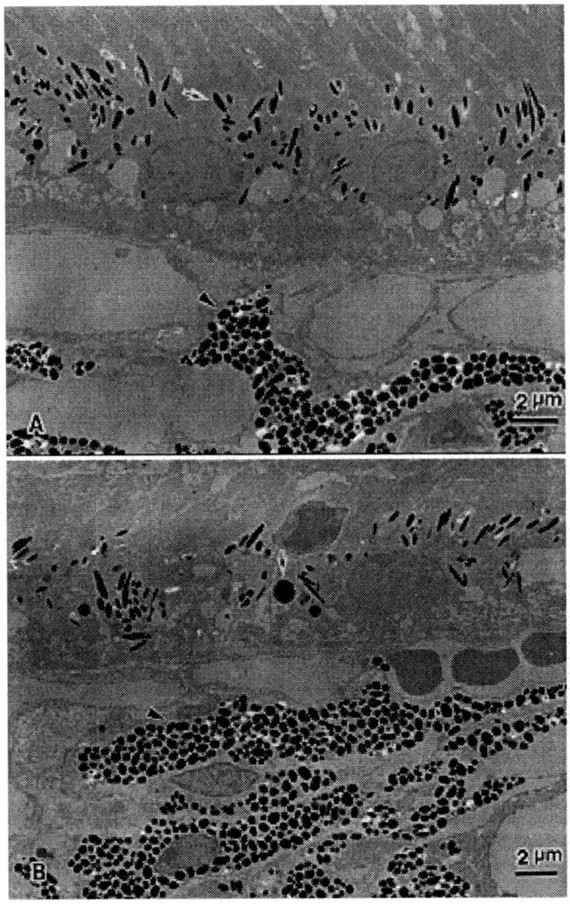

Figure 3.4.5. Electron micrographs of the RPE and choroid of 1-month-old normal littermate and hemizygote macular mouse. In normal littermate, many melanin granules in the RPE are spindle-shaped, and in the choroid. They are small oval or round (arrows) (A). In the hemizygote macular mouse, the melanin granules in the RPE are round or spindle-shaped, and those in the choroid are small, oval or round. The round melanin granules in the RPE seem to be larger than those in each control group and are almost the same as those in 14-day-old macular mice (B). Bar: 2μm (A, B).

The number of melanin granules in the RPE of 12-day-old hemizygote macular mice was 37.4±6.3 per 75μm^2 and of 14-day-old mice 36.3±6.8 per 75μm^2; in the normal littermates the numbers were 42.0±8.5 per 75μm^2 and 41.8±6.2 per 75μm^2, respectively. The difference is statistically significant ($p<0.05$) (Fig. 3.4.5) (Table 3.4.2). The computed image analyzer showed that the melanin granules in the RPE occupied 17.9±4.4% of a 75μm^2 field in the 12-day-old and 17.5±2.7% of such as a field in the 14-day-old hemizygote macular mice: in the normal littermates the figures were 19.9±4.4% and 19.4±2.7%, respectively. The percentage granule content was significantly lower in the macular mice than in the normal littermates (Table 3.4.3). There was no statistically significant difference in percentage of melanin granule content between the normal and fasting littermates (Table 3.4.3).

Table. 3.4.2. Number of melanin granules in retinal pigment epithelium (n: number of electron micrographs at an original magnification of 2000).

	Examined fields (n)	Melanin granules (/75μm²)
12-day-old macular mouse	50	37.40±6.34*,**
12-day-old normal mouse	50	42.04±8.52*
12-day-old nonmacular fasting mouse	50	40.84±8.12***
14-day-old macular mouse	50	36.32±6.85**,****
14-day-old normal mouse	50	41.76±6.17**
14-day-old nonmacular fasting mouse	50	40.12±7.45****
Unpaired t-test, *p<0.04; **p<0.05; ***p<0.1; ****p<0.07		

Table 3. 4. 3. Density of melanin granules (/75μm²) in retinal pigment epithelium (n: number of electron micrographs at an original magnification of 2000).

	Fields examined (n)	granule content (%)
12-day-old Macular mouse	50	17.85±4.35*,***
12-day-old normal mouse	50	19.90±4.35*
12-day-old nonmacular fasting mouse	50	19.14±3.00***
14-day-old macular mouse	50	17.51±2.67**,****
14-day-old normal mouse	50	19.37±2.69**
14-day-old nonmacular fasting mouse	50	19.07±2.67****
Unpaired t-test, *p<0.02; **p<0.001; ***p<0.08 (nonsignificant), ****p<0.05		

The melanin granules were spindle-shaped or small and round in the RPE and small or round on the choroid in normal litter mates (Fig. 3.4.5A). There were fewer melanin granules in the RPE and choroids of macular mice than in those of normal litter mates. Spindle-shaped melanin granules were more frequently seen in macular mice than in normal litter mates. The round melanin granules in RPE seemed larger than those in each control group and were almost the same size as those in 14-day-old macular mice (Fig. 3.4.5B).

Regarding the cytochrome oxidase activity (% area) in the retinal photoreceptor inner segments, quantitative analysis with a computed analyzer showed a statistically significant difference in reactive products between the control mice (55.42±18.36%, n=50) and the hemizygote macular mice (32.86±15.09%, n=50; $P<0.01$).

Discussion

In experiment I, swollen or enlarged mitochondria in the photoreceptor inner segment of 22-week-old nutritionally copper-deficient rats was characteristic and the activity of cytochrome oxidase, a copper-containing enzyme, was decreased in the mitochondria in their photoreceptor inner segment. In experiment II, the same findings were seen. Swollen and deformed mitochondria, as in patients with Menkes' disease are usually observed in animals with the nutritional or hereditary copper deficiency.

Cattle retina contains the second highest amount of copper in ocular tissue measuring with dry tissue by Tauber and Krause (1943). Hirayama (1990) also demonstrated with histochemical methods using rubeanic acid or rhodanine that trace metal copper is commonly located in the retina. Important copper metalloenzymes include cytochrome oxidase, superoxide dismutase, uricase, and DOPAmine β-hydroxylase. Copper and cytochrome oxidase coexist in the retinal photoreceptor inner segment. On the other hand, no cytochrome oxidase is demonstrated histochemically in the retinal pigment epithelium, choroid, sclera, or optic nerve (Hirayama, Dake and Amemiya 1992). The coexistence of copper and cytochrome oxidase suggests that copper plays a role in this copper metalloenzyme, while the non-coincidence of localization of copper and cytochrome oxidase may be attributed to histochemical problems or to some unknown function of copper.

According to the principle of histochemical demonstration for cytochrome oxidase activity (Seligman, Karnovsky, Wasserkrug et al, 1968), the reaction products resulting from the oxidation of DAB by cytochrome oxidase are present on the inner membranes of mitochondria and tend to grow into the intracristal spaces of mitochondria with strong cytochrome oxidase activity. Because of higher mitochondrial activity in nerve cells, cytochrome oxidase activity is a good metabolic and functional marker for neurons (Wong-Riley and Kageyama, 1986).

In the current study, a lower than normal osmium black precipitation was seen on the inner membranes and in the intracristal spaces of mitochondria in copper deficient rats, indicating low cytochrome oxidase activity. On the other hand, osmium black precipitate in the control rats were diffusely located on the inner membranes and completely occupied the intracristal spaces of mitochondria. These findings suggest that the copper deficiency may reduce cytochrome oxidase activity and decrease the function of photoreceptor inner segments.

Biochemical studies have shown that cytochrome oxidase in the mitochondria of copper deficient rats is reduced and that the amount of cytochrome a and a_3 is 30-40% of the control value (Lawrence, Davies, Mills et al, 1985). In addition, Prohaska and Wells (1975) demonstrated enlarged mitochondria in the brains of dietary copper deficient rats with a 25% reduction in cytochrome a and a_3 activities and 20% reduction in cytochrome oxidase activity. These findings are in accord with the current histochemical findings that copper deficiency reduces cytochrome oxidase activity.

Morphological alterations such as increased numbers of mitochondria and enlarged mitochondria containing tubulovesiculated cristae and dense body formation seen in Menkes' disease, brindled mice and experimental dietary copper deficient rats were not observed in 11-week-old copper deficient rats, although swollen mitochondria were seen in 22-week-old copper deficient rats (Dake and Amemiya, 1991). Since not only the swollen mitochondria but also the majority of normal-looking mitochondria showed very faint cytochrome oxidase activity in the brains of brindled mice, morphological changes in the mitochondria may be secondary to functional changes, such as reduced cytochrome oxidase activity (Yoshimura, 1988).

Morphological changes of mitochondria in photoreceptor inner segments appear to occur under conditions of severe or long-term copper deficiency (Mishima, Dake, Amemiya et al, 1996a). Swollen mitochondria have also been reported in ischemic cells (Ghadially, 1988). Cytochrome oxidase reduction may induce mitochondrial swelling (Prohaska and Wells, 1974; Prohaska and Wells, 1975), and mitochondria may increase in number to maintain mitochondrial function. Since the hemizygote macular mouse has a suckling disturbance and loses weight with age, we must consider the possibility that malnutrition reduces the production of melanins and anoxia causes mitochondrial swelling in the photoreceptor inner segment and cortical neurons. However, the findings in fasting littermates ruled out such possibilities.

The electron microscopic findings in the RPE in patients with Menkes' disease are: reduced numbers of melanin granules, absence of large spindle-shaped melanin bodies and presence of small and irregular melanin granules in electron-dense inclusion bodies (Wray, Kuwabara, Sanderson, 1976). In the current study, the melanin granules seemed larger in the RPE and choroid of macular mice than in those of normal littermates, and there were fewer melanin granules in the RPE of macular mice than in normal littermates. The author assumes that the decreased number of melanin granules in the RPE of the hemizygote macular mouse could be related to reduced tyrosinase activity, because tyrosinase is also a copper-containing enzyme. No melanin granules in the RPE of the nutritionally copper-deficient rat experiment has been found, because Wistar Kyoto albino rats without tyrosinase activity in the RPE were used. Furthermore, the function of the mitochondria in the RPE may be reduced by the lowered activity of cytochrome oxidase, although abnormal mitochondrial features were not seen in the RPE. It is assumed that in the macular mouse the activities of copper-containing enzymes – cytochrome oxidase, superoxide dismutase, tyrosinase etc – are decreased. Melanin production in the RPE might be affected, starting in the embryonic period, by lowered activities of copper-containing enzymes, such as tyrosinase, related to melanin production, since tyrosinase activity in the RPE usually disappears after birth (Mishima, Hasebe and Fujita, 1978). The decreased number of melanin granules in the RPE of the hemizygote macular mouse is not incompatible with the findings in patients with Menkes' disease. Large melanosomes, which have been referred to as giant melanosomes, have been reported in pigmentary disorders (Martuza, Philippe, Fitzpatrick, et al, 1985; Weis and Zelickson, 1977). The author assumes that the large melanin pigment in the RPE and choroid of macular mice is associated with hereditary copper deficiency (Mishima, Amemiya and Takano, 1999).

V. The Optic Nerve

Results

Electron microscopic findings

Experiment I

The number of myelinated axons from rats 3-, 5- and 7-week-old is demonstrated in Table 3.5.1. The difference between the deficient and control groups at each week was statistically significant by a Chi-square test ($P<0.01$).

Table 3.5.1. The number of myelinated axons in the postlaminar portion of the optic nerve (100 μ m^{-2}).

Group	Age (weeks)		
	3*	5*	7*
Control	46.0±16.5	56.5±12.8	48.7±11.6
Copper-deficient	24.1±12.6	22.0±9.9	38.9±20.2
*p<0.01			

In the postlaminar part of the optic nerve of rats fed a copper-deficient diet for 7 weeks, unmyelinated axons were more numerous than in the control rats (Fig. 3.5.1, 2). In the initial stage of the deficiency, destruction of myelin and proliferation of glial cells and their processes were local changes and were not observed diffusely in the optic nerve. However, this tendency became more prominent with age. The optic nerve in the deficient rats had few axons and many glial cells, mainly astrocytes, and their well-developed processes occupied the space between the axons. In comparison with the control group, the myelin in the copper-deficient rats were thinner and its lamellae were detached with many vacuoles. Swollen axons and vacuoles in the axonal cytoplasm were seen in the deficient group. After 7 weeks on a copper-deficient diet, swollen neurons were frequently observed in the prelaminar portion of the optic nerve (Fig. 3.5.2,3). Swollen axons contained few neurofilaments and many vacuoles. The control group revealed no abnormal findings.

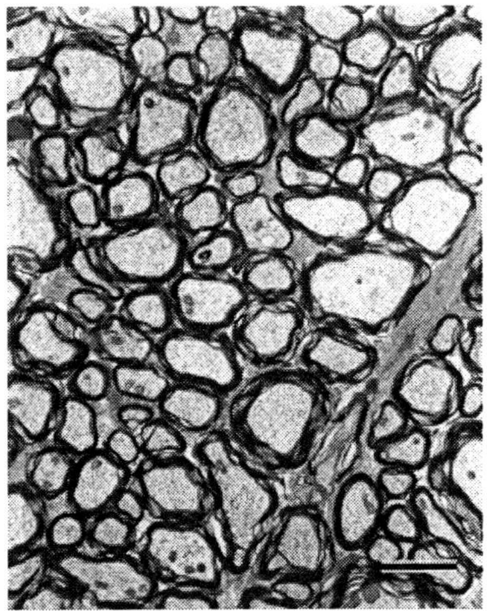

Figure 3.5.1. Electron micrograph of the postlaminar portion of the optic nerve of a rat fed a normal diet for 7 weeks. Bar: 2μm.

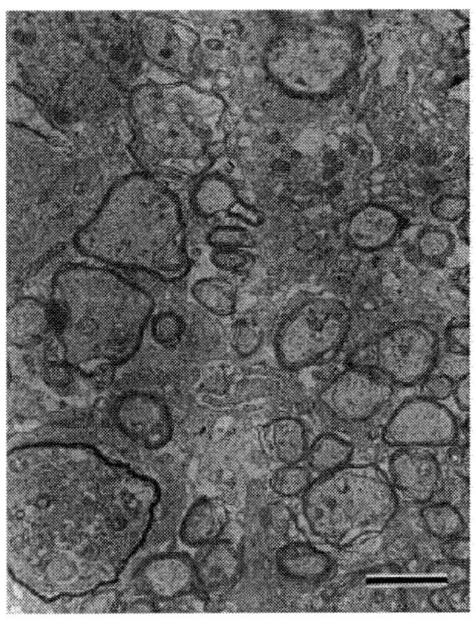

Figure 3.5.2. Electron micrograph of the postlaminar portion of the optic nerve of a rat fed a copper deficient diet for 7 weeks. Several unmyelinated axons and damaged myelin are seen. Glial cells with well-developed processes occupy the spaces between axons. Bar: 2μm.

Experiment II

Normal littermates had many axons and much myelin in the optic nerves at 14 days of age and they still had well-developing axons and myelin at 1 month of age (Figs. 3.5.4, 5). Fourteen-day-old heterozygote macular mice had fewer axons and more maldeveloped myelin in the optic nerve than did 14-day-old normal littermates (Figs. 3.5.6,7). One-month-old heterozygote macular mice had more axons and myelin in the optic nerve than did 14-day-old mice, but less than normal littermates. The optic nerve of 1-month-old heterozygote mice had focally demyelinated axons, but treated hemizygote macular mice had no demyelinated axons. Fourteen-day-old hemizygote macular mice had fewer axons than did normal littermates heterozygotes and much hypomyelination and unmyelinated axons (Fig. 3.5.8). But, at least 1 month of age, they had many well-developed axons, much myelin and no demyelineted axons (Fig. 3.5.9). The microtubules of the axons in hemizygote and heterozygote macular mice decreased in number. The numbers of myelinated axons in 14-day-old and 1-month-old hemizygote macular mice and normal littermates are listed in Table 3.5.2. The difference in number of axons between the normal littermates and hemizygote and heterozygote macular mice groups at 14 days and 1 month of age was statistically significant by the t-test ($P<0.01$). The difference in the number of axons between hemizygote and heterozygotes at 14-days of age was also statistically significant ($P<0.01$) (Table 3.5.2). The difference in the number of myelinated axons between hemizygote and heterozygote macular mice was not statistically significant at 1 month of age.

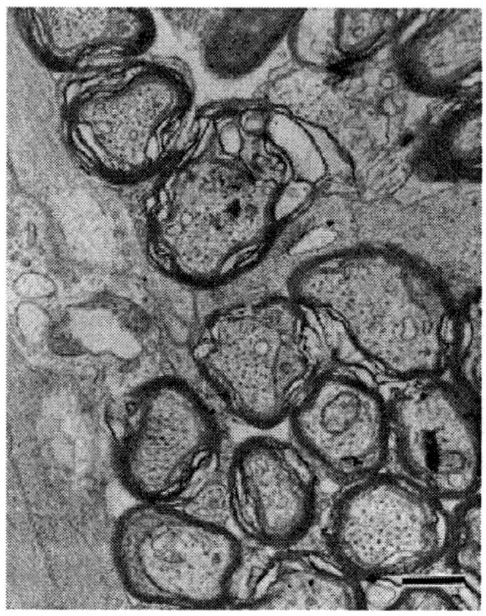

Figure 3.5.3. Electron micrograph of the postlaminar portion of the optic nerve of a rat fed a copper deficient diet for 7 weeks. Thin lamellae are seen. Axons with vacuoles are swollen. Bar: 0.5μm.

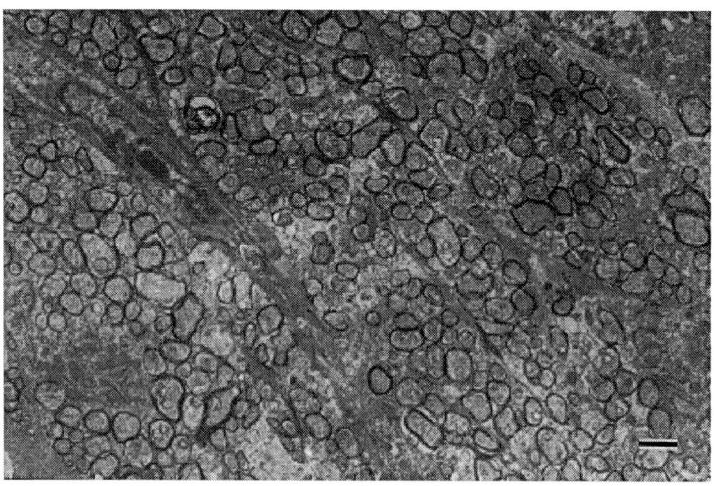

Figure 3.5.4. Electron micrograph showing optic nerve of a 14-day-old control mouse. Many axons and well-developed myelin are seen. Bar: 2μm.

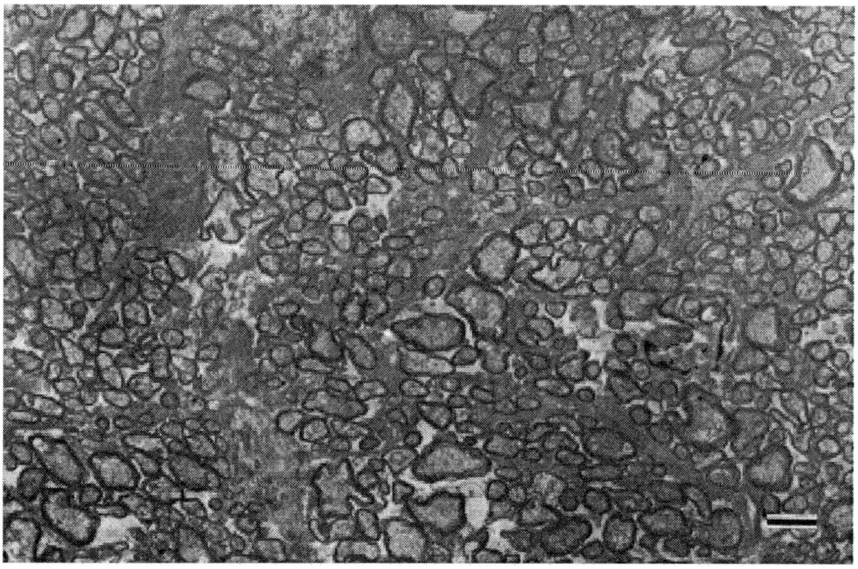

Figure 3.5.5. Electron micrograph of optic nerve of a 1-month-old control mouse. Many well-developed myelinated axons are seen. Bar: 2μm.

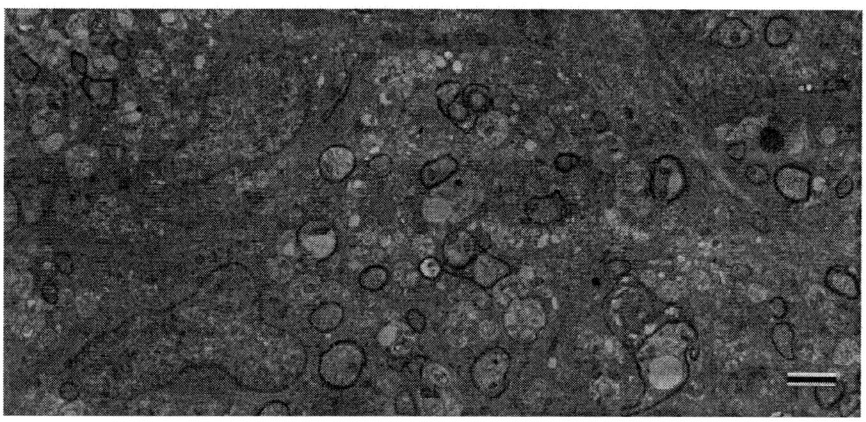

Figure 3.5.6. Electron micrograph showing optic nerves of a 14-day-old heterozygote macular mouse. Fewer axons and undeveloped myelin are seen, and glial cells with undeveloped processes occupy the spaces between axons. Bar: 2μm.

Table 3.5.2. Myelinated axons in optic nerve ($100\mu m^{-2}$).

	14 days after birth	1 month after birth
Hemizygotes (Ml/y)	9.7±3.8	38.3±8.3
Heterozygotes (Ml +)	15.5±4.0	38.4±8.4
Normal mice (+/y)	26.6±6.5	52.7±8.1

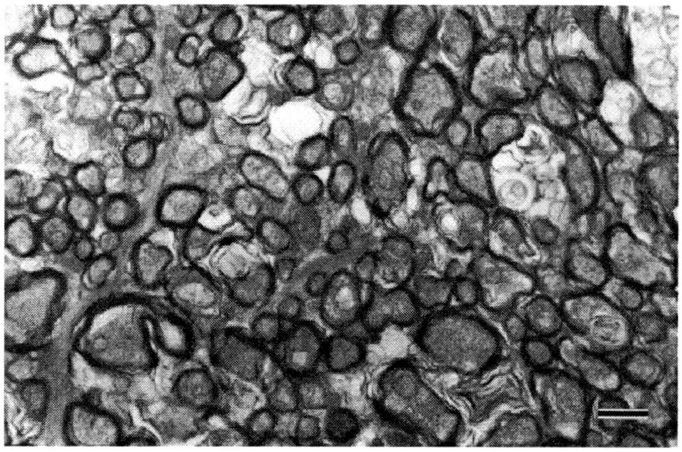

Figure 3.5.7. Electron micrograph showing optic nerve of a 1-month-old heterozygote macular mouse. Myelinated axons are increased, but demyelinated axons (arrows) are also seen. Bar: 1μm.

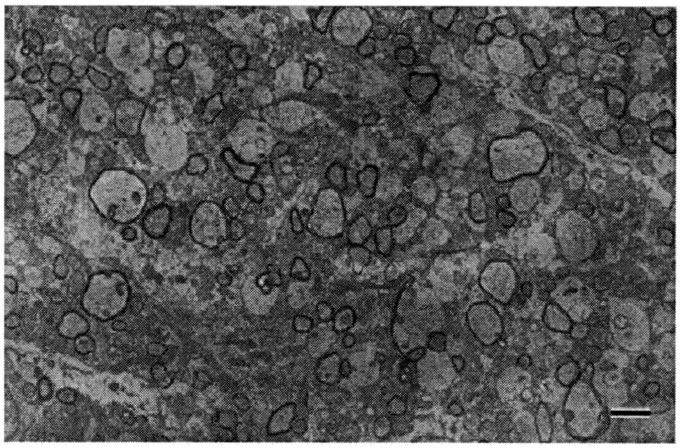

Figure 3.5.8. Electron micrograph showing optic nerve of a 14-day-old hemizygote macular mouse. Fewer axons, undeveloped myelin and unmyelinated axons (arrows) are present, and glial cells with developed processes occupy the spaces between axons. Bar: 2μm.

Discussion

In the brain, copper deficiency decreases cytochrome oxidase activity, perhaps by altering mitochondria (Yoshimura, 1988). The optic nerve has never been studied in relation to copper deficiency. A series of authors' studies (Dake and Amemiya, 1991; Mishima, Dake, Amemiya et al, 1996b) showed swollen axons with many vacuoles and scarce organelles, but normal-looking mitochondria. Pathogenesis of these alterations has not been established but would appear to be a biochemical disturbance. Reduction of cytochrome oxidase activity (Carlton and Kelly, 1967) has been observed in swollen mitochondria and unswollen normal-looking mitochondria (Yoshimura, 1988). Copper deficiency may affect not only cytochrome oxidase activity but also other metalloenzymes involved in protein metabolism.

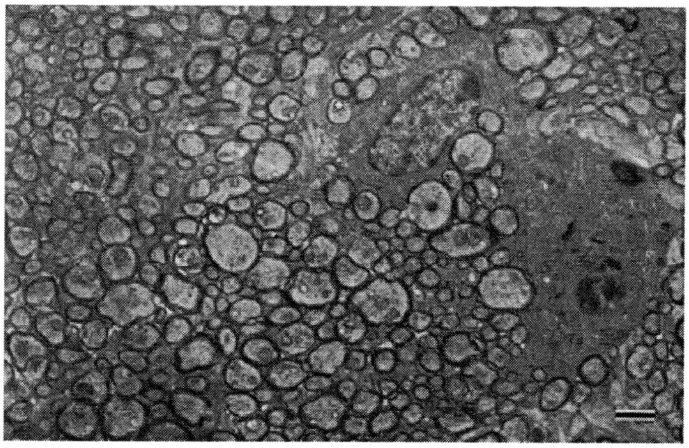

Figure 3.5.9. Electron micrograph showing optic nerve of a 1-month-old hemizygote macular mouse. Myelinated axons are increased, but are still fewer than in control mice. Bar: 2μm.

According to Skoff et al (1976 a, b), myelination in the optic nerve of rats begins about 6 days after birth with the appearance of oligodendrocytes, and is accompanied by increasing 2, 3-cyclic nucleotide 3-phosphohydrolase (CNP) activity in the initial stage and, later, an increase in basic protein and proteolipid protein levels (Sprinkle, Zoruba and Mcklann, 1978). It has been shown that CNP activity is depressed in demyelinating disorders. Prohaska (1974) reported that CNP activity was decreased in the central nervous system in copper deficiency and indicated that copper deficiency caused hypomyelination. In this dietary copper-deficient experiment, 3-week-old rats were used, and the myelin in their optic nerves was therefore still developing. These experimental results suggest that the development of myelin in the optic nerve was apparently delayed or disturbed in the early stage of copper deficiency and that myelin structure was damaged in the later stage. Since CNP was considered to be associated with the outer and inner surfaces of the myelin sheath and oligodendroglial plasma membrane, Zimmerman et al (1976) suggested that hypomyelination was partially due to dysfunction of oligodendroglia caused by copper deficiency. Moreover, essential components of myelin such as phospholipid and protein were found to be reduced in copper deficiency.

The macular mouse is known as a model of Menkes' disease, and is characterized by black eyes, white hair, frizzy whiskers, dermatolysis, convulsions and ataxia (Nishimura, 1989). It has disturbed copper metabolism and abnormal copper distribution in various organs (Tsurui and Sugie, 1990). It was confirmed that the hemizygote macular mouse stops nursing at 10 days of age and dies at 14 or 15 days of age. Nishimura (1989) reported that in this mouse the copper content of the liver and cerebrum is low and that of the kidney is high. We could not measure the amount of copper in the eyes of hemizygote macular mice and normal littermates because the amount of ocular tissue was too small. Furthermore, they reported that copper accumulates in organs with a high affinity for copper when this mouse is given copper either by mouth or by injection (Nishimura, 1989). Since it is difficult for a macular mouse with disturbed copper absorption by the small intestine to increase their serum copper levels by oral administration, we injected 50μg $CuCl_2$ per 0.1ml distilled water into the abdomens of 7-day-old hemizygote macular mice (Mann, Camakaris, Danks et al, 1979; Nagara, Yajima and Suzuki, 1981; Meguro, Kodama and Abe et al, 1991). These mice could then survive. The heterozygote macular mice also has disturbed copper metabolism and abnormal copper distribution in various organs (Nishimura, 1989).

The ocular pathology of Menkes' disease shows progressive degeneration of retinal ganglion cells, loss of nerve fibers, and optic atrophy. The electron microscopic findings of the optic nerve in Menkes' disease show markedly reduced numbers of myelinated nerve fibers, thin myelin sheaths, disappearance of microtubules in the axons and markedly increased astrocytic cytoplasm (Sleelenfreund, Gartner and Vinger, 1968; Wray, Kuwabara and Sanderson, 1976; Cotineau, Rozelle and Treppoz, 1979). In the current study, axon and myelin in the optic nerves in 14-day-old hemizygote and heterozygote macular mice were almost similarly decreased. These findings are similar to those of the nutritionally copper-deficient rats. That is, optic nerve changes in the nutritional and hereditary copper deficiencies are almost the same as those in Menkes' disease. Neural degeneration cannot be reduced in patients with Menkes' disease treated with copper after birth (Grover and Scrutton, 1975; Garnica, Frias, Rennert et al, 1977; Johnson, Coleman and Poe, 1991). In contrast, hemizygote macular mice are known to survive and show almost normal growth when they are treated with copper at 7 days of age (Nishimura, 1989; Tanaka, Kobayashi, Fujita et al, 1990; Meguro, Kodama, Abe et al, 1991), and neuropathological findings and cuproenzyme activity have been improved (Yamano, Shimada, Onaga et al, 1988; Meguro, Kodama, Abe et al. 1991). Actually, in the current experiment, the myelinated axons in the 1-month-old hemizygotes developed rather well after the administration of copper at 7 days of age. However, the optic nerves of hemizygote macular mice contained fewer axons than did those of normal littermates. The optic nerves of heterozygote macular mice also contained fewer axons. As described above, the heterozygote macular mouse also has a copper metabolism disorder with hypomyelination, demyelination and poorly developed axons in the optic nerve. Optic nerve development in hemizygote macular mice treated with copper did not recover completely until 1 month of age. This may be due to a congenitally disturbed copper transport system or the effects on the optic nerve of chronic copper deficiency from the embryonal period on. Treated hemizygote macular mice did not have demyelinated axons in the optic nerve, but the heterozygote macular mice did. Thus, copper treatment is effective in the restoration of optic nerve development. Skoff et al (1976a, 1976b) reported that myelination in the optic nerve of rats begins about 6 days after birth with the appearance of oligodendrocytes and is accompanied by increasing 2', 3'-cyclic nucleotide 3'-phosphodiesterase (CNP) activity in the initial stage and later, an increase in basic protein and proteolipid protein levels (Sprinkle, Zaruba and Machann, 1978). Prohaska (1974) reported that CNP activity was decreased in the CNS in copper deficiency and indicated that copper deficiency caused hypomyelination. Cuproenzymes, such as cytochrome c oxidase, are reduced in the brains of hemizygote macular mice (Meguro, Kodama, Abe et al, 1991), and their astrocytes cannot transport copper to neurons because an excessive amount of copper accumulates in the astrocytes as copper-metallothionein (Kodama, Meguro, Abe et al, 1991). Zimmerman et al (1976) suggested that hypomyelination is caused by the dysfunction of oligodendrocytes with abnormal mitochondria and decreased activity of cuproenzymes such as cytochrome c oxidase and superoxide dismutase, due to copper deficiency. Thus, hypomyelination in the optic nerves of hemizygote and heterozygote macular mice may be caused by oligodendrocyte dysfunction due to disturbed cuproenzyme activities related to copper deficiency.

PART II. EXCESS COPPER (COPPER INTOXICATION)

I. Significance

Copper is a heavy metal whose unbound ions are toxic. Almost all of the copper in the body is present as a component of copper proteins, thereby reducing the in vivo concentration of unbound copper ions to almost zero (Harris, 1997). Genetic mechanisms control the processes by which copper is incorporated into apoproteins and toxic accumulations of copper are avoided (Sternlieb, Morell and Scheinberg, 1973).

Wilson's disease, intraocular foreign body, and dietary chronic copper poisoning cause excess copper in ocular tissues. Although there have been many reports on these diseases in recent years (Nittis and Gitlin, 2002; Ogra and Suzuki, 2002; Ozawa and Aoki, 1996), the mechanism of homeostasis in conditions of copper excess is not clear.

Wilson's disease is known to be due to high copper levels and abnormal copper metabolism. Patients show the characteristic Kayser-Fleischer corneal ring and sunflower cataract. Although many pathological studies of the cornea and the lens in Wilson's disease have been reported (Tso, Fine and Thorpe, 1975; Johnson and Campbell, 1982; Innes, Strachan, Triger et al, 1986), the effect of copper on the retina has not been studied well.

II. Excess Copper Experiment

Materials and Methods

One-month-old and 10-month-old normal Wistar Kyoto rats were injected intraperitoneally with 5mg/ml of $CuCl_2$/kg body weight once a week for 4 weeks. Age-equivalent control rats were injected with 1ml of distilled water/kg body weight once a week. The rats were weighed at the time of each injection. After 4 weeks the eyeballs were enucleated under pentobarbital anesthesia after blood had been drawn from the heart for the determination of serum copper and ion levels.

Clinical Features of Copper Excess Animals

Of the 1-month-old rats treated with $CuCl_2$ 29% died within 3 weeks. All the 10-month-old rats treated with $CuCl_2$ survived for 1 month. Fig. 3.6.1 shows the body weight changes. There was a significant difference in weight gain between 1-month-old Cu-injected and 1-month-old control rats ($p<0.05$) (Fig. 3.6.1A). There was no significant difference in weight gain between 10-month-old Cu-injected and control rats ($p=0.90$) (Fig. 3.6.1B).

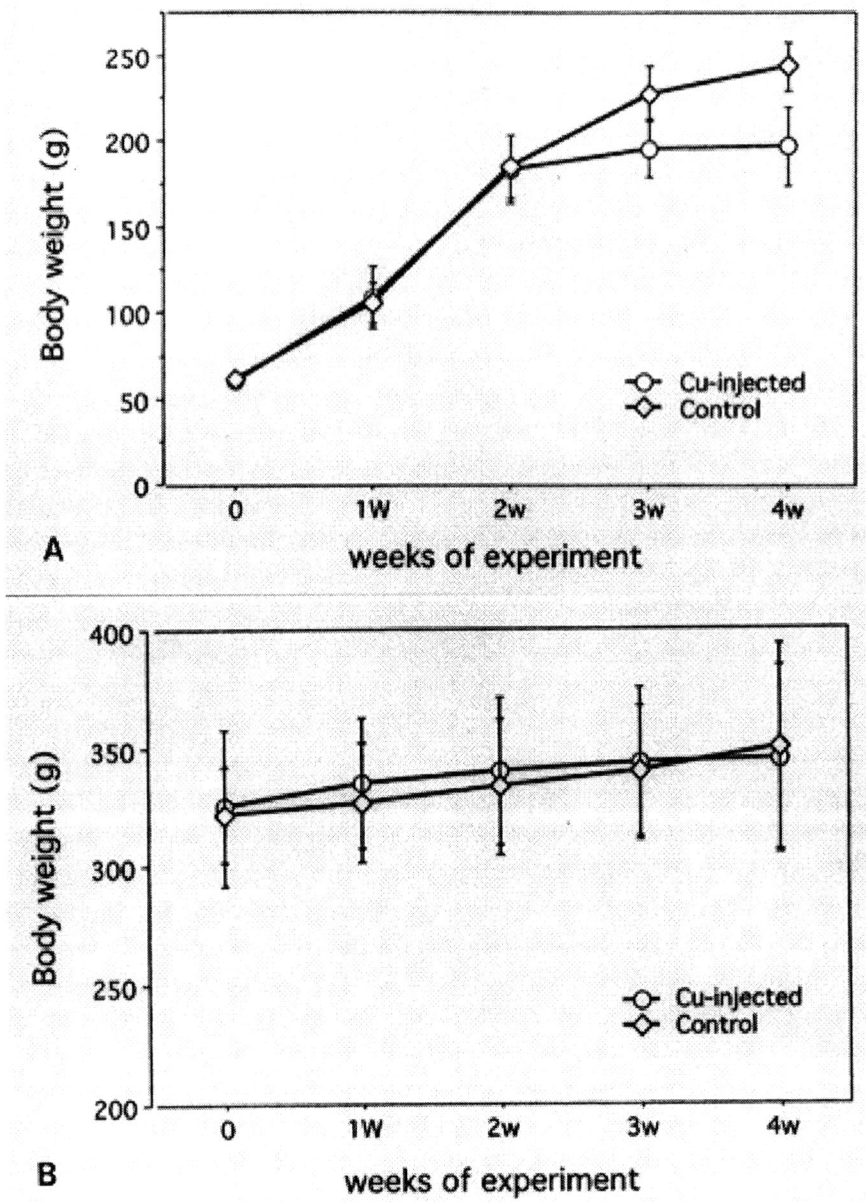

Figure 3.6.1. The body weight changes of 1-month-old (A) and 10-month-old (B) Cu-injected and control rats.

The serum copper and ion levels are shown in Table 3.6.1. In the 1-month-old rats, there was no detectable difference in the serum copper level. In the 10-month-old rats, the serum copper level was significantly higher in the Cu-injected rats than in the controls ($p<0.01$). There was no significant difference in the serum ion level between Cu-injected rats and control rats in both age groups.

Table 3.6.1. Serum copper and iron levels (Mean±SD).

		Serum copper	Serum iron
	n	μg/100ml	μg/100ml
1-month-old rats			
Cu-injected	5	107.6±8.7	157.0±1.7
control	7	98.3±3.8	194.7±30.1
10-month-old rats			
Cu-injected	5	169.7±16.8*	265.5±72.2
Control	5	114.7±9.1*	214.0±29.5
In 10-month-old rats the copper level in the serum is significantly			
higher in the Cu-injected rats than in the controls (*p<0.01)			

III. The Retina

Results

Light microscopic findings

In the 1-month-old Cu-injected rats, there was no obvious abnormality (Fig. 3.6.2). The 10-month-old Cu-injected rats showed a decreased number of cells in the inner nuclear layer (Fig. 3.6.3) and the difference between the 10-month-old Cu-injected and control rats was significant ($p<0.001$) (Table. 3.6.2). In the 1-month-old Cu-injected rats, on the other hand, there was no significant difference in the number of cells in the inner nuclear layer between Cu-injected and control rats.

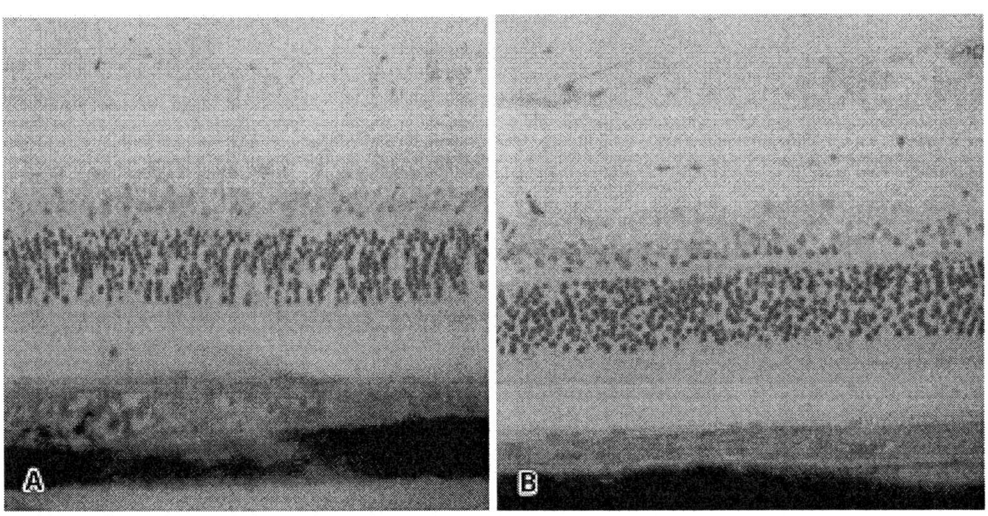

Figure 3.6.2. Light micrographs of retinas of 1-month-old (A) and 10-month-old (B) Cu-injecteds and control rats. There is no obvious difference between a Cu-injected (A) and a control rat (B). Toluidine blue, × 400.

Table 3.6.2. Number of cells in the inner nuclear layer per 1600 μm^2 field at the posterior pole of the retina (mean±SD).

	n	Cu-injected	Control
1-month-old rats	5	75.0±8.2	79.6±5.0
10-month-old rats	5	45.0±7.2*	73.6±4.5*
There is a significant difference between 10-month-old Cu-injected and control rats (*$p<0.001$).			

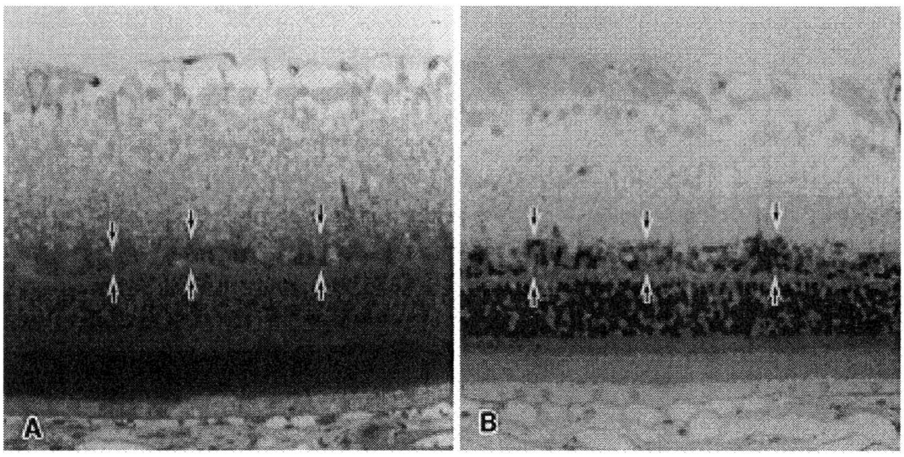

Figure 3.6.3. Light micrographs of retinas of 10-month-old rats. (A) The retina of a Cu-injected rat shows a decrease of cells in the inner nuclear layer (arrows). (B) The retina of a control rat is ticker than that of a Cu-injected rat (arrows). Toluidine blue. × 400.

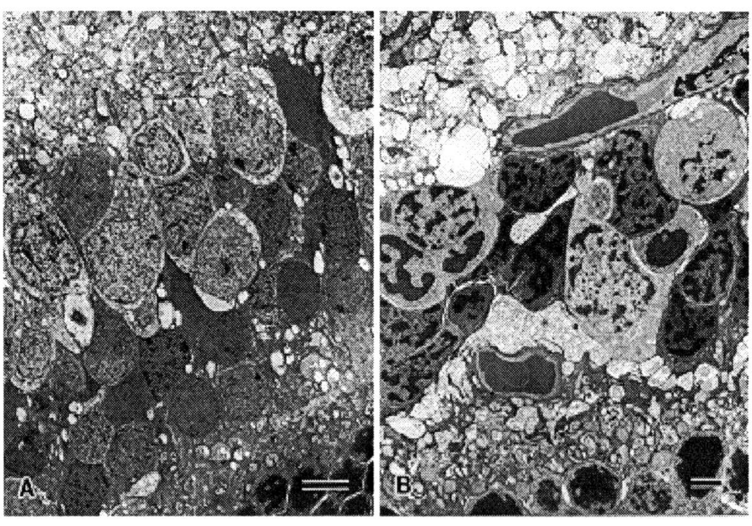

Figure 3.6.4. (A) TEM of inner nuclear layer of a 1-month-old Cu-injected rat. There are no abnormal changes in the nuclei in the inner nuclear layer. (B) TEM of inner nuclear layer of a 10-month-old Cu-injected rat. The number of cells is definitely decreased and the nuclei show irregularly shaped clumps of chromatin and pyknosis (arrows). Bar: 5μm (A), 2μm (B).

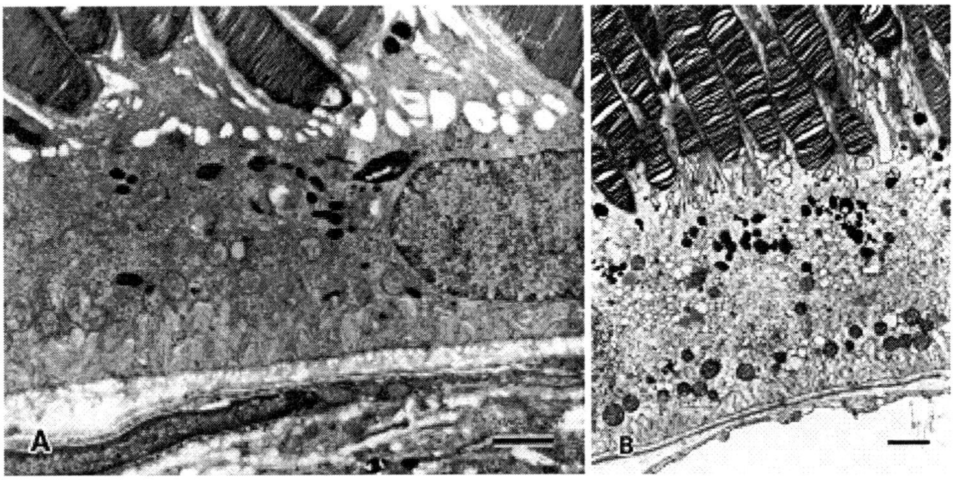

Figure 3.6.5. (A) TEM of the RPE of a 1-month-old Cu-injected rat. Although high density secondary lysosomes are seen in the RPE, no iron peaks were detected with EDXA (Fig. 3.6.6A). (6B) TEM of the RPE of a 10-month-old Cu-injected rat. High density deposits are seen in secondary lysosomes in the aptical portion of the RPE and show iron peaks with EDXA (Fig. 3.6.6C). Bar: 2μm (A, B).

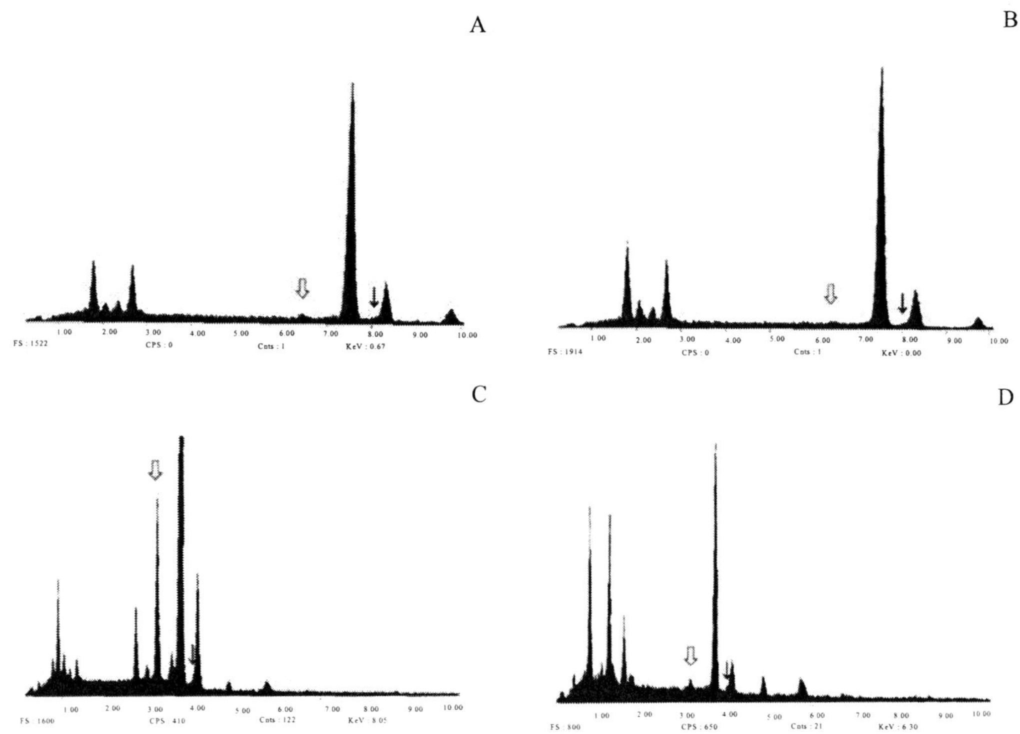

Figure 3.6.6. (A) Representative spectrum of deposits in the RPE of a 1-month-old Cu-injected rat, (B) a 1-month-old control rat, (C) a 10-month-old Cu-injected rat, and (D) a 10-month-old control rat. Arrows show the iron and copper peaks. ⇓: Fe; ↓: Cu.

Electron microscopic findings

In the inner nuclear layer of the 10-month-old Cu-injected rats, TEM showed clumps of chromatin and pyknosis in the nuclei (Fig. 3.6.4B). High density deposits were present in secondary lysosomes in the apical portion of the retinal pigment epithelium (RPE) (Fig. 3.6.5B). These deposits in the 10-month-old Cu-injected rats were analyzed with EDXA and were found to contain ion, but not copper (Fig. 3.6.6C). No significantly high copper and ion peaks were detected in the 1-month-old Cu-injected rats (Fig. 3.6.6A, B, D). Photoreceptor cells showed no abnormal ultrastructural changes in either of the Cu-injected groups.

Discussion

In this experiment, regardless of the dose of copper administered to rats for 4 weeks, copper accumulation was not evident in the retina. Normal hepatocytes eliminate the extra copper in the bile and can store the copper with metallothionein if the dose is reasonable (Owen and Hazelrig, 1964; Owen, 1964). Although the Cu-injected rats in this experiment seemed clearly to have copper poisoning because of weight loss and a high death rate at 1 month of age, copper was not detected in the retina with EDXA but iron was evident. We cannot explain this discrepancy, but we can present a hypothesis (Takehara, 2003). In the current experiment EDXA detected iron, not copper, in the RPE. It is known that copper catalyzes a free-radical reaction which leads to the decomposition of fatty acids of membrane phospholipids and thus to oxidative damage to red blood cells (Sayato, Nakamura and Hasegawa, 1991; Sansinanea, Cerone and Najle, 1994; Saenko,Skoroboga'ko and Yaropolov, 1990; Forman, Kumar, Redeker et al. 1980). Hypercupremia may induce hemolysis and lead to iron accumulation. Toyokuni et al (1989) reported hemolysis and liver damage in rats treated with copper doses equivalent to the authors'. The loss of ceruloplasmin synthesized in the liver may have influenced iron accumulation. Ceruloplasmin contains more than 95% of the copper in human plasma. It is synthesized mainly in the liver. Ceruloplasmin can oxidise ferrous iron to ferric iron. In some experiments, ceruloplasmin was shown to play a role in the mobilization and oxidation of iron from tissue stores with subsequent incorporation of ferric iron into transferrin (Frieden and Hsieh, 1976). Recent studies have shown that aceruloplasminemia characterized by mutations in the ceruloplasmin gene and iron accumulation in the basal ganglia as well as in parenchymal tissues in the CNS is caused by a total deficiency of ceruloplasmin ferroxidase activity (Harris, Klomp and Gitlin, 1998; Miyajima, 2000; Miyajima, Fujimoto, Kohno et al, 1998; Getlin, 1998; Okamoto, Wada, Oga et al, 1996). In this experiment, the loss of ceruloplasmin might have been caused by liver damage which prevented iron transfer and led to iron accumulation, because the retina is part of the CNS.

Iron accumulation only in the RPE may be due to the following: TEM studies on ocular siderosis in animals and humans have demonstrated iron accumulation in the secondary lysosome as a siderosome (Virata, Kylstra and Peiffer, 1995; Welch, 1976). This is in accord with the current findings. According to these reports, histochemistry showed diffuse iron in the sensory retina as well as in the RPE. EDXA can detect elements only in high electron dense deposits. Thus, fine iron accumulations may be present in other layers of the retina. TEM showed deformed nuclei in the inner nuclear layer. The author and his associate speculate that the free radical reaction induced by iron may provoke such a nuclear change.

Ferrous iron is the electron donor in the presence of hydrogen peroxide and generates a hydroxyl radical. The retinal damage of siderosis and aceruloplasminemia have been considered to share the same mechanism. Thus, the retinal changes may be due to secondary iron accumulation induced by Cu excess.

It is not clear why the retinal changes occurred only in 10-month-old Cu-injected rats, but not in 1-month-old rats receiving the same dose. Takehara (2003) speculated that young rats died prior to a great amount of iron accumulation in the RPE because of the lower 50% lethal dose in young rats. In spite of $CuCl_2$ injection, the surviving one-month-old rats might be resistant to Cu toxicity. In addition, Cu intoxication occurs suddenly after long-term administration of Cu and the effects of Cu exposure might be indirect rather than direct due to Cu accumulation.

Although free radicals tend to impair the photoreceptor outer segment first which is rich in unsaturated fatty acids, the inner nuclear layer receives the greater damage, so the number of cells in the current experiment was decreased. Generally speaking, toxic effects appear first at the photoreceptor outer segment discs. For instance, siderosis and aluminium toxicity (Lu, Gong and Amemiya, 2002) destroy the outer segment discs severely. However, secondary siderosis due to Cu excess presents another aspect of morphological damage. Although we cannot describe the mechanism completely, we assume that the retinal damage in the current experiment is due to iron accumulation, probably affected in part by long-term Cu excess. Experimental hypercupremia may induce secondary siderosis in the rat retina.

REFERENCES

American Institute of Nutrition. Report of the American Institute of Nutrition Ad Hoc Committee on standards for nutritional studies. *J Nutr.* 1977;107:140-148.

Bowness JM, Morton RA, Shakir MH, Stubbs AL. Distribution of copper and zinc in mammalian eyes. Occurrence of metals in melanin fractions from eye tissues. *Biochem J.* 1952;51:521-530.

Carlton WW, Kelly WA. Neural lesion in the offspring of female rats fed a copper-deficient diet. *J Nutr.* 1967;97:42-97.

Cotineau J, Rozelle A, Treppoz M. La maladie de Menkes: a propos d'une nouvelle observation. *J Fr Ophthalmol.* 1979;2:33-37.

Dake Y, Amemiya T. Electron microscopic study of the optic nerve in copper deficient rats. *Exp Eye Res.* 1991;52:177-181.

Dake Y. Electron histochemical examination of cytochrome oxidase in the retinal photoreceptor cell of copper deficient rats. *Acta Histochem Cytochem.* 1992;25:371-378.

Danks DM, Cartwright E. Menkes' kinky hair disease: further definition of the defect in copper transport. *Science.* 1973;179:1140-1142.

Danks DM. Copper deficiency in humans. *Annu Rev Nutr.* 1988;8:235-257.

Dipaolo RV, Kanfer JN, Newberne JN. Copper deficiency and the central nervous system. *J Neuropathol Exp Neurol.* 1974;33:226-236.

Eckert CD. Elemental concentrations in ocular tissues of various species. *Exp Eye Res.* 1983;37:639-647.

Everson GJ, Tsai H-C C, Wang T-I. Copper deficiency in the guinea pig. *J Nutr.* 1967;93:533-540.

Forman ST, Kumar KS, Redeker AG, Hochstein P. Hemolytic anemia in Wilson disease: clinical findings and biochemical mechanisms. *Am J Hematol.* 1980;9:269-275.

Frieden E, Hsieh HS. The biological role of ceruloplasmin and its oxidase activity. *Adv Exp Med Biol.* 1976;74:505-529.

Gallager CH, Reeve VE. Copper deficiency in the rats. Effect on synthesis of phospholipids. *Aust J Exp Biol Med Sci.* 1970;49:21-31.

Garnica AD, Frias IL, Rennert OM. Menkes kinky hair syndrome: is it a treatable disorder? *Clin Gent.* 1977;11:154-161.

Ghadially FN. *Ultrastructural pathology of the cell and matrix.* Vol. 1. London: Butterworths;1988:240-249.

Gitlin JD. Aceruloplasminemia. *Pediatr Res.* 1998;44:271-276.

Grover WD, Scrutton MC. Copper infusion therapy in trichopoliodystrophy. *J Pediatr.* 1975;86:216-220.

Harris FD. Copper. In: O'Dell BL, Sunde RA, ed. *Handbook of Nutritionally Essential Mineral Elements.* New York: Marcel Dekker Inc;1997:231-241.

Harris ZL, Klomp LW, Gitlin JD. Aceruloplasminemia: an inherited neurodegenerative disease with impairment of iron homeostasis. *Am J Clin Nutr.* 1998;67:972-977.

Hayashi K, Kenyon KR. Increased cytochrome oxidase activity in alkali burned corneas. *Curr Eye Res.* 1988;7:131-138.

Hirai K, Ogawa K, Wang GY, Ueda T. Varied cytochrome oxidase activities of the alveolar tye I, type II and type III cells in rat lungs: Qualitative cytochemistry. *J Electron Microsc.* 1989;38:449-456.

Hirayama Y. Histochemical localization of zinc and copper in rat ocular tissues. *Acta Histochem.* 1990;89:107-111.

Hirayama Y, Dake Y, Amemiya T. Cytochrome oxidase in rat ocular tissues with special reference to copper. *Acta Histochem.* 1992;93:307-312.

Innes JR, Strachan IM, Triger DR. Unilateral Kayser-Fleischer ring. *Br J Ophthal-mol.* 1986;70:469-470.

Johnson RE, Campbell RJ. Willson's disease. Electron microscopic, x-ray energy spectroscopic and atomic absorption spectroscopic studies of corneal copper deposition and distribution. *Lab Invest.* 1982;46:564-569.

Johnson DE, Coleman L, Poe L. MR of progressive neurodegenerative changes in treated Menkes' kinky hair disease. *Neuroradiology.* 1991;33:181-182.

Johnson MA, Fisher JG, Kays SE. Is copper an antioxidant nutrient? *Crit Rev Food Sci Nutr.* 1992;32:1-31.

Kageyama GH, Wong-Riley M. The histochemical localization of cytochrome oxidase in the retina and lateral geniculate nucleus of the ferret, cat, and monkey, with particular reference to retinal mosaics and on/off center visual channels. *J Neurosci.* 1984;4:2445-2459.

Kageyama GH, Meyer RL. Hitochemical localization of cytochrome oxidase in the retina and optic tectum of normal goldfish; a combined cytochrome oxidase-horseradish peroxidase study. *J Comp Neurol.* 1988;270:354-371.

Kitano S. Membrane and contactile properties of rat vascular tissue in copper-deficient conditions. *Circ Res*. 1980;46:681-689.

Kodama H, Meguro Y, Abe T, Rayner MH, Suzuki KT, Kobayashi S, Nishimura M. Genetic expression of Menkes disease in cultured astrocytes of the macular mouse. *J Inher Metab* Dis. 1991;14:896-901.

Lachica EA, Condo GJ, Gasagrande VA. Development of cytochrome oxidase staining in the retina and lateral geniculate nucleus: a possible correlate of on- and off-center channel maturation. *Dev Brain Res*. 1987;34:298-302.

Lawrence CV, Davies NT, Mills CF, Nicol F. Studies on the effect of copper deficiency on rat liver mitochondria. I. Changes in mitochondrial composition. *Biochem Biophy Acta*. 1985;809:351-361.

Lu ZY, Gong H, Amemiya T. Aluminium chloride induces retinal changes in the rat. *Toxicol Sci.* 2002;66:253-260.

Mann JR, Camakaris J, Danks DM, Walliczek EG. Copper metabolism in mottled mouse mutants. Copper therapy of brindled (Mo^{br}) mice. *Biochem J.* 1979;180:605-612.

Martuza RL, Philippe I, Fitzpatrick TB, Zwaan J, Seki Y, Lederman J. Melanin macroglobules as a cellular marker of neurofibromatosis: a quantitative study. *Invest Dermatol.* 1985;85: 347-350.

Meguro Y, Kodama H, Abe T, Kobayashi S, Kodama Y, Nishimura M. Changes of copper level and cytochrome c oxidase activity in the macular mice with age. *Brain Dev.* 1991;13:184-186.

Mishima H, Hasebe H, Fujita H. Melanogenesis in the retinal pigment epithelial cell of the chick embryo. Dopa-reaction and electron microscopic autoradiography of ^{3}H-Dopa. *Invest Ophthalmol Vis Sci*. 1978;17:403-411.

Mishima K, Dake Y, Amemiya T、Nishimura M. Electron microscopic study of retinas of macular mice. *Graefes Arch Clin Exp Ophthalmol.* 1996a;234:S101-105.

Mishima K, Dake Y, Amemiya T, Nishimura M. Electron microscopic study of optic nerves of macular mice. *Exp Eye Res.* 1996b;63:85-98.

Mishima K, Amemiya T, Takano K. X-ray microanalysis of melanin granules of retinal pigment epithelium and choroid in hereditary copper deficient mice (macular mice). *Exp Eye Res.* 1999;68:59-65.

Miyajima H Fujimoto M, Kohno S, Kaneko E, Gitlin JD. CSF abnormalities in patients with aceruloplasminemia. *Neurology*. 1998;51:1188:1190.

Miyajima H. Aceruloplasminemia. *Rinsho Shinkeigaku*. 2000;40:1290-1292.

Morgan RF, O'Dell BL. Effect of copper deficiency on the concentration of catecholamines and related enzyme activities in the rat brain. *J Neurochem*. 1977;28:207-213.

Nagara H, Yajima K, Suzuki K. The effect of copper supplementation on the brindled mouse. A clinico-pathological study. *J Neuropathol Exp Neurol.* 1981;40:428-446.

Nishimura M. Animal model for trace metal element deficient disease (particularly, mouse models for Menkes' syndrome) (in Japanese). *Med Immunol.* 1989;17:725-733.

Nittis T, Getlin ID. The copper-iron connection: Hereditary aceruloplasminemia. *Semin Hematol.* 2002;39:282-289.

Ogura Y, Suzuki K. Intracellular trafficking and regulation of copper in mammalian cells. *Biomed Res Trace Elements*. 2002;13:3-10.

Okamoto N, Wada S, Oga T, Kuwabara Y et al. Hereditary ceruloplasmin deficiency with hemosiderosis. *Hum Genet.* 1996;97:755-758.

Owen CA Jr,. Absorption and excretion of Cu^{64} labelled copper by the rat. *Am J Physiol.* 1964;210:1203-1206.

Owen CA Jr, Hazelrig JB. Metabolism of Cu^{64} labelled copper by the isolated rat liver. *Am J Physiol.* 1964;210:1059-1064.

Ozawa M, Aoki T. Inherited neurological disease-relationship between an essential trace elements and Wilson/Menkes' disease. *Nippon Rinsho.* 1996;54:117-122.

Prohaska JR, Wells WW. Copper deficiency in the developing rat brain: a possible model for Menkes' steely-hair disease. *J Neurochem.* 1974;23;91-98.

Prohaska JR, Wells WW. Copper deficiency in the developing rat brain: Evidence for abnormal mitochondria. *J Neurochem.* 1975;25:221-228.

Prohaska JR. Changes in tissue growth, concentrations of copper, cytochrome oxidase and superoxide dismutase subsequent to dietary or genetic copper deficiency in mice. *J Nutr.* 1983:113:2148-2158.

Prohaska JR. Biochemical changes in copper deficiency. *J Nutr Biochem.* 1990;1:452-461.

Redmond TM, Duke DJ, Coles WH, Simons JA、Crouch RK. Localization of corneal superoxide dismutase by biochemical and histocytochemical techniques. *Exp Eye Res.* 1984;38:369-378.

Saenko EL, Skorubogat'ko OV, Yaropolow AI. Interrelation between structure and protective action of normal and pathological ceruloplasmins during copper-induced lysis of red blood cells. *Biochem Int.* 1990;22:749-757.

Sansinanea A, Cerone S, Najle R. Lipid peroxidation in erythrocyte membrane of sheep with chronic copper poisoning. *J Clin Biochem Nutr.* 1994;17:65-72.

Sayato Y, Nakamura K, Hasegawa T. Lipid peroxidation induced by copper in rat erythrocytes. *Eisei Kagaku.* 1991;37:137-142.

Seelenfreund MH, Gartner S, Vinger PF. The ocular pathology of Menkes' disease. *Arch Ophthalmol.* 1968;80:718-720.

Seligman AM, Karnovsky MJ, Wasserkrug HL, Hanker TS. Nondroplet ultra-structural demonstration of cytochrome oxidase activity with a polymerizing osmiophilic reagent, diaminobenzidine (DAB). *J Cell Biol.* 1968;38:1-14.

Siegel CR, Pinnel SR, Martin GR. Crosslinking of collagen and elastin. Properties of lysyl oxidase. *Biochemistry.* 1970;23:4486-4492.

Skoff RP, Price DL, Stocks A. Electron microscopic autoradiographic studies of gliogenesis in rat optic nerve. I. Cell proliferation. *J Comp Neurol.* 1976a;169:291-312.

Skoff RP, Price DL, Stocks A. Electron microscopic autoradiographic studies of gliogenesis in rat optic nerve. II. Time of origin. *J Comp Neurol.* 1976b;169:313-334.

Sprinkle TJ, Zaruba ME, Mackhann GM. Activity of 2',3'-cyclic nucleotide 3'-phosphodiesterase in regions of rat brain during development: quantitative relationship to myelin basic protein. *J Neurochem.* 1978;30:309-314.

Sternlieb I, Morell AG, Scheinberg IH. The remarkable selectivity of hepatocytes in the update of glycoproteins. *Gastroenterology.* 1973;64:1049-1052.

Takehara A. Ultrastructural and analytical study of retinas of rats with excess copper. *Acta Med Nagasaki.* 2003;48:9-14.

Tanaka K, Kobayashi K, Fujita Y, Fukuhara C, Onosaki S, Min K. Effect of chelators on copper theory of macular mouse, a model animal of Menkes' kinky disease. *Res Commun Chem Pathol Pharmacol.* 1990;266:217-227.

Tauber FW, Krause AC. The role of iron, copper, zink and manganese in the metabolism of the ocular tissues, with special reference to the lens. *Am J Ophthalmol.* 1943;26:260-266.

Toyokuni S, Okada S, Hamazaki S, Fujioka M, Li JL, Midorikawa O. Cirrhosis of the liver induced by cupric nitrilotriacetate in Wistar rats. An experimental model of copper toxicosis. *Am J Pathol.* 1989;134:1263-1274.

Tso MO, Fine BS, Thorpe HE. Kayser-Fleisher ring and associated cataract in Wilson's disease. *Am J Ophthalmol.* 1975;79:479-488.

Tsurui S, Sugie H. A pathophysiological study of macular mutant mouse as a model of human Menkes' kinky hair disease. I. Copper contents and copper dependent enzyme activities in various organs (in Japanese). *No to Hattatsu.* 1990;22:560-565.

Tuberville AW, Wood TO, McLaughlin BJ. Cytochrome oxidase activity of Fuchs' endothelial dystrophy. *Curr Eye Res.* 1986;5:939-947.

Tuberville AW, Wood TO, McLaughlin BJ. Cytochrome oxidase activity of postsurgical bullous keratopathy endothelium. *Curr Eye Res.* 1987;6:1057-1063.

Virata SR, Kylstra JA, Peiffer RL. The ocular effects of intralenticular iron foreign bodies in rabbits. *Ophthalmic Surg.* 1995;26:142-144.

Weiss LW, Zelickson AS. Giant melanosomes in multiple lentigines syndrome. *Arch Dermatol.* 1977;113:491-494.

Welch RB. Two remarkable events in the field of intraocular foreign body: (1) The reversal of siderosis bulbi. (2) The spontaneous extrusion of an intraocular copper foreign body. *Trans Am Ophthalmol Soc.* 1976;73:187-203.

Wong-Riley MTT, Kageyama GH. Localization of cytochrome oxidase in the mammalian spinal cord and dorsal root ganglia, with quantitative analysis of ventral horn cells in monkeys. *J Comp Neurol.* 1986;245:41-61.

Wray SH, Kuwabara T, Sanderson P. Menkes' kinky hair disease: a light and electron microscopic study of the eye. *Invest Ophthalmol.* 1976;15:128-138.

Yamano T, Shimada M, Onaga A, Kawasaki H, Iwane S, Ono K, Nishimura M. Electron microscopic study on brain of macular mutant mouse after copper therapy. *Acta Neuropathol.* 1988;76:574-580.

Yoshimura N. Neuronal degeneration in the brain of the brindled mouse. Histo-chemical demonstration of decreased cytochrome oxidase activity in the cerebellum and brain stem. *Acta Pathol Jpn.* 1988;38:705-712.

Zimmerman AW, Matthieu JM, Quarles RH, Brady RO, Hsu JM. Hypomyelination in copper-deficient rat. Prenatal and postnatal copper replacement. *Arch Neurol.* 1976;33:111-119.

Chapter 4

SELENIUM

I. SIGNIFICANCE

Since Schwarz and Foltz (1957) showed that traces of selenium (Se) prevent liver necrosis in vitamin E-deficient rats. Se is not only a toxin, but also an essential trace element. In 1979, a Chinese research group reported that Se supplementation prevents development of a cardiomyopathy in Keshan disease in children living in low-Se area.

The glutathione peroxidases are selenium-containing enzymes and reduce equivalents from glutathione to catabolize hydroperoxides. Se deficiency causes a decrease in the activity of all glutathione peroxidases. But the effect varies from tissue to tissue. The glutathione peroxidases catabolize hydrogen peroxide and fatty acid-derived hydroperoxides. They protect cells from these oxidant molecules.

Pure Se deficiency usually causes no clinical illness in free-living humans or animals. Only when laboratory animals are raised through several generations on a Se-deficient regimen do they exhibit pathologic changes from Se deficiency alone (Burk and Levander, 1999).

Very few experimental studies of Se deficiency alone have been reported. Se deficiency causes cataracts in the second generation in rats (Spinkfer, Harr, Newferne et al, 1971) and Se toxicity also causes cataracts in rats during the suckling period (Osládalová, Babicky´ and Obenberger, 1977).

II. SE-DEFICIENT EXPERIMENT

Materials and Methods

Female Wistar Kyoto rats were fed a Se-deficient diet (Hafeman, Sunde, Hoekstra, 1974) starting 20 days after birth. Rats were killed late in the afternoon by luxation of the neck after 3, 6, 9, 10, 12, 18 or 24 months.

As controls, normal female Wistar Kyoto rats were fed a usual diet for 10, 12, 18 or 24 months. Then the rats were killed.

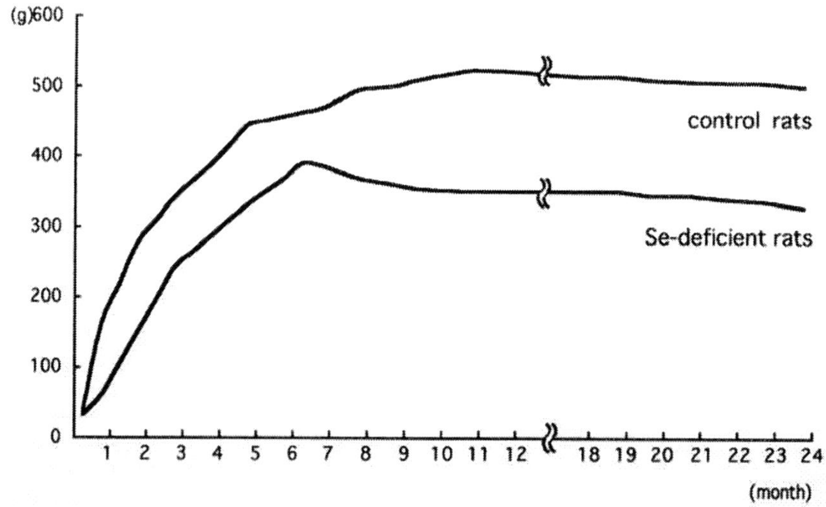

Figure 4.2.1. Growth curve.

Clinical Features of the Se-Deficient animal

Rats that were fed a Se-deficient rats showed coarsening of hair, and no growth retardation (Fig. 4.2.1) ($p<0.001$ at 18 months after fed a Se-deficient diet).

The serum Se level was 0 after 6 months on a Se-deficient diet, while the serum vitamin E level was always more than 5 mg/dl.

III. The Cornea

Results

Scanning Electron Microscopic (SEM) Findings

The most superficial epithelial cells had many microvilli and microplicae and showed light cells in majority in the cornea of rats fed on a Se-deficient diet for 18 or 24 months (Fig. 4.3.1).

Transmission Electron Microscopic (TEM) Findings

The most superficial epithelial cells of rats fed a Se-deficient diet for 18 months showed many microvilli and microplicae and almost intact basal cells with well-developed hemidesmosomes and basement membrane (Fig. 4.3.2). The stroma, Descemet's membrane and endothelial cells showed no abnormalities.

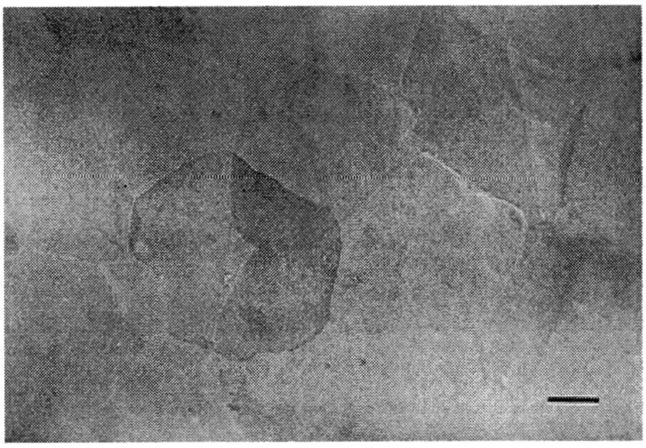

Figure 4.3.1. SEM micrograph of the corneal surface of a rat fed a Se-deficient diet for 18 months. Many microvilli and microplicae are seen. Bar: 10μm.

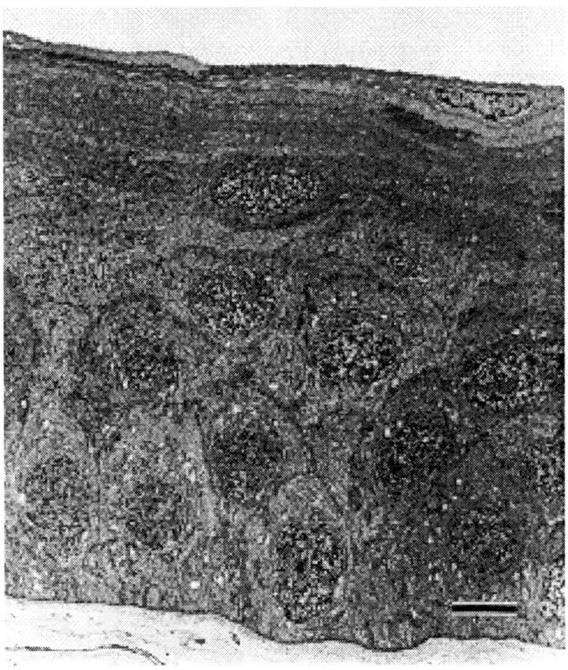

Figure 4.3.2. TEM micrograph of the corneal epithelium of a rat fed a Se-deficient diet for 18 months. There are no abnormalities in intercellular junctions, hemidesmosomes and basement membrane of basal epithelial cells and cytoplasmic components. No deposits are seen at the subepithelial portion. Bar: 5μm.

Discussion

The corneal structures are damaged due to vitamin deficiency such as vitamin A, B_2 (Takami, Gong and Amemiya, 2004), C and E and trace element deficiency such as Zn (Mizoguchi and Amemiya, 1992; Gong, Takami, Amemiya et al, 2004), Cu, Mn (Gong and Amemiya, 1999) and Mg (Gong, Takami, Kitaoka et al, 2003). The deficiency of these essential trace elements may lead to cell degeneration as well as lowered activity of the superoxide dismutases (SOD), Zn·Cu-SOD and Mn-SOD (Keen and Zindenberg-Cherr, 1994). Vitamin A, C and E have strong antioxidant action (Keen and Zindenberg-Cherr, 1994) which prevents peroxidation of lipid membranes in the tissues. The antioxidant action of vitamin B_2 is performed through the reduced activity of flavoenzyme and glutathione reductase (Batey and Eckhert, 1991). On the other hand, antioxidant action of Se is considered to be similar to that of vitamin E and to be related to glutathione peroxidase. However, the cornea was not affected by Se deficiency.

IV. The Retina

Results

Light Microscopic Findings

In the retina of rats fed a Se-deficient diet for 18 months, the decrease of the inner nuclear layer was prominent (Fig. 4.4.1).

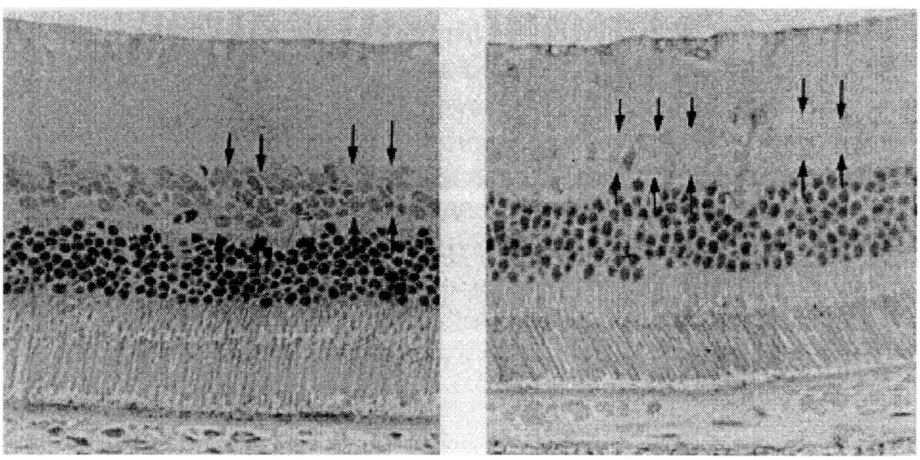

Figure 4.4.1. Light micrographs of the retina of an 18-month-old control rat (left) and that of a rat fed a Se-deficient diet for 18 months (right). The decrease of the inner nuclear layer (arrows) is prominent. H.E. stain, × 400.

Electron Microscopic Findings

During 9 months on a Se-deficient diet, the retina showed no abnormality, but in rats fed a Se-deficient diet for 10 months starting 20 days after birth, the retina was a little thin, especially the inner nuclear layer, of which nuclei formed 3 or 4 layers. In 10-month-old control rats, the inner nuclear layer consisted of 4-5 layers. In rats fed a Se-deficient diet for 12 months, the inner nuclear layer consisted of 3 layers. Amacrine and horizontal cells had decreased. However, bipolar and Müller cells were seen, and photoreceptor cell nuclei were normal in number, i.e. 8-9 layers, and the outer and inner segments looked normal. The retinal pigment epithelium showed no abnormal accumulation of lipofuscin granules.

In rats fed a Se-deficient diet for 18 or 24 months starting 20 days after birth, the retina was thin. The inner nuclear layer showed 2 layers which consisted mainly of bipolar and Müller cells (Fig. 4.4.2). The photoreceptor cell nuclei were markedly decreased in number; the outer nuclear layer became 4 or 5 layers (Fig. 4.4.2). The photoreceptor cell outer segment was decreased in number (Fig. 4.4.3). The retinal pigment epithelium had scarce lipofuscin granules (Fig. 4.4.4). The mitochondria looked normal. In 24-month-old control rats, the inner nuclear layer consisted of 4 layers, while photoreceptor cell nuclei formed 8-9 layers. No abnormal changes were found in the retinal capillary.

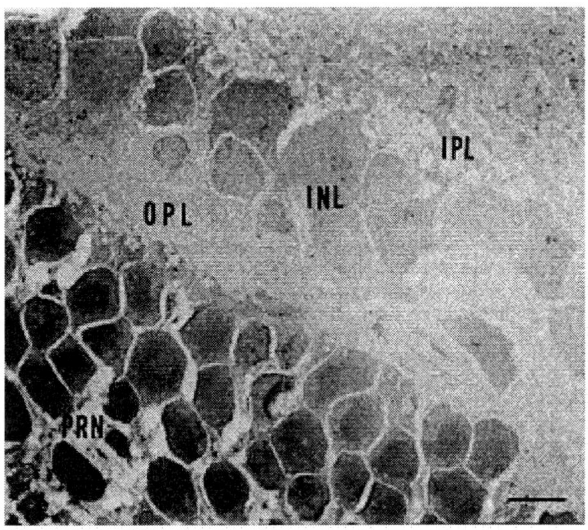

Figure 4.4.2. Electron micrograph of the retina of an 18-month-Se-deficient rat. The inner nuclear layer (INL) shows 1-2 nuclear lines, chiefly bipolar and Müller cell nuclei, while photoreceptor nuclei (PRN) are also decreased to 4-5 lines. OPL: Outer plexiform layer, IPL: Inner plexiform layer. Bar: 5μm.

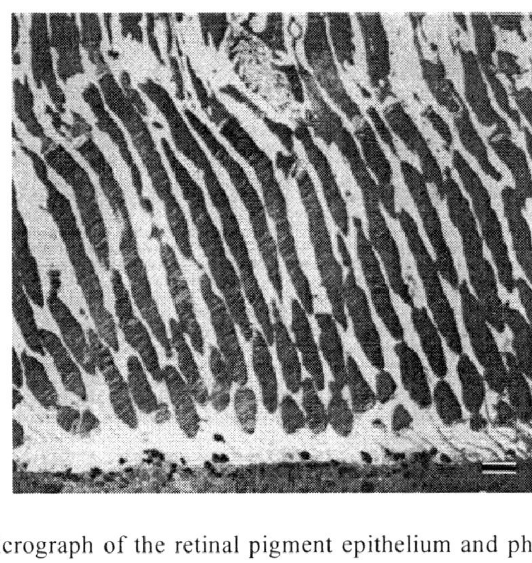

Figure 4.4.3. Electron micrograph of the retinal pigment epithelium and photoreceptor outer segments of a rat fed a Se-deficient diet for 18 months. Photoreceptor outer segments elongate well to the retinal pigment epithelium, but inter-outer segement spaces are wide. The retinal pigment epithelium contains scarce lipofuscin granules and looks normal. Bar: 5μm.

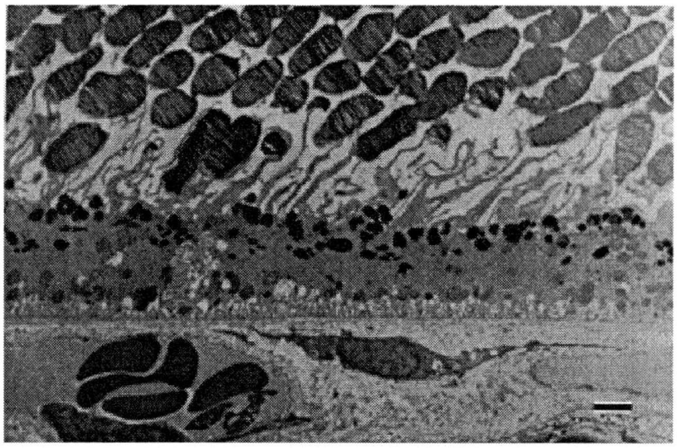

Figure 4.4.4. Electron micrograph of the retinal pigment epithelium of an 18-month-Se-deficient rat. The retinal pigment epithelium contains scarce lipofuscin granules. Bar: 2μm.

Discussion

In the eye the iris contains the highest concentration of Se followed by the retina and lens (Shearer, McCormack, DeSart et al, 1980). Many investigators have suggested that Se deficiency and a subsequent lack of adequate levels of glutathione peroxidase could lead to peroxidative damage of lipid membranes by H_2O_2 (Lawrence, Sunde, Schwartz et al, 1974).

Se has long been considered to have an antioxidant action like that of vitamin E, although these two chemicals were always used simultaneously in the experiment. Se-vitamin E deficiency induces a wide variety of morphologic changes which include hepatic necrosis, degeneration, and necrosis of cardiac and skeletal muscles (Grant, 1961; Obel, 1953, Schwarz and Folty, 1957; Van Vleet, 1970) and are associated with vascular lesions, edema, yellow discoloration of body fat, and anemia (Grant, 1961; Mahan, Jones, Cline et al, 1973; Obel 1953). Vitamin E is another antioxidant functioning in association with Se. Glutathione peroxidase activity can be stimulated with the use of this vitamin. This effect is related to additional dietary Se intake, but the effect of Se is independent of dietary vitamin E intake (Scott, Kellemer, Monty et al, 1977). Although combined Se and vitamin E deficiency, induced in growing rats or pigs, causes massive hepatic necrosis as mentioned above, Se deficiency alone causes no abnormalities of liver histology (Burk, Lawrence and Lane, 1980). Similar experimental results were obtained in the retina. In rats fed a vitamin E and Se deficient diet, the retinal pigment epithelium shows an intense yellow autofluorescent pigment (Katz, Stone and Dratz, 1978; Stone, Katz, Lurie et al, 1979). Rats fed a vitamin E deficient diet show numerous lipofuscin deposits in the retinal pigment epitheliun (Amemiya, 1978;Amemiya, 1981; Hayes, 1974; Robison, Kuwabara and Bieri, 1979). The retinal pigment epithelium seems to be more sensitive to physiological antioxidant deficiencies than do the testes, kidneys, intestines and heart (Katz, Stone and Dratz, 1978). However, our study revealed that Se deficiency alone caused no cytological abnormalities in rat retinal pigment epithelium. In the retina, Se deficiency alone caused the decrease of horizontal and amacrine cells (Amemiya, 1985). This suggests that the role of Se in vivo may be different from that of vitamin E.

The main organization of the retina is on a vertical basis, that is, activity in the rods and cones is transmitted through the bipolar cells to the ganglion cells, then out of the eye into higher neural centers. On the other hand, the horizontal and amacrine cells may play roles in the horizontal spread and interaction of activity. This basic concept on the transmission of light excitation suggests that Se deficiency in the eye first damages the horizontal connections such as the amacrine and horizontal cells in the retina and has less effect on the vertical excitation system through the rods and bipolar and ganglion cells. The rods seem to be rather resistant to selenium deficiency, but finally decrease in numbers. Little is known, however, of the mechanisms involved. Müller cells show neither a decrease in the number of their nuclei in the inner nuclear layer nor proliferation. Thus, the retina becomes thin as the retinal cells, mainly horizontal and amacrine cells and decrease in number due to Se deficiency.

V. The Rectus Muscle

Results

Electron Microscopic Findings

No abnormal changes were found in the recti muscles at any period of the experiment (Fig. 4.5.1).

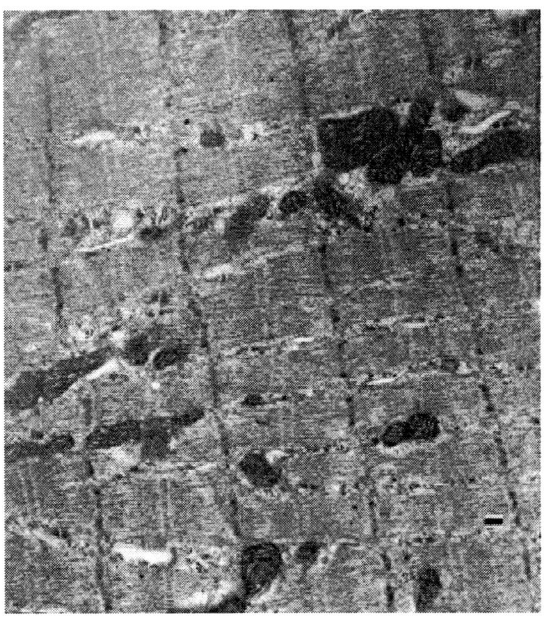

Figure 4.5.1. Electron micrograph of the rectus muscle of an 18-month-Se-deficient rat. No deposit of lipofuscin granules is present in the cytoplasm of a myocyte. Bar: 1μm.

Discussion

Se has been assumed to act as an antioxidant similar to vitamin E, but morphological differences in the retina and recti muscles between vitamin E (Amemiya, 1981; Amemiya, 1987) and selenium deficiencies (Amemiya, 1988) suggests that Se acts as an antioxidant unlike vitamin E. The current study revealed that Se deficiency alone caused no abnormality in recti muscles. Glutathione peroxidase is a selenoenzyme (Rotruck, Pope, Ganther et al, 1973). Although it has been suggested that Se deficiency and a subsequent lack of adequate levels of glutathione peroxidase can lead to peroxidative damage of lipid membranes by H_2O_2, the effect of Se deficiency on the retina and recti muscles was different from that of vitamin E deficiency. However, Se might interrupt the activity of vitamin E.

References

Amemiya T. Effect of vitamin E deficiency on photoreceptor outer segment and pigment epithelium of the rat retina. *Acta Soc Ophthalmol Jpn.* 1978;82:822-826.

Amemiya T. Effect of vitamin E administration on photoreceptor outer segment and retinal pigment epithelium of vitamin E deficient rats. *Int J Vit Nutr Res.* 1981;51:114-118.

Amemiya T. Retinal changes in the selenium deficient rat. *Int J Vit Nutr Res.* 1985:55:233-237.

Amemiya T. Differences in muscular changes in rats with vitamin E and with selenium deficiency. *Int J Vit Nutr Res.* 1987;57:139-143.

Amemiya T. Effects of vitamin E and selenium deficiencies on rat capillaries. *Int J Vit Nutr Res.* 1988;59:122-126.

Batey DW, Eckhert CD. Analysis of flavins in ocular tissues of the rabbit. *Invest Ophthalmol Vis Sci.* 1991;32:1981-1985.

Burk RF, Lawrence RA, Lane JM. Liver necrosis and lipid peroxidation in the rat as the result of paraquat and diquat administration. Effect of selenium deficiency. *J Clin Invest.* 1980;65:1024-1031.

Burk RF, Levander OA. Selenium. In Shils ME, Olson JA, Shike M, Ross AC, ed. *Modern Nutrition in Health and Disease.* 9th ed. Philadelphia:Lippincott Williams;1999:265-276.

Gong H, Amemiya T. Corneal changes in manganese-deficient rats. *Cornea.* 1999;18:472-482.

Gong H, Takami Y, Kitaoka T, Amemiya T. Corneal changes in magnesium-deficient rats. *Cornea.* 2003;22:448-456.

Gong H, Takami Y, Amemiya T, Tozu M, Ohashi Y. Ocular surface in Zn-deficient rats. *Ophthalmic Res.* 2004;36:129-138.

Grant CA. Morphological and etiological studies of dietetic microangiopathy in pigs (mulberry heart'). *Acta Vet Scand.* 1961;2(Suppl 3):1-107.

Hafeman DG, Sunde RA, Hoekstra WG. Effect of dietary selenium on erythrocyte and liver glutathione peroxidase in the rat. *J Nutr.* 1974;104:580-587.

Hayes KC. Retinal degeneration in monkeys induced by deficiencies of vitamin E or A. *Invest Ophthalmol Vis Sci.* 1974;13:499-510.

Hoekstra WG. Biochemical function of selenium and its relation to vitamin E. *Fed Proc.* 1975;34:2083-2089.

Katz ML, Stone WL, Dratz EA. Fluorescent pigment accumulation in retinal pigment epithelium of antioxidant-deficient rats. *Invest Ophthalmol Vis Sci.* 1978;17:1049-1058.

Keen Cl, Zindenberg-Cherr S. Trace element and vitamin interactions in free radical defence. In Wahlqvist ML, Truswell AS, Smith R, Nestel PJ, ed. Nutrition in a Sustainable Environment. *Proceedings of the XV International Congress of Nutrition.* Adelaide, London:Smith-Gordon and Company Ltd;1994:799-803.

Keshan Disease Research Group. Observations on effect of sodium selenite in prevention of Keshan disease. *Chin Med J.* 1979;92:471-476.

Lawrence RA, Sunde RA, Schwartz GL, Hoekstra WG. Glutathione peroxidase activity in rat lens and other tissues in relation to dietary selenium intake. *Exp Eye Res.* 1974;18:563-569.

Mahan DC, Jones JE, Cline JH, Cross RF, Teague HS, Grifo AP Jr. Efficacy of selenium and vitamin E injections in the prevention of white muscle disease in young swine. *J Am Sci.* 1973;36:1104-1108.

Mizoguchi T, Amemiya T. Ultrastructure of the corneal epithelium of zinc deficient rats--deficiency and recovery. *Trace Ele Med.* 1992;9:84-89.

Obel AL. Studies on the morphology and etiology of so-called toxic liver dystrophy (hepatosis dietetica) in swine. *Acta Pathol Microbiol Scand.* 1953;94(Suppl):1-87.

Ostádalová I, Babicky′ A, Obenberger J. Cataract induced by administration of a single dose of sodium selenite to suckling rats. *Experientia.* 1978;34:222-223.

Robison WG, Kuwabara T, Bieri JG. Vitamin E deficiency and the retina: photoreceptor and pigment epithelial changes. *Invest Ophthalmol Vis Sci.* 1979;18:683-690.

Rotruck JT, Pope AL, Ganther HE, Swenson AB, Hafeman DG, Hoekstra WG. Selenium: Biochemical role as a component of glutathione peroxidase. *Science.* 1973;179:588-590.

Schwarz K, Foltz CM. Selenium as an initial part of α-factor 3 against dietary necrotic liver degeneration. *J Am Chem Soc.* 1957;79:3292-3293.

Scott DL. Kellemer J, Monty S, Lobowsky M. Influence of dietary selenium and vitamin E or glutathione peroxidase and glutathione in the rat. *Biochim Biophys Acta.* 1977;497:218-224.

Shearer TR, McCormack DW, De Sart DJ, Britton JL, Lopez MT. Histological evaluation of selenium induced cataracts. *Exp Eye Res.* 1980;31:327-333.

Sprinker LH, Harr JR, Newberne PD, Whanger PD, Weswig PH. Selenium deficiency lesions in rats fed vitamin E supplemented rations. *Nutr Rep Int.* 1971;4:335-340.

Stone WL, Katz ML, Lurie M, Marmor MF, Dratz EA. Effects of dietary vitamin E and selenium on light damage to the rat retina. *Photochem Photobiol.* 1979;29:725-730.

Takami Y, Gong H, Amemiya T. Riboflavin deficiency induces ocular surface damage. *Ophthalmic Res.* 2004;36 :156-165.

Van Vleet JF, Carlton W, Olander HJ. Hepatosis dietetica and mulberry heart disease associated with selenium deficiency in Indian swine. *J Am Med Assoc.* 1970;157:1208-1219.

Chapter 5

CHROMIUM

I. SIGNIFICANCE

In 1959, chromium (Cr) was identified as an element related to insulin action and glucose tolerance in the rat and clinical reports were subsequently published, showing the effect of Cr on diabetic symptoms in malnourished infants and patients receiving total parenteral nutrition (Stoecker, 1999). Cr has been shown to be involved in the metabolism of glucose (Schwarz and Mertz, 1958; Anderson, 1995) and lipid (Anderson, Bryden, Evock-Clover et al, 1997). However, nothing is known about the role of Cr in ocular tissues. Nutritional significance of Cr has been studied at the aspects of mainly symptomatology (Anderson, 1998; Schroeder 1966), serology and chemistry (Riales and Albrink, 1981; Schwarz and Mertz, 1959), but not at the morphological aspects.

Trivalent chromium was identified as the biologically active metal component of glucose tolerance factor by Schwarz and Mertz (1959). Patients on total parenteral nutrition (TPN) developed severe diabetic symptoms that were refractory to insulin (Aderson, 1995). After the addition of Cr to TPN fluids, diabetic symptoms were alleviated, and exogenous insulin was no longer required. In rats, severe chromium deficiency produced by strict elimination of dietary chromium and environmental chromium contamination produces a syndrome that is indistinguishable from diabetes mellitus with elevated serum cholesterol levels (Schwarz and Mertz, 1959, Schroeder, 1966). Thus Cr is an essential trace element for the maintenance of normal glucose tolerance (Mertz, 1998). Cr has been studied in relation to the glucose metabolism with diabetic syndrome (Anderson, 1998; Anderson, Cheng, Bryden et al, 2000) and lipid metabolism with lipoprotein (Abraham, Brooks and Flyath, 1992; Offenbacher, Rinko and Pi-Sunyer, 1985; Riales and Abbrink, 1981).

II. Chromium-Deficient Experiment

In experimental animals, dietary concentrations below 50μg (0.96μmol) chromium/kg diet are necessary to produce symptoms associated with chromium deficiency (Stoecker, 1999). However, at the present time, it is difficult to induce a clear-cut Cr deficiency syndrome in most animal species (Offenbacher、Pi-Sunyer and Stoecker, 1997). To avoid contamination with Cr, animals must be housed in plastic cages and exposure to any adventitious Cr must be prevented. Semipurified laboratory diets must be formulated to contain <0.1μmol/kg to demonstrate Cr depletion (Seaborn and Stoecker, 1989). In addition, an additional metabolic stress may be required for symptoms of Cr deficiency to be apparent (Nielsen, 1988; Hambidge and Rodgerson, 1969; Pekarek, Hauer, Rayfield et al, 1975).

Material and Methods

Twenty-one-day-old male Wistar Kyoto rats weighing 35.5 to 45.0g were divided into a Cr-deficient and a control group. The Cr-deficient rats were fed a low Cr powdered diet made by ourselves. The low Cr diet is the AIN-93G formula-based diet containing sucrose without added Cr. It contains no Cr and is complete in all other nutrients. The Cr-deficient and control groups received the diet ad libitum. Distilled deionized water was given freely to the Cr-deficient group. Control rats were fed the AIN-93G formula-based diet containing 0.9295mgCr/100g of diet and all other nutrients. The concentrations of the low Cr and usual diet were measured by graphite furnace atomic absorption analysis. The Cr content was 0.03mg/100g in the low Cr diet and 0.8mg/100g in the control diet. After 3 months on a low Cr diet, the eyes were enucleated rapidly under Nembutal anesthesia, just before light exposure, and 1, 2, 3, 4, 7, 11 and 12h after the start of light exposure and 1 and 3h after the start of darkness, and blood was drawn from the abdominal aorta for measurement of blood sugar, cholesterol and Cr levels

The rats were killed after 3, 7, 12 and 18 months on a low Cr diet.

Clinical Features of the Cr-Deficient Animal

There was no significant difference in body weight between Cr-deficient and control rats throughout the experiment ($p>0.05$), i.e. 512.5±17.5g (n=10) in the control rats and 508.5±17.0g (n=10) in the rats fed the low Cr diet for 3 months and 810±71g (n=5) in the control rats and 850±83g (n=5) in the rats fed the low Cr diet for 18 months. The rats fed a low Cr diet for 18 months exhibited normal health with no hair loss.

There was a statistically significant difference in the serum Cr level between the control and Cr-deficient rats ($p=0.0036$), i.e. 0.056±0.01μg/l (n=4) in the controls and 0.024±0.003μg/l (n=5) in the rats fed the deficient diet for 12 months.

The blood sugar levels of control and Cr-deficient rats are shown in Table 5.2.1. After the 7th month of the experiment, there were statistically significant differences in blood sugar levels between the control and the Cr-deficient rats.

The cholesterol levels of age-equivalent control and Cr-deficient rats were not significantly different at any time during the experiment ($p>0.05$) (Table 5.2.2).

The Cr-deficient diet made by ourselves was proved by inductively coupled plasma atomic emission spectrometry to contain less than 0.03mgCr/100g despite of 0.8mg Cr/100g in the usual diet. On the other hand, the serum level of Cr was confirmed to be less than 0.2 μg/l in both Cr deficient and control rats because of the limit of sensitivity for Cr measurement. However, no morphological changes were found in the retina of rats fed a usual diet containing Cr. In addition, the fact that the serum level of blood sugar was higher in rats fed on Cr-deficient diet should be due to Cr deficiency.

The blood glucose level in the rats fed a Cr-deficient diet for more than 7 months was significantly higher than that in the control rats. This was probably due to Cr deficiency because impaired glucose tolerance has been attributed to Cr depletion in a number of species (Mertz, 1969) and Cr deficiency induces increased serum cholesterol and plaque formation in rats (Schroeder, 1968). In addition, pathological changes appeared in the corneas and retinas of the rats fed a Cr-deficient diet, but not in the control rats. Thus the abnormal findings in the corneas and retinas of the Cr-deficient rats were probably due to Cr deficiency.

Table 5.2.1. The blood sugar levels of the rats fed on a Cr-deficient diet (mg/dl).

Groups	7-month-deficient rat	12-month-deficient rat	18-month-deficient rat
Cr deficiency	112.3±31.6 (n=8)*	134.3±32.0 (n=6)**	140.5±36.5 (n=6)***
Control	74±16.1 (n=5)*	83.3±14.3 (n=7)**	90.4±24.4 (n=5)***

*P=0.03, ** P=0.003 and ***P=0.023; n=the number of the specimens.

Table 5.2.2. The serum cholesterol levels of the rats fed on a Cr-deficient diet (mg/dl).

Groups	7-month-deficient rat	12-month-deficient rat	18-month-deficient rat
Cr deficiency	66±17 (n=8)	84 (n=1)	103 (n=1)
Control	66 (n=1)	79(n=1)	98 (n=1)

There are no significant differences of the serum cholesterol levels in the 7-, 12-, and 18- month-Cr-deficient groups compared to their control rats, n: the number of the specimens. P>0.05.

III. The Conjunctiva and Cornea

Results

The Conjunctiva

Scanning Electron Microscopic (SEM) Findings

In 12-month-Cr-deficient rats, SEM showed no abnormalities in the conjunctival surface. In 18-month-Cr-deficient rats, however, the conjunctival surface revealed many goblet cells with numerous microvilli, but secretory granules looked scarce (Fig. 5.3.1).

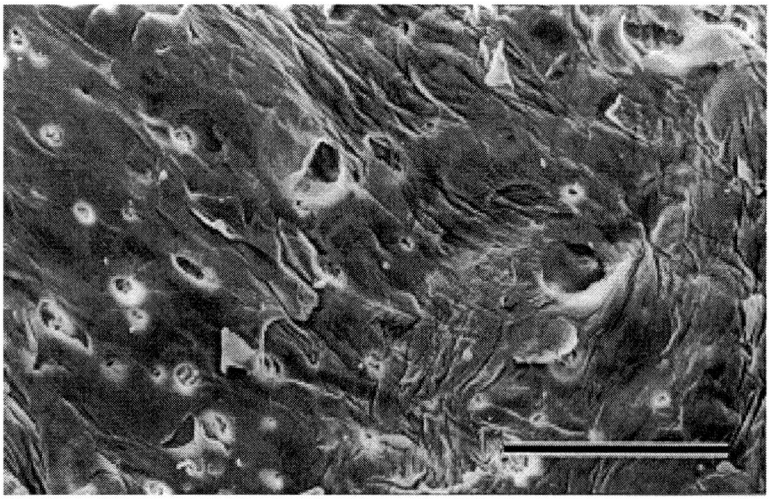

Figure 5.3.1. SEM micrograph of the conjunctiva of rats fed a Cr-deficient diet for 18 months. Many goblets cells are seen, but secretory granules appear ambiguously. Bar: 10 μm.

Transmission Electron Microscopic (TEM) Findings

Twelve-month-Cr-deficient rats showed many goblet cells filled with secretory granules and numerous microvilli and microplicae. On the other hand, 18-month-Cr-deficient rats showed many goblet cells which had the narrow orifice and vacant cavity (Fig. 5.3.2). But epithelial cells had normal features in the cytoplasm.

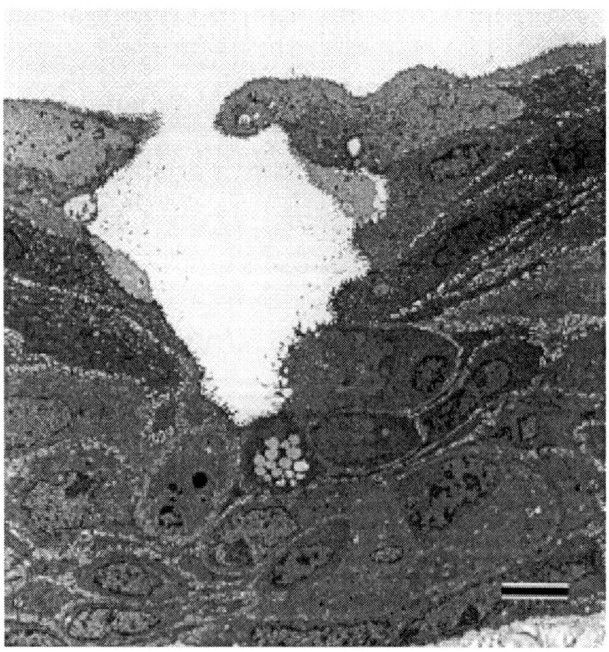

Figure 5.3.2. TEM micrograph of the conjunctiva of a rat fed a Cr-deficient diet for 18 months. The conjunctiva shows a narrow orifice of a goblet cell with empty cavity and normal fine structures of the epithelial cell. The epithelial surface has many microvilli. Bar: 5μm.

The Cornea

SEM Findings

Microvilli and microplicae in the most superficial epithelial layer looked a little bit scarce in 7-month-Cr-deficient rats and further scarce in 12-month-deficient rats. In 18-month-deficient rats, microvilli and microplicae were prominently decreased (Fig. 5.3.3), while SEM showed pentagonal endothelial cells as well as hexagonal ones (Fig. 5.3.4).

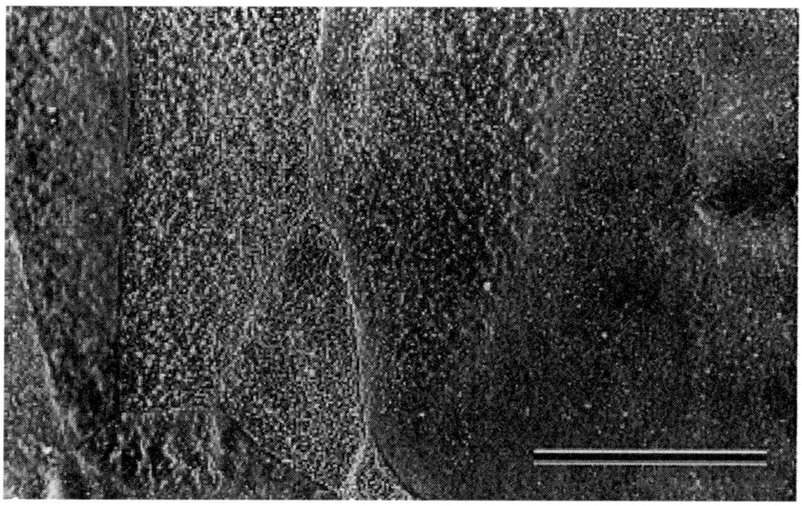

Figure 5.3.3. SEM micrographs of the cornea of a rat fed a Cr-deficient diet for 18 months, showing scarce microvilli and microplicae on the surface. Bar: 10μm.

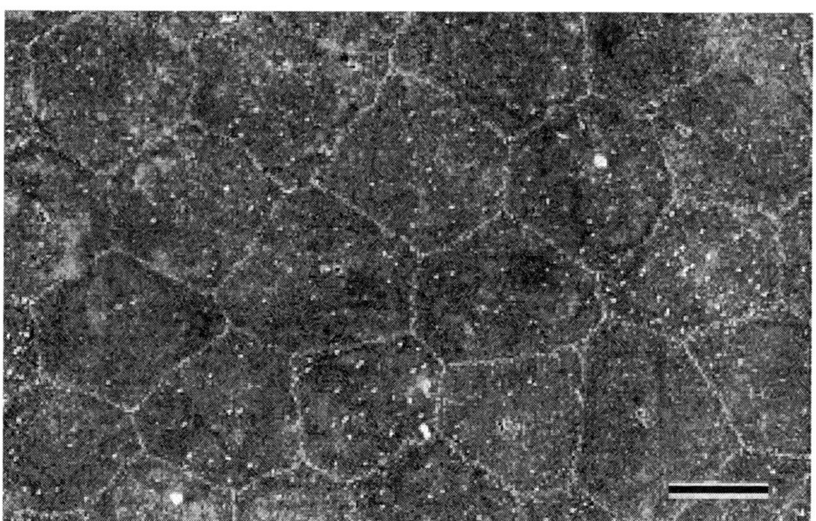

Figure 5.3.4. SEM micrograph of endothelial cells of a rat fed a Cr-deficient diet for 18 months. The endothelial cells are almost the same in size and some show pentagonal. Bar: 10μm.

TEM Findings

TEM of the corneas of the 7-, 12- and 18- month-old control rats showed normal features: many microvilli, well-developed intercellular junctions with many fibrils, ribosomes, no vacuoles, many hemidesmosomes in the basal epithelial cells and basement membranes. Neither apoptotic findings nor abnormal dense bodies were found.

In the corneas of rats fed the deficient diet for 7 months, the cytoplasmic components in the epithelial cells were reduced and empty spaces were seen. The epithelial cell nuclei showed scattered chromatin granules and a sparse nuclear matrix (Fig. 5.3.5). The basement membranes of the basal cells were thick, but the hemidesmosomes looked normal. The thickness of the Descemet membrane was 1.05±0.32μm. The endothelial cells looked normal.

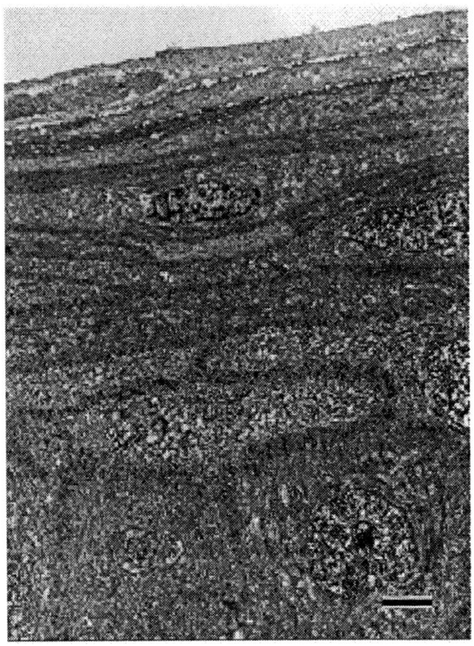

Figure 5.3.5. TEM micrograph of the cornea of a rats fed a Cr-deficient diet for 7 months, showing decreased microvilli in the most superficial epithelial cell, but epithelial cells have well-developed fibrils and desmosome-like intercellular junctions and many ribosomes. Bar: 2μm.

In the corneas of the rats fed the Cr-deficient diet for 12 months, TEM showed slightly more abnormalities than in those of the rats fed the deficient diet for 7 months: fewer microvilli and microplicae in the most superficial epithelial cells, scarce cytoplasmic components, ill-developed intercellular junctions with decreased fibrils and nuclei with scarce matrix. At the basal portion of basal cells, cellular debris was released from the cytoplasm (Fig. 5.3.6). The corneas of the control rats were normal.

In the corneas of the rats fed the Cr-deficient diet for 18 months, TEM showed a prominent decrease of cytoplasmic components in the epithelial cytoplasm, reduction of fibrils and poorly developed intercellular junctions with fewer fibrils. The basal cells had specific features: appearance of apoptotic nucleus (Fig. 5.3.7), thickened basement membrane, disappearance of hemidesmosomes, and membrane-bound amorphous dense material with a core in the basal portion (Fig. 5.3.8). In the subepithelial stroma there were numerous irregular dense deposits. The Descemet membrane was 1.03±0.25μm thick, n=30 in the Cr-deficient rats and 1.38±0.45μm, n=27 in the controls. The endothelial cells had a flat nucleus but almost normal features.

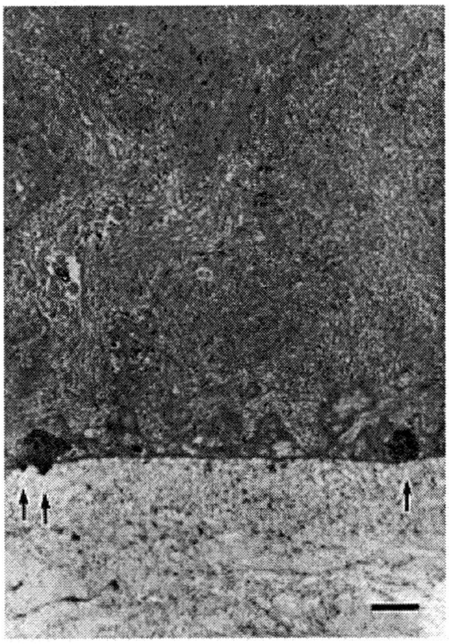

Figure 5.3.6. TEM micrograph of the cornea of a rat fed a Cr-deficient diet for 12 months, showing dense materials (arrows) releasing from the bottom of a basal cell to the subepithelial stroma and abnormal basal infoldings. Hemidesmosomes disappear, but the basement membrane remains. Bar: 1μm.

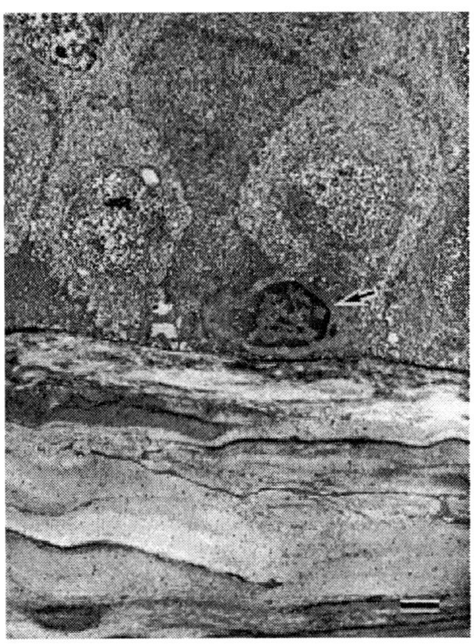

Figure 5.3.7. TEM micrograph of the cornea of a rat fed a Cr-deficient diet for 18 months. A basal cell contains a pyknotic nucleus (arrow) and condensed cytoplasmic components. Bar: 2μm.

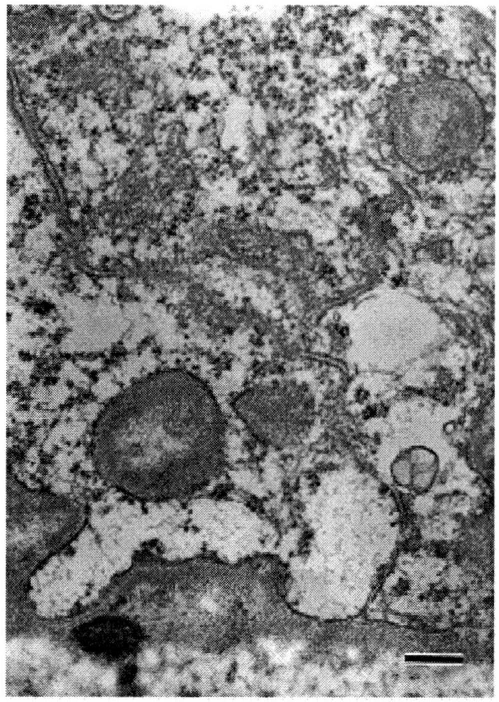

Figure 5.3.8. TEM micrograph of the cornea of an 18 month-Cr-deficient rat. At the bottom of a basal cell, clusters of fine granules partially enveloped by a membrane are seen. The basal cytoplasmic membrane is infolded and the infolded part contains thickened basement membrane, fine granules and cellular debris. Bar: 200μm.

Discussion

Measurements of serum Cr levels are very few (Seaborn and Stoecker, 1989), but the present experiment showed 0.065 μg/dl of serum Cr in the controls and less than 0.024μg/dl in the Cr-deficient group at 7 months; the difference is significant. Body weight was not a factor in Cr deficiency because it did not differ between the Cr-deficient and the control rats. However, the blood glucose level in the rats fed a Cr-deficient diet for more than 7 months was significantly higher than that in the control rats. This was probably due to Cr deficiency because impaired glucose tolerance has been attributed to Cr depletion in a number of species (Mertz, 1969) and Cr deficiency induces increased serum cholesterol and plaque formation in rats (Schroeder, 1968; Mertz, 1969). In addition, pathological changes appeared in the corneas and retinas of the rats fed a Cr-deficient diet, but not in the control rats. Thus the abnormal findings in the corneas and retinas of the Cr-deficient rats were probably due to Cr deficiency.

The effect of Cr deficiency on the conjunctiva was the decrease of secretory granules despite no reduction of goblet cells. This finding is different from that of goblet cells in deficiencies of other micronutrients. In deficiencies of vitamins A (Kanazawa, Kitaoka, Ueda et al, 2002), B_2 (Takami, Gong and Amemiya, 2004) and C (Chapter 12) and Zn (Gong, Takami, Amemiya et al, 2004), goblet cells decrease in number and have scarce secretory granules. This finding was also different from that of deficiencies of other micronutrients. Why these differences are caused is unclear. Cr might not be related to the production of secretory granules.

The most prominent change in the cornea is the scarcity of chromatin granules and matrix in the nuclei of epithelial cells. Chromatin granules are scarce and scattered and stainability with osmic acid is low. However, the nuclei of the endothelial cells show no such tendencies. An in vitro experiment showed that Cr^{3+} binds preferentially to DNA in chromatin and causes an increase in initiation sites, thus enhancing RNA synthesis (Oba, Suketa and Okada 1986). Therefore, Cr deficiency may induce chromatin damage and reduction of ribosomes.

Cell attachments such as those between desmosomes and hemidesmosomes and fibrous components in the cornea are poorly developed. Intercellular junctions are not decreased in number but have lost clear fine structures; a few fibrils are attached to the dense plate. The basement membranes of the basal cells are thick, but hemidesmosomes have disappeared. These changes of fibrous components suggest that Cr is related to collagen and to protein metabolism although biochemical studies of Cr have so far shown no evidence of such a relationship. Reduction of microvilli in the most superficial layer of the epithelium suggests that the production of protein for actin filaments, which form the core of microvilli, is disturbed.

A series of studies by the authors on deficiencies of trace elements and vitamins in ocular tissues revealed that Cr deficiency induced specific changes in the rat cornea. One of the specific changes is a prominent decrease of cytoplasmic components and the karyoplasm, which never appear in deficiencies of other micronutrients. Inadequate fixation makes the matrix substances soluble and the ultrastructural figures show vacuoles and empty spaces in the cytoplasm as artifacts. In the current experiments every specimen showed a decrease of the cytoplasmic and nuclear matrices which became more prominent as the Cr deficiency continued. Therefore we consider that the decrease of cytoplasmic and nuclear matrices contains low-molecular amino acids, soluble proteins, enzymes, etc. Since the role of Cr in the living body remains unclear, it is very difficult to explain the changes in the cytoplasmic and nuclear matrices. Cr might be related to soluble products in the matrix through Cr-associated metabolism. The appearance of membrane-bound amorphous dense structures with cores in the subepithelial layer of the cornea is also specific for Cr deficiency, because deficiencies of Zn, Cu, Mg, Mn, and vitamins A and C induce no such changes. However, riboflavin deficiency induces the same abnormal structures in the subepithelial layer of the cornea (Takami, Gong and Amemiya, 2004). These structures may represent debris of epithelial cells released from the basal epithelial cells to the subepithelial stroma similar to debris from the basal portion of retinal pigment epithelial cells to Bruch's membrane, because they are seen at various sites: cytoplasmic matrix, openings in the cytoplasmic membrane, basal infolding and subepithelial stroma.

IV. The Retina

Results

Electron Microscopic Findings

In both rats on the low Cr diet for 4 months and age-equivalent control rats, the maximum number of phagocytized lamellar structures in the retinal pigment epithelium (RPE) appeared 2h after the start of light exposure (Figs. 5.4.1A and 5.4.2). In the control rats 7h after the start of light exposure the number of phagocytized lamellar structures in the RPE was almost zero (Figs. 5.4.1D and 5.4.2). On the other hand, many phagocytized lamellar structures in the RPE were found in the Cr-deficient rats even 7h after the start of light exposure (Figs. 5.4.1B and 5.4.2). There were significiently more phagocytized lamellar structures in the RPE of Cr-deficient rats 1, 2, 7, 11 and 12h after the start of light exposure than in that of control rats (Fig. 5.4.1C, Fig. 5.4.2) ($p<0.05$). However, no morphological abnormalities were found in the outer and inner segments of the photoreceptor and nuclei of Cr-deficient rats on.

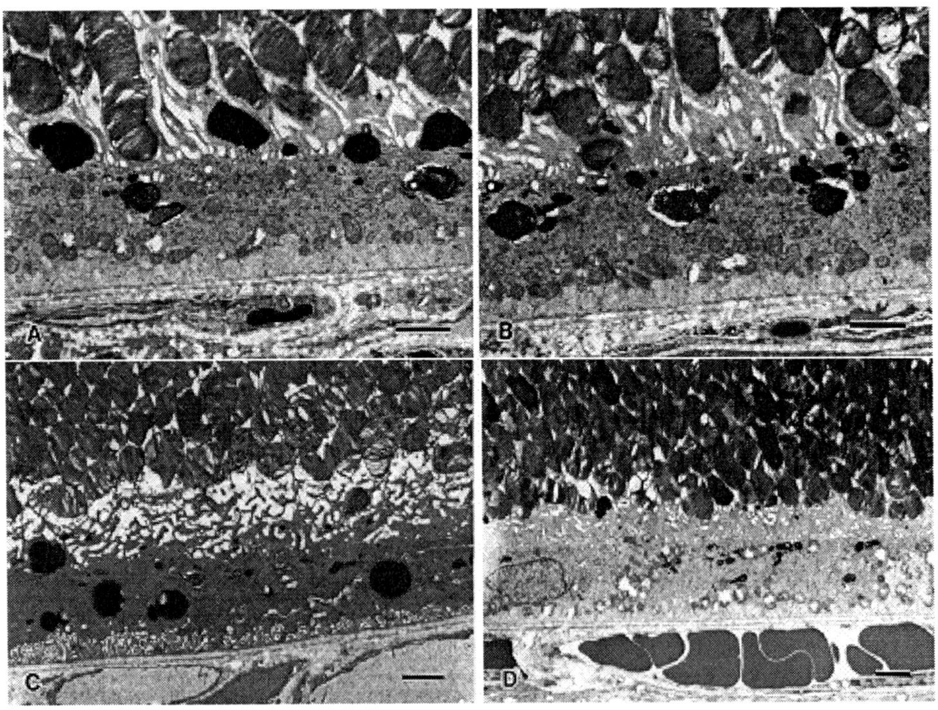

Figure 5.4.1. TEM micrographs of the RPE of Cr-deficient rats. A 4-month-Cr-deficient rat shows many discs separated from the tip of photoreceptor outer segments and phagocytized lamellar structures in the retinal pigment epithelium at 2h after the start of exposure to light (A). A 7-month-Cr-deficient rat also has many phagocytized lamellar structures in the retinal pigment epithelium at 7h after the start of light exposure (B). Phagocytized lamellar structures are still seen at 12h after light exposure (C), but no lamellar structures at 7h after light exposure in a control rat (D). Bar: 2μm (A-D).

In rats that were fed a Cr-deficient diet for 7 months, the RPE cells contained many lamellar structures, dense bodies and ribosomes. The outer segment had discs with various electron densities and the part of outer segment tips were segmented as masses between the outer segment tips and cytoplasmic processes of RPE cells. In rats fed the Cr-deficient diet for 12 months, the retina was a little bit thin, and RPE cells contained only a few lamellar structures. Between the outer segment and retinal pigment epithelial cells unidentified cells appeared near the apical portion of the RPE cells (Fig. 5.4.3). The photoreceptor cell nuclei were decreased in 2 to 6 lines and Müller cells were destructed (Fig. 5.4.4). The inner nuclear layer nuclei were reduced to 2 to 3 lines (Fig. 5.4.4). In rats fed on the Cr-deficient diet for 18 months, the retina further became thin. The retinal changes varied between sites. The RPE cells were severely degenerated: the basal infoldings were high and contained fine amorphous materials (Fig. 5.4.5). Many destructed mitochondria and dense granules remained (Fig. 5.4.5). The cytoplasmic processes were long and slender and looked atrophic (Fig. 5.4.6). Between the RPE cells and outer segments were numerous cellular debris (Fig. 5.4.6). The outer and inner segments were severely degenerated (Fig.5.4.6,7) and the outer nuclear layer showed decreased nuclei accompanied by the disappearance of Müller cells among nuclei (Fig. 5.4.7). The inner nuclear layer nuclei were prominently decreased in number (Fig. 5.4.7). At some site the outer plexiform layer, inner nuclear layer and photoreceptor cell were lost. The RPE was in contact with the dendrites and neurons in the inner plexiform layer (Fig. 5.4.8A). Ganglion cells disappeared. Neurons lost synapsis (Fig. 5.4.8B).

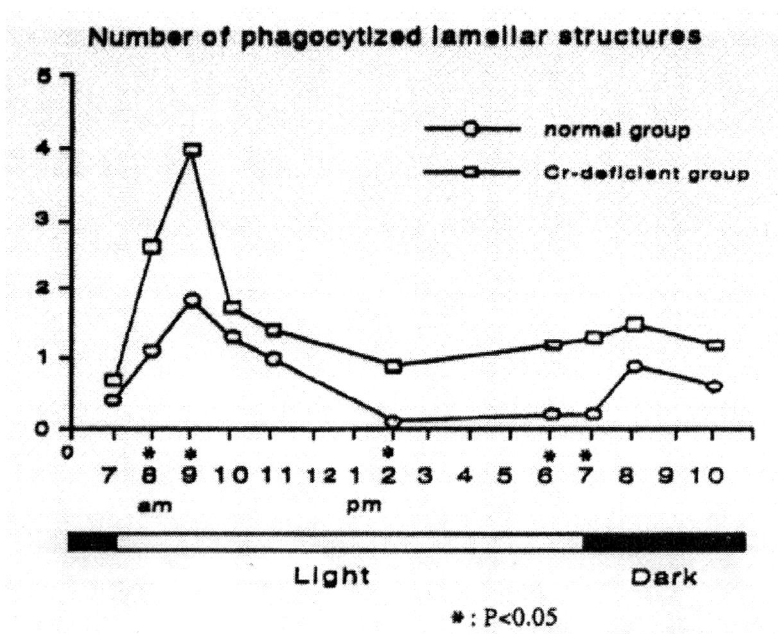

Figure 5.4.2. The number of phagocytized lamellar structures in the retinal pigment epithelium after the start of light exposure and darkness (per 15μm base line).

Discussion

The RPE cells of rats fed a Cr-deficient diet for 4 months contained many lamellar structures phagocytized OS discs, although the normal rat showed maximal amount of lamellar structures at 2h after light exposure and almost none 6h after light exposure (Ueda, Kanazawa, Gong et al, 2002). This phenomenon was found in a 7 month experiment and suggests the accelerated phagocytosis of the RPE cells is probably due to degeneration of the OS.

The photoreceptor outer segment discs are composed of polyhydric unsaturated fatty acids, and their metabolism is well balanced by various vitamins and trace elements. There have been no descriptions of the retinas of animals with a deficiency of Cr only. Rats deprived of the antioxidant nutrients such as vitamin E, selenium, methionine and chromium had severe changes in the retina and RPE: swollen, disoriented and vesiculated disc membranes of the photoreceptor outer segments and many lipofuscin granules and lipid droplets in the RPE (Katz, Parker, Handelman et al, 1982). In the current study, the single deficiency of Cr induced no visible disc membrane abnormalities, lipofuscin granules or lipid droplets in the RPE of rats fed a low Cr diet for 7 months.

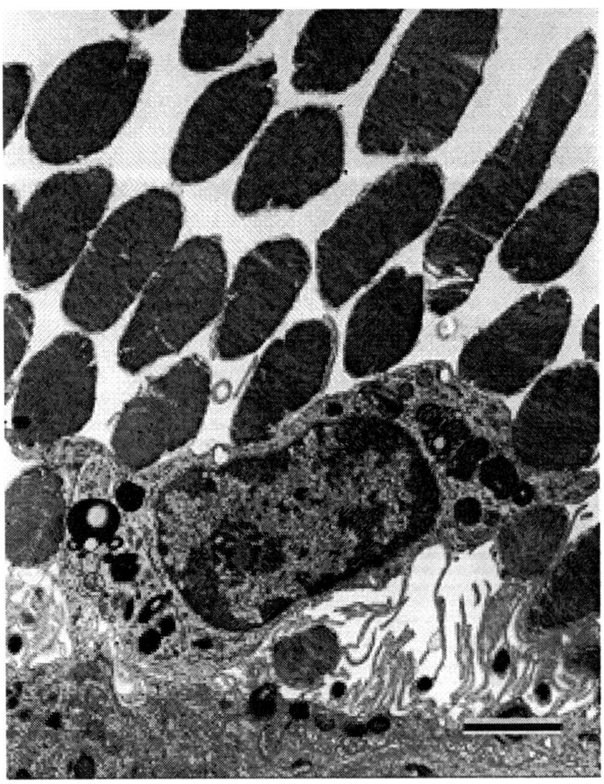

Figure 5.4.3. TEM micrograph of the photoreceptor outer segment and RPE of a rat fed a Cr-deficient diet for 12 months. An unidentified cell is about to be phagocytized by the RPE and secondary lysosomes are inside the cell. Bar: 2μm.

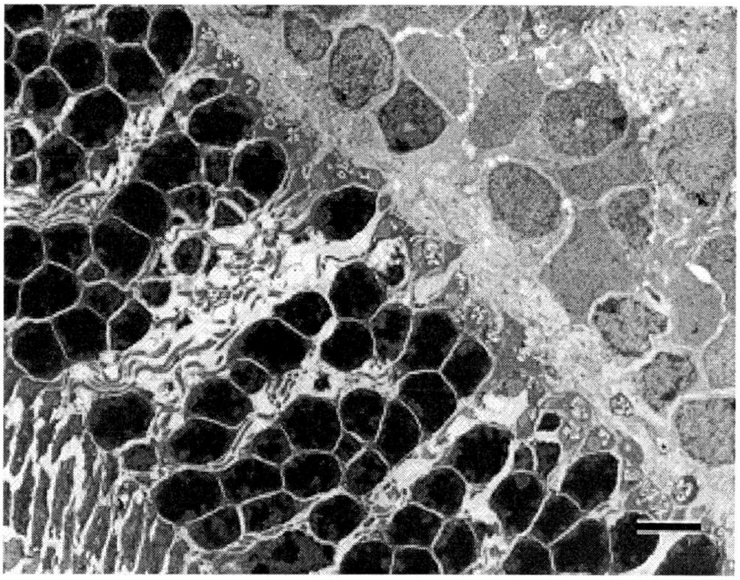

Figure 5.4.4. TEM micrograph of retina of a rat fed a Cr-deficient diet for 12 months. The outer nuclear layer nuclei are decreased to 6-7 lines and Müller cells are destroyed. The inner nuclear layer nuclei are decreased to 1-3 lines. Bar: 5μm.

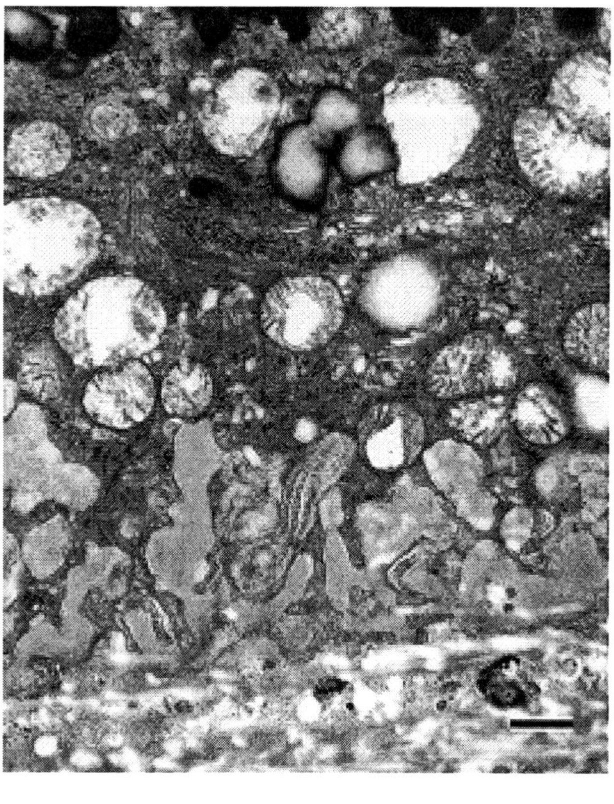

Figure 5.4.5. In the RPE of a 18-month-Cr-deficient rat, basal infoldings are high and contain much amorphous substances. The basement membrane disappears. Mitochondrial cristae are destroyed. Bar: 500nm.

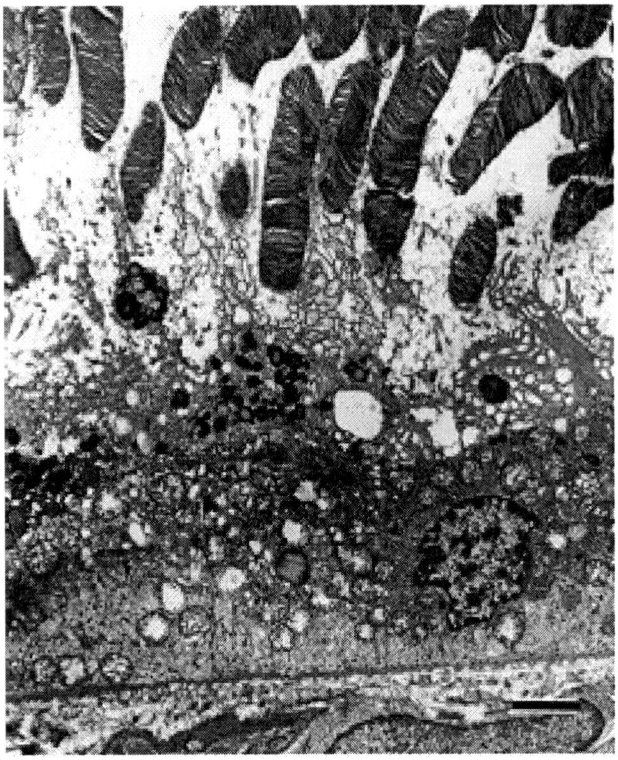

Figure 5.4.6. TEM micrograph of retinas of rats fed a Cr-deficient diet for 18 months. In some site photoreceptor outer segments remain, but are degenerated and the RPE with condensed cytoplasmic components shows destroyed mitochondria and elongated microvilli. Bar: 2μm.

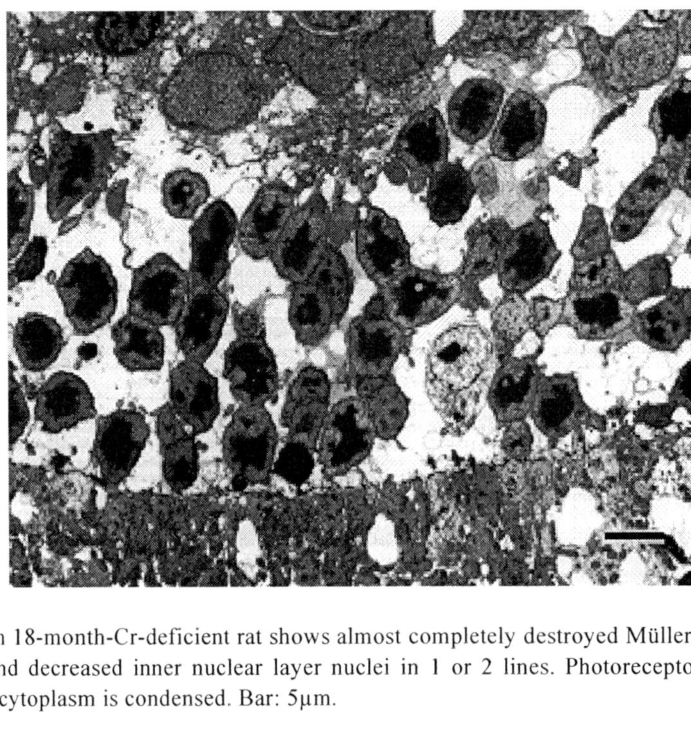

Figure 5.4.7. An 18-month-Cr-deficient rat shows almost completely destroyed Müller cells in the outer nuclear layer and decreased inner nuclear layer nuclei in 1 or 2 lines. Photoreceptor inner segments remain, but the cytoplasm is condensed. Bar: 5μm.

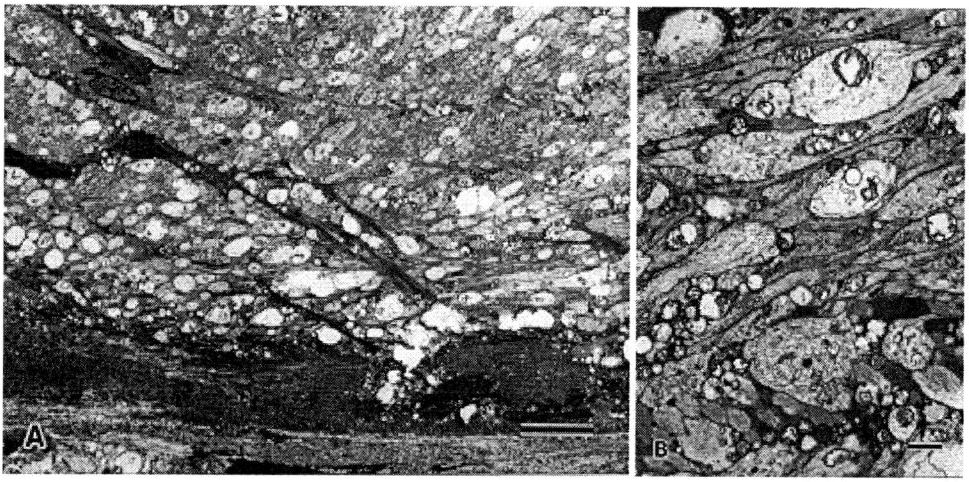

Figure 5.4.8. TEM micrographs of the retina of 18-month-Cr-deficient rats. In some site the RPE is in direct contact with the inner plexiform layer (A). The RPE is necrotic. In the inner plexiform layer neurons and dendrites are vacuolated and no synapses are seen (B). Bar: 10μm (A), 1μm (B).

Since trivalent Cr lowers the blood level of low density lipoproteins, because Cr inhibits hydroxy-methylglutaryl-CoA reductase on the cell surface (Zima, Mestek, Tesarova et al, 1998), while it raises that of high density lipoproteins (Riales and Albrink, 1981). Cr deficiency might affect lipid metabolism in the retina, especially in the photoreceptor outer segment. But there is no report that Cr affects the metabolism of polyhydric unsaturated fatty acids.

The retinal changes induced by Cr deficiency are different from those seen in a series of our nutritional deficient studies such as Zn, Mn (Gong and Amemiya, 1996), Mg (Gong, Amemiya and Takaya, 2001), Cu (Mishima, Dake, Amemiya et al,1996), Se (Amemiya, 1985) and vitamins A (Dowling and Gibbons, 1961; Amemiya, 1968), B_{12} (Amemiya, Kawada and Maekawa, 1987), C and E (Robison, Kuwabara and Bieri, 1979; Amemiya, 1978, 1981a,b). In most deficiencies, the degeneration begins at the OS discs and extends to the IS and photoreceptor nuclei, but the inner plexiform and ganglion cell layers scarcely disappear. However, Cr deficiency induces severe degeneration from the inner plexiform layer to the RPE layer, and the ganglion cell and nerve fiber layers disappear. The OS changes reflect the RPE cell. In vitamin A deficiency, lamellar structure disappear in the RPE cells due to loss of OS (Dowling and Gibbons, 1961; Amemiya, 1968), while vitamin E deficiency makes lipofuscin granules increase in the RPE cells due to lysosomal dysfunction (Robison, Kuwabara and Bieri, 1979; Amemiya, 1978, 1981a,b). Vitamin B_{12} deficiency affects the circadian rhythm of phagocytosis in the RPE cells without any morphological changes of the OS. Although deficiencies of Zn, Cu (Mishima, Dake, Amemiya et al, 1996) and Mn (Gong and Amemiya, 1996) may damage the OS first due to decreased activity of Zn-Cu, and Mn superoxide dismutases or antioxidant enzyme, the damages are limited in the photoreceptor cell. Even if the damages include the decrease of inner nuclear layer nuclei, such damages are considered to be secondary following the photoreceptor cell degeneration.

The severer degeneration due to Cr deficiency compared to that due to other micronutrient deficiencies can not be clearly explained because Cr function still remains unclear. Cr has mainly been studied by biochemistry and symptomatology. In patients and animals under Cr deficiency, Cr deficiency is found to induce hyperglycemia and hypercholesterolemia. That is, Cr is found to be related in some metabolic processes as Cr-containing enzymes in the glucose and cholesterol metabolisms. In the current study, Cr-deficient rats show no abnormal clinical signs such as weight gain and abnormal fur and behaviour. However, they show hyperglycemia. The retinal changes in Cr-deficient rats are a little bit similar to those in spontaneously diabetic rats (Lu, Bhutto and Amemiya, 2003) and diabetic patients. Non-vascular retinal changes are not clearly described in the current textbook, probably because the main causative factors are vascular, but described in the old literature. In effect, the diabetic human retina shows a thinned nerve fiber layer and a decrease in number of ganglion cells; light microscopic findings show decreased nuclei in the outer and inner nuclear layer (Bek, 1994). These resemble the retinal changes of Otsuka Long-Evans Tokushima Fatty (OLETF) rats including vascular changes such as microaneurysms, narrow capillary lumen and thick basement membranes (Lu, Bhutto and Amemiya, 2003). Cr-deficient rats in the current study also show similar retinal changes. However, microaneurysms are not proven without vascular cast technique. Since OLETF rats and Cr-deficient rats show neither hemorrhages nor exudates in the retina, animal diabetes mellitus is unsatisfactory in this respect. It seems to be difficult for rats to have retinal hemorrhages and exudates. For instance, the spontaneously hypertensive rat never shows hemorrhages or exudates in the retina, although retinal capillaries are typical for hypertension. Cr-deficient rats may be a new model of experimental diabetic retinopathy. On the other hand, hypercholesterolemia has never shown such retinal changes. RICO rats and inherited hypercholesterolemic rats showed retinal changes different from Cr-deficient rats (Yamakawa, Bhutto, Lu et al, 2001). No one knows how abnormal activity of Cr-related enzymes has a relation to the retinal lipid metabolism. The destruction of a whole retinal architecture in the Cr-deficient rat might be due to the abnormality of lipids forming the retinal architecture. In addition, the coexistence of hyperglycemia and hypercholesterolemia may accelerate the retinal damage so that Cr deficiency is more destructive than the other micronutrient deficiencies.

References

Abraham AS, Brooks BA, Elath U. The effects of chromium supplementation on serum glucose and lipids in patients with and without non-insulin-dependent diabetes. *Metabolism*. 1992;41:768-771.

Amemiya T. Cytochemical and electron microscopic examination of the retina of rats with hypovitaminosis A. *Acta Soc Ophthalmol Jpn*. 1968;72:1074-1099.

Amemiya T. Retinal changes in the selenium deficient rat. *Int J Vit Nutr Res*. 1985;55:233-237.

Amemiya T, Kawata T, Maekawa A. Ocular pathology in vitamin B_{12} deficient rat. In: Uchino H, Takaku H, ed. *Symposium on Vitamin B_{12} in Kyoto*. Tokyo:Kyowa Kikaku Tsushin;1987:80-85.

Anderson RA. Chromium and parenteral nutrition. *Nutrition*. 1995;11:83-86.

Anderson RA, Bryden NA, Evock-Clover CM, Steele NC. Beneficial effects of chromium on glucose and lipid variables in control and somatotropin-treated pigs are associated with increased tissue chromium and altered tissue copper, iron, and zinc. *J Anim Sci*. 1997;75:657-661.

Anderson RA. Nutritional factors influencing the glucose/insulin systems: chromium. *J Am Coll Nutr*. 1997;16:404-410.

Anderson RA. Effects of chromium on body composition and weight loss. *Nutr Rev*. 1998;56:266-270.

Anderson RA, Cheng N, Bryden NA, Polansky MM, Cheng N, Chi J, Feng J. Elevated intakes of supplemental chromium improve glucose and insulin variables in individuals with type 2 diabetes. *Diab Metab*. 2000;26:22-27.

Dake Y. Electron histochemical examination of cytochrome oxidase in the retinal photoreceptor cell of copper deficient rats. *Acta Histochem Cytochem*. 1992;25:371-378.

Dowling JE, Gibbons IR. The effect of vitamin A deficiency on the fine structure of the retina. In: Smelser GK, ed. *The Structure of the Eye*. New York:Academic Press Inc;1961:85-99.

Gong H, Amemiya T. Ultrastructure of retina of manganese-deficient rats. *Invest Ophthalmol Vis Sci*. 1996;37:1967-1974.

Gong H, Amemiya T, Takaya K. Retinal changes in magnesium-deficient rats. *Exp Eye Res*. 2001;72:23-32.

Gong H, Takami Y, Amemiya T, Tozu M, Ohashi Y. Ocular surface in Zn-deficient rats. *Ophthalmic Res*. 2004;36:129-138.

Hambidge KM, Rodgerson DO. Comparison of hair chromium levels of nulliparous and parous women. *Am J Obstet Gynecol*. 1969;103:320-321.

Kanazawa S, Kitaoka T, Ueda Y, Gong H, Amemiya T. Interaction of zinc and vitamin A on the ocular surface. *Graefes Arch Clin Exp Ophthalmol*. 2002;240:1011-1021.

Katz ML, Parker KR, Handelman GJ, Bramel TL, Dratz EA. Effects of antioxidant nutrient deficiency on the retina and retinal pigment epithelium of albino rats; a light and electron microscopic study. *Exp Eye Res*. 1982;34:339-369.

Lu ZY, Bhutto IA, Amemiya T. Retinal changes in Otsuka Long- Evance Tokushima Fatty rats (spontaneously diabetic rat)---Possibility of a new experimental model for diabetic retinopathy. *Jpn J Ophthalmol*. 2003;47:28-35.

Mertz W. Chromium occurrence and function in biological systems. *Physiol Rev*. 1969;49:163-239.

Mertz W. Chromium research from a distance: from 1959 to 1980. *J Am Coll Nutr*. 1998;17:544-547.

Mishima K, Dake Y, Amemiya T, Nishimura M. Electron microscopic study of retinas of macular mice. *Graefes Arch Clin Exp Ophthalmol*. 1996;234:S101-S105.

Nielsen FH. Nutritional significance of the ultratrace elements. *Nutr Rev*. 1988;46:337-341.

Oba H, Suketa Y, Okada S. Enhancement of in vitro ribonucleic acid synthesis on chromium (III)-bound chromatin. *J Inorg Biochem*. 1986;27:179-189.

Offenbacher E, Rinko C, Pi-Sunyer FX. The effects of inorganic chromium and brewer's yeast on glucose tolerance, plasma lipids, and plasma chromium in early subjects. *Am J Clin Nutr*. 1985;42:454-456.

Pekarek RS, Hauer EC, Rayfield EJ, Wannemacher RW Jr, Beisel WR, Maryland E. Relationship between serum chromium concentrations and glucose utilization in normal and infected subjects. *Diabetes*. 1975;24:350-353.

Riales RA, Abbrink MJ. Effect of chromium chloride supplementation on glucose tolerance and serum lipids including high-density lipoprotein of adult men. *Am J Clin Nutr*. 1981;134:2670-2678.

Robison WG, Kuwabara T, Bieri JG. Vitamin E deficiency and the retina: Photoreceptor and retinal epithelial changes. *Invest Ophthalmol Vis Sci*. 1979;18:683-690.

Schroeder HA. Chromium deficiency in rats:A syndrome simulating diabetes mellitus with retarded growth. *J Nutr*. 1966;88:439-445.

Schroeder HA. The role of chromium in mammalian nutrition. *Am J Clin Nutr*. 1968;21:230-244.

Seaborn CD, Stoecker BJ. Effect of starch, sucrose, fructose, and glucose on chromium absorption and tissue concentrations in obese and lean mice. *J Nutr*. 1989;119:1444-1451.

Shwarz K, Mertz W. Chromium (III) and the glucose tolerance factor. *Arch Biochem Biophys*. 1959;85:292-295.

Takami Y, Gong H, Amemiya T. Riboflavin deficiency induces ocular surface damage. *Ophthalmic Res*. 2004;36:156-165.

Ueda Y, Kanazawa S, Gong H, Miyamura N, Kitaoka T, Amemiya T. The retinal pigment epithelium of Cr-deficient rats. *Life Sci*. 2002;71:1569-1577.

Yamakawa K, Bhutto IA, Lu ZY, Watanabe Y, Amemiya T. Retinal vascular changes in rats with inherited hypercholesterolemia---Corrosion cast demonstration. *Curr Eye Res*. 2001;22:258-265.

Chapter 6

MANGANESE

I. SIGNIFICANCE

Manganese (Mn) is one of the essential trace elements for humans and animals. It is present only in trace amounts in animal tissue.

An old South African folk remedy calls for the use of alfalfa as a treatment for diabetes. Rubenstein, Levin and Elliot et al (1962) found that alfalfa extract contains a high concentration of manganese. They described a patient with diabetes who was resistant to insulin therapy but responded to the oral administration of manganese chloride and, hence, had a consistent drop in blood glucose levels. Histologic studies have shown that Mn-deficient guinea pigs have hypertrophied pancreatic islet tissues with degranulated ß-cells and an increased number of Langerhans' cells (Everson and Shrader, 1968).

In spite of low concentration of Mn in animal tissues and its essential participation in several biologic functions (Orent and McCollum, 1931; Kemmerer, Elvehjem and Hart, 1931), its precise biochemical role remains unclear. Mn has something to do with certain enzymes involved in carbohydrate metabolism (Hurley, Keen and Baly, 1984; Baly, Curry, Keen et al, 1985), some amino acid metabolizing pathways (Wedler and Muenster, 1982), and mucopolysaccharide synthesis (Leach, Muenster and Wien, 1969, Leach, 1971; Leach and Lilburn, 1978; Bolze, Reeves, Lindbeck et al 1985). Mn itself seems to be a mutagenic initiator of cancer in some tumors (Flessel, 1979). However, except for the pancreas, Mn specificity for tissues or organs is little known.

The clinical expressions of Mn deficiency include neurologic problems as well as growth retardation, abnormal skeletal development, and loss of reproductive capacity (Shils and McCollum, 1943). Maternal Mn deficiency during pregnancy induces ataxia, skeletal abnormalities, and high infant mortality (Erway, Hurley and Fraser, 1970; Hurley, 1981). In humans, Mn deficiency is thought to be rare because of its relative abundance in food. However, long-term parenteral nutrition and enteral tube feeding can induce deficiencies of some trace elements. A Japanese girl with short intestine syndrome – 2 years and 5 months of age – who was treated with enteral tube feeding showed catch-up growth after manganese administration (Norose and Araki, 1987). Mn deficiency in humans also might be induced by some drugs, such as hydrazine and anti-hypertensive drugs with chelating properties

(Comens, 1956; Borg and Cotzias, 1962; Mehta and Reilly, 1990). Although Mn has been detected chemically in various parts of the eye, its significance in ocular tissues is unclear.

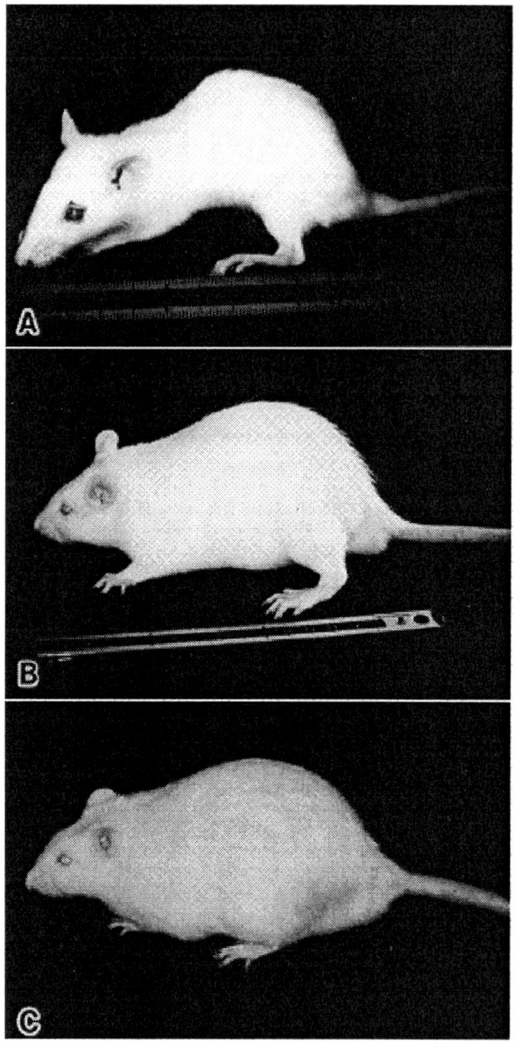

Figure 6.2.1. Gross appearance of the animals. There are obvious differences in a 2-month-old Mn-deficient rat (A), an age-equivalent control rat (B), and a rat that has recovered from Mn deficiency (C):A exhibits emaciation, hair loss, and conjunctival secretion (arrows).

II. Mn-Deficient Experiment

Material and Methods

When Wistar Kyoto rats were fed a Mn-deficient diet, they hardly showed Mn-deficient signs and symptoms. Then, during gestation and delivery, pregnant female rats are given deionized and distilled water and a Mn-deficient solid diet containing 0.23mg of Mn/100g diet and all other nutrients, obtained from Nippon Clea Incorporated, Tokyo, Japan. The male and female infant rats were given free access to an Mn-deficient diet. When they reached the age of 3 months, Mn-deficient females were mated with Mn-deficient males, and their offspring (second generation of Mn-deficient rats) continued to be given free access to an Mn-deficient diet. Corneas from second generation of Mn-deficient rats were examined at the age of 2 months. For a recovery experiment, after being fed an Mn-deficient diet for 3 months, the second generation of Mn-deficient rats were given free access to the normal diet containing 5.53mg of Mn/100g and all other nutrients, obtained from Oriental Yeast Co. Ltd., Tokyo, Japan for 3months. In the recovery experiment corneas were examined 3 months after the start of the normal diet.

Clinical Features of the Mn-Deficient Animal

Overt characteristics: The Mn-deficient rats exhibited characteristics typically seen in Mn-deficient animals (Fig.6.2.1): growth retardation, inability to right themselves from a supine position, hair loss, and high mortality during the first week of life. Compared with the values in the control group, the plasma manganese levels of the deficient group were obviously decreased in every experimental month; the difference between the two groups was statistically significant (Table 6.2.1). Body weights were not significantly different between the two groups at the beginning of the experiment. In manganese-deficient rats, however, the rate of weight gain gradually decreased (Table 6.2.2). Conjunctival secretions were seen in some of the Mn-deficient rats. However, the cornea was clear.

Table 6.2.1. Plasma manganese levels (μg/l).

	Months after start of experiment			
Groups	6*	12*	18*	30*
Mn-deficient	1.56±0.43 n=5	1.20±0.10 n=5	1.02±0.08 n=5	0.88±0.08 n=5
Control	4.21±1.26 n=5	4.18±0.08 n=5	4.14±0.19 n=5	3.92±0.13 n=5

n: number of animals. * p<0.0001 (Fisher's protected least significant difference).

Table 6.2.2. Body weight (g).

	Months after start of experiment			
Group	6	12*	18*	30
Mn-deficient	356±6.5 n=5	424±37 n=5	528±24 n=5	396±10 n=5
Control	369±18 n=5	603±13 n=5	717±25 n=5	425±76 n=5

n: number of animals. * p<0.0001 (Fisher's protected least significant difference).

III. THE CORNEA

Rats from second generation of Mn-deficient rats at age 2 months were used.

Results

In Mn-deficient rats, the whole corneas were significantly thin, especially the stroma ($p<0.05$: Table 6.3.1) (Fig.6.3.1). The stroma contained many keratocytes. In the recovery experiment, the corneas became almost as thick as the control corneas.

Table 6.3.1. Thickness of corneal stroma.

Groups	Size (μm)	Number of eyes
2-month-old Mn-deficient rat	78±13.6[a]	16
Equivalent-age control rat	96±11.4[ab]	12
Recovery rat	91±9.3[ab]	14

a: Significant difference as determined by Fisher's Protected Least Significant Difference. The corneal stromas are significantly different in thickness between Mn-deficient and control groups and between Mn-deficient and recovery groups ($p<0.05$).
b: There is no significant difference between the control and recovery groups ($p>0.05$).

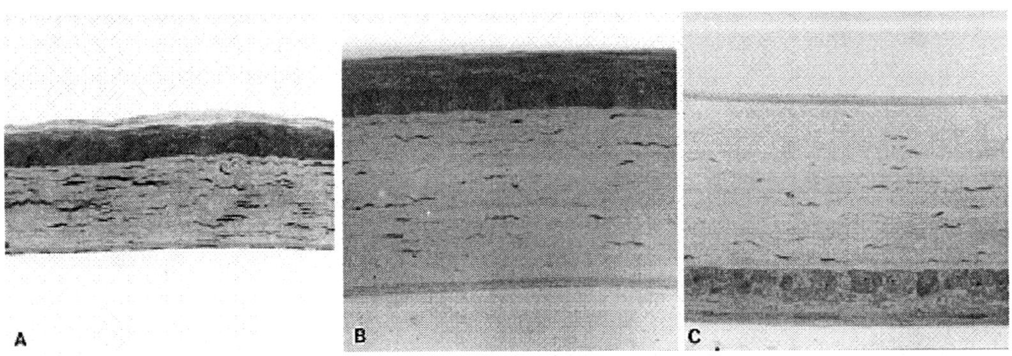

Figure 6.3.1. Light micrograph of cornea. A 2-month-old Mn-deficient rat (A), a control rat (B), and a recovered rat (C). A: A general thinness of the whole cornea, especially the stroma, in which many keratocytes remain, as compared with control cornea (B). The corneal stroma in C is almost as thick as in the control (B). Toluidine blue, × 200.

Transmission Electron Microscopy (TEM) Findings

The corneal epithelial cells of Mn-deficient rats had very few microvilli and bundles of tonofibrils (Fig. 6.3.2). In the basal layer of the epithelium, abnormal mitochondria were present in the cytoplasm of the dark cells. Mitochondria were more numerous, abnormal in shape, and lacked electron density. Basal epithelial cells had little chromatin in the nuclei (Fig. 6.3.3). The diameter of collagen fibers in the corneal stroma was significantly decreased (Table 6.3.2, Fig. 6.3.4), and the number of keratocytes was increased. Descemet's membrane was significantly thinner than that in the control group ($p<0.0001$) (Table 6.3.3); it had less-uniform electron density, and there were microcracks between the endothelium and Descemet's membrane (Fig. 6.3.5). The endothelial surface in the Mn-deficient rats seemed rough and contained small pit-like structures, 0.65±0.39μm in diameter, most of which were in cytoplasmic processes located near a neighboring cell (Fig. 6.3.5).

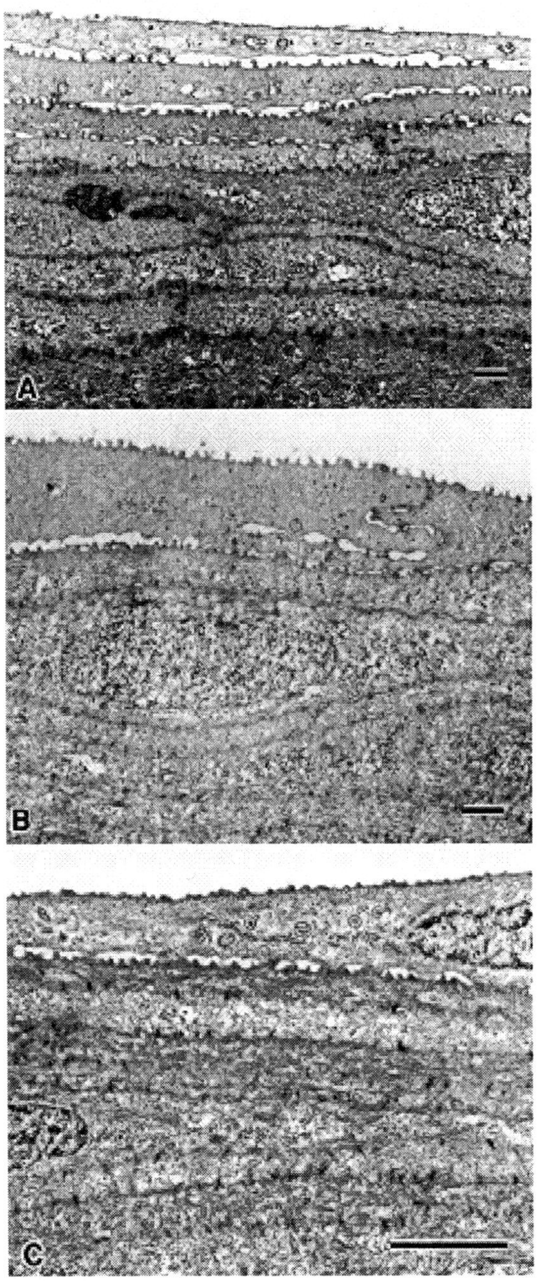

Figure 6.3.2. TEM micrographs of corneal epithelial cells. A 2-month-old Mn-deficient rat (A), a control rat (B), and a recovered rat (C). A: A decreased number of microvilli in the most superficial layer and decreased bundles of tonofibrils in the epithelial cell cytoplasm. B: The corneal epithelium of an age-equivalent control rat. C: Almost the same appearance as B. Bar: 1μm (A-C).

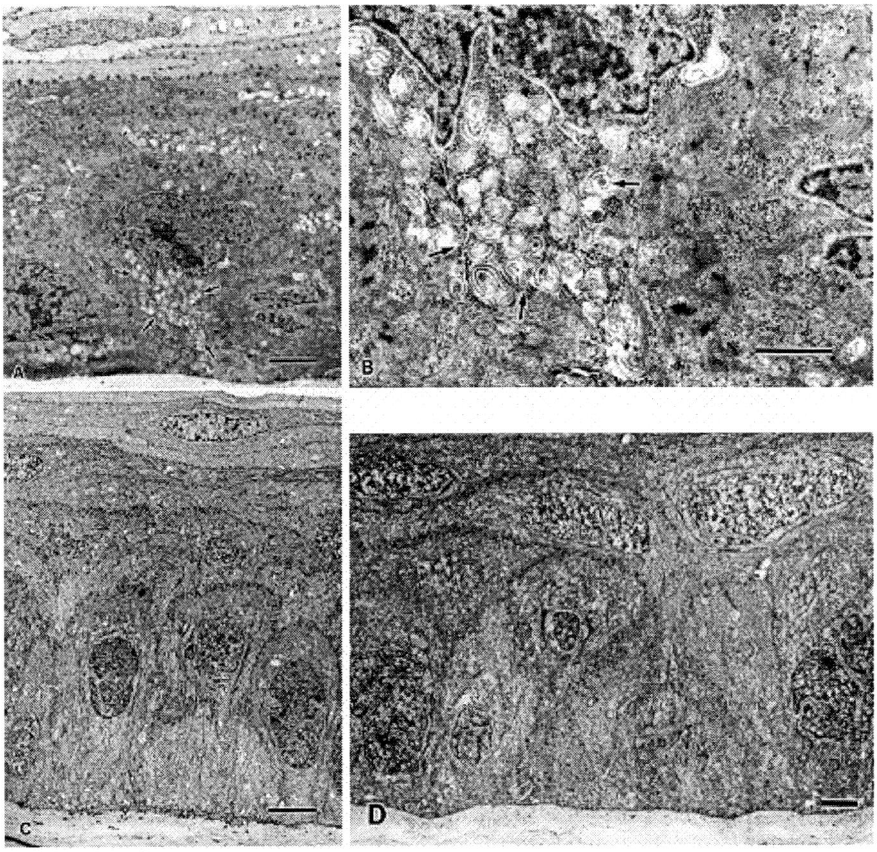

Figure 6.3.3. TEM micrographs of corneal epithelium. A, B: A 2-month-old Mn-deficient rat; a pair fed control rat (C), and a recovered rat (D). Destroyed mitochondria (arrows) are seen in A and B. C: The corneal epithelium of an age-equivalent pair-fed control rat. D: Normal mitochondria are seen. Bar: 5μm (A,C), 500nm (B), 2μm (D).

Table 6.3.2. Number and diameter of collagen fibers in corneal stroma.

Groups	Number of fields examined	Number of fibers/0.16μm^2	Number of diameters measured	Diameter (nm)
2-month-old Mn-deficient rat	52	49.5±12.8[a]	242	33.6±10.5[a]
Equivalent-age control rat	38	60.4±5.6[ab]	194	45.4±5.3[ab]
Recovery rat	36	59.3±4.3[ab]	190	45.1±4.7[ab]

a: Significant difference as determined by Fisher's Protected Least Significant Difference. There are significant differences in the number of collagen fibers between the Mn-deficient and control groups ($p<0.005$) and between the Mn-deficient and recovery groups ($p<0.001$), respectively, and there are also significant differences in diameters of collagen fibers between the Mn-deficient and control groups ($p<0.005$) and between the deficient and recovery groups ($p<0.001$).

b: There are no significant differences in the number of collagen fibers or the diameter between the control and recovery groups.

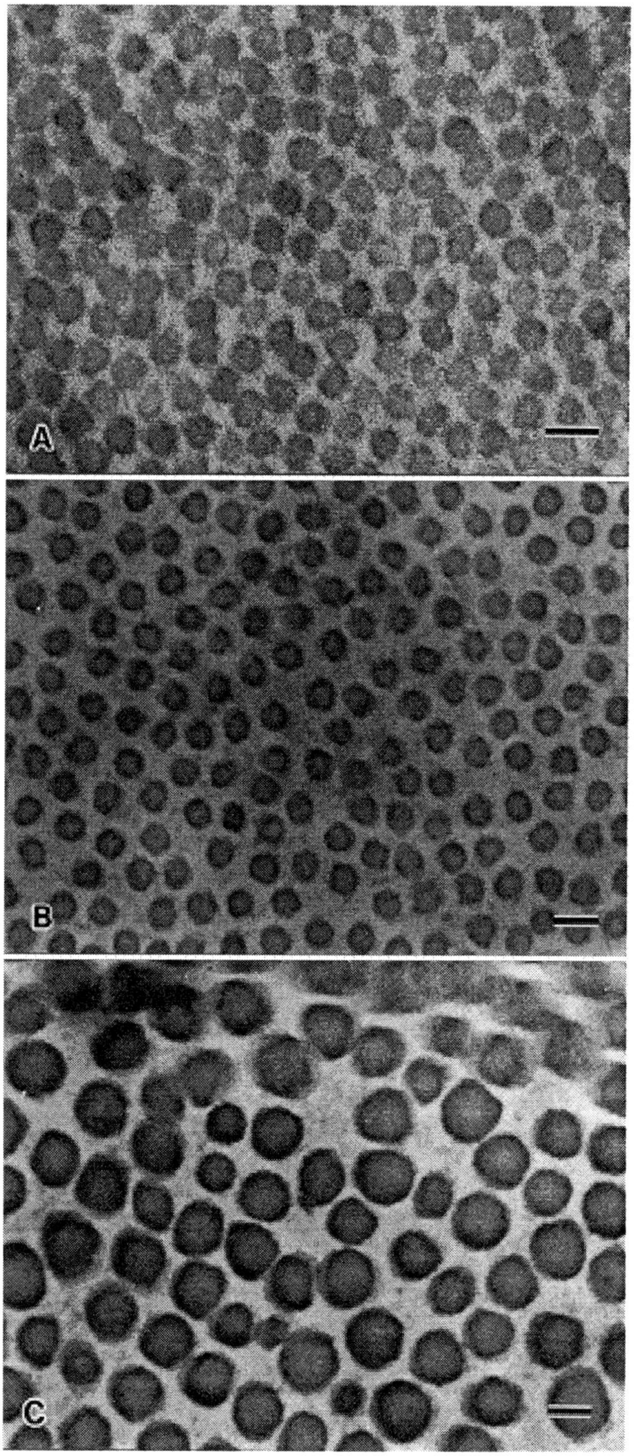

Figure 6.3.4. TEM micrographs of the corneal collagen fibers. Two-month-old Mn-deficient rat (A), a control rat (B), and a recovered rat (C). A: Irregular diameters and arrangement of collagen fibers. B: The collagen fibers of an age-equivallent control rat.C: Almost the same features as B. Bar: 50nm (A, B), 100nm (C).

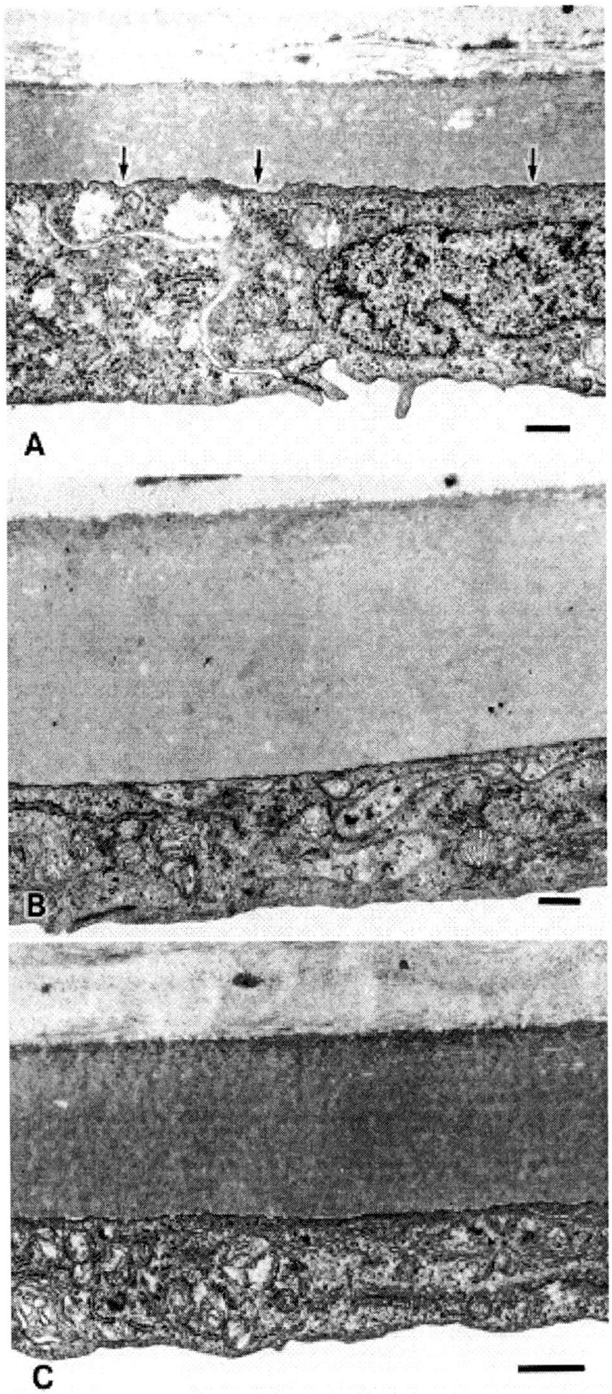

Figure 6.3.5. TEM micrographs of Descemet's membrane. A 2-month-old Mn-deficient rat (A), a control rat (B), and a recovered rat (C). A: Descemet's membrane has less uniform density; there are microcracks (arrows) between the endothelium and Descemet's membrane, and Descemet's membrane is significantly thinner than that of the control. B: Descemet's membrane in an age-equivalent control rat. There is no significant difference between the control and a recovered rat. Bar: 500nm (A, B), 1μm (C).

Table 6.3.3. Thickness of Descemet's membrane.

Groups	Fields examined (n)	Thickness (μm)
2-month-old Mn-deficient rat	46	1.5±0.2[a]
Equivalent-age control rat	39	2.9±0.6[ab]
Recovery rat	30	3.2±0.3[ab]

a: Significant difference as determined by Fisher's Protected Least Significant Difference. Descemet's membrane shows significant difference in thickness between the Mn-deficient and control groups ($p<0.001$) and between the Mn-deficient and recovery groups ($p<0.001$).

b: There is no significant difference between the control and recovery groups ($p>0.05$).

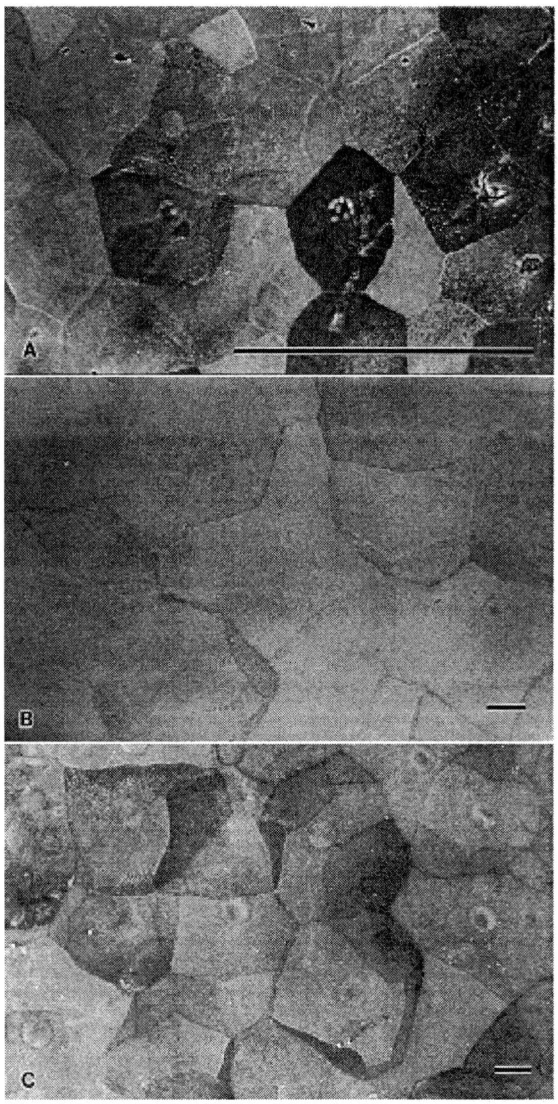

Figure 6.3.6. SEM micrographs of corneal epithelium. A 2-month-old Mn-deficient rat (A), a control rat (B), and a recovered rat (C). There are obviously more dark cells in A than in B and C. Bar: 100μm (A), 10μm (B, C).

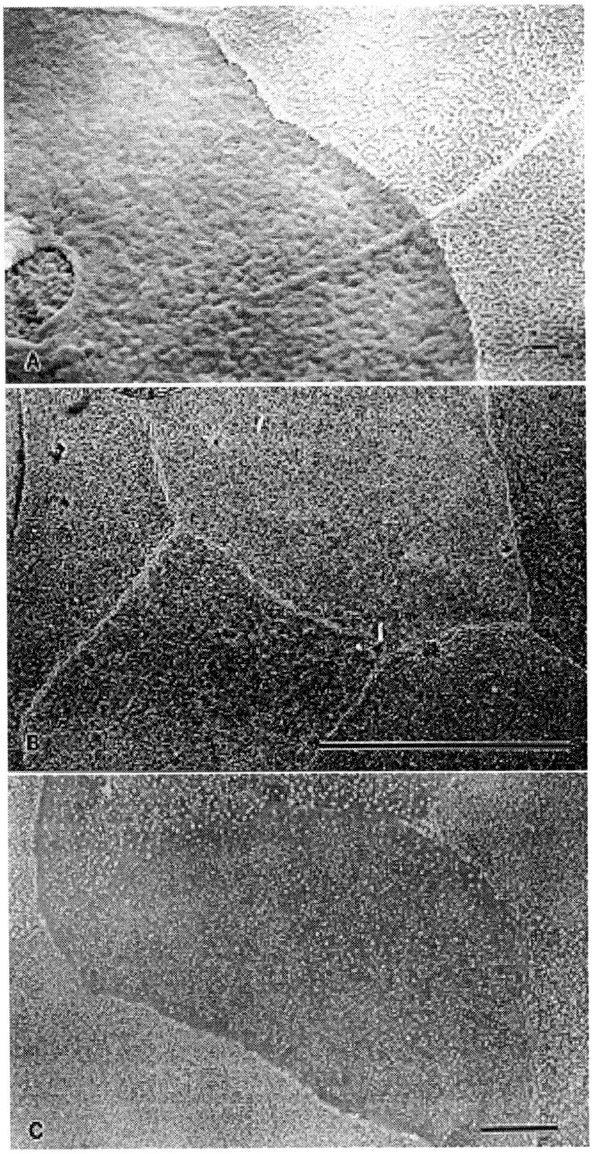

Figure 6.3.7. High magnification of corneal dark cells. Microvilli on the corneal epithelial surface of a rat on a Mn-deficient diet for 2 months (A) are scattered and changed in shape, as compared with a control cornea (B). In the recovered rat (C), microvilli resemble those in the control rat. Bar: 1μm (A,C), 20μm (B).

In the recovery experiment, the epithelial cells showed increased numbers of fibrils and normal-appearing mitochondria (Figs 6.3.3,3). The stroma was almost as thick as that of the control rats, and their diameter was almost the same as in the controls (Table 6.3.2); the microcracks between the stroma and Descemet's membrane disappeared. Descemet's membrane in rats recovered from Mn deficiency was as thick as that in the controls and showed uniform density (Fig. 6.3.5). The endothelial cell surface in the recovered rats were smooth, and the small pit-like structures in the cytoplasmic processes disappeared (Fig. 6.3.5).

Scanning Electron Microscopy (SEM) Findings

SEM micrographs of epithelium from the Mn-deficient rats showed more dark cells than in the controls (Fig. 6.3.6). There were many fewer microvilli in the dark cells than in the light cells (Fig. 6.3.7). The surface of the corneal endothelium in the Mn-deficient rats contained many irregular pentagon-shaped cells instead of the normal regular hexagon-shaped cells. Small holes with a diameter of 0.78±0.26μm were scattered over the cell surface near the adjacent endothelial cell (Fig. 6.3.8). The diameter of the endothelial pit-like structures seen with SEM was not significantly different from that of those seen with TEM ($p=0.10$).

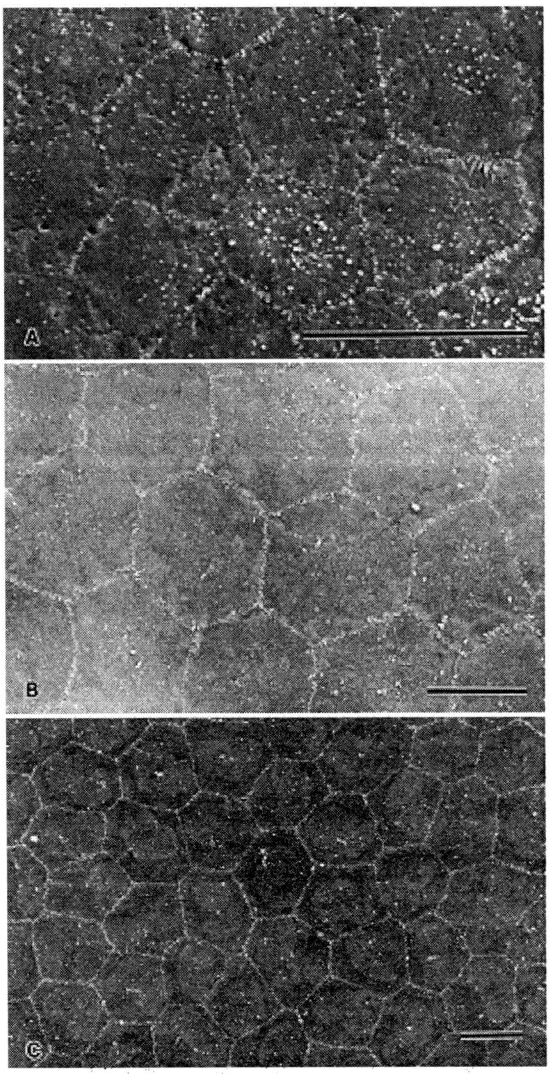

Figure 6.3.8. SEM micrographs of corneal endothelium. A 2-month-old Mn-deficient rat (A), a control rat (B), and a recovered rat (C). A: Many pit-like structures on the endothelial surface of the cornea, especially near a neighboring cell and most of the endothelial cells are pentagon-shaped. Endothelial cells are hexagonal in B. In the recovered rat (C), the endothelial cells have the same appearance as in the control rat. Bar: 20μm (A, C), 10μm (B).

In rats recovered from Mn deficiency, the epithelial surface was made up of many light cells and fewer dark cells (Fig. 6.3.6). Microvilli and microplicae were increased (Fig. 6.3.7). The endothelial surface showed many normal regular hexagon-shaped cells, and small holes were scarce (Fig. 6.3.8).

Discussion

Tauber and Krause (1943) showed that the corneal epithelium contains more manganese (4.61µg/100g wet tissue and 231µg/100g dry tissue) than other ocular tissues. TEM and SEM showed that the number of microvilli in Mn-deficient rats is obviously decreased. SEM showed an increased number of dark cells in the most superficial layer of the epithelium, in which microvilli were scattered and had changed shape. It has been hypothesized that the dark cells are the "oldest" cells on the ocular surface, indicating that they are about to desquamate (Klyce and Beuerman, 1988; Smolin and Thoft, 1994). Thus the increase of dark cells in the corneal epithelium of Mn-deficient rats may suggest accelerated desquamation. However, morphologic findings alone cannot indicate whether the increase of dark cells means a loss of corneal epithelial barrier function, dehydrating capacity of the epithelium or accelerated aging.

TEM revealed many abnormal mitochondria in the epithelial cells at the base of the corneal epithelium. One of the effects of Mn deficiency on enzymes is a decrease of SOD activity, which is present in the mitochondrial matrix.

The function of SOD is believed to be associated in part with the protection of cells from the toxic effects of free superoxide radicals. Mn-SOD could scavenge the O_2-generated by mitochondrial respiratory activity. A Mn-deficient diet decreased Mn-SOD activity in the kidneys and heart of Sprague-Dawley rats (Paynter, 1980). In humans the cornea contains much more Mn-SOD activity than does the retina (Bebndig, Syensson, Marklund et al, 1998) and may be more susceptible to photochemical injury. The corneal changes, especially in the mitochondrial membrane in the current study may be due to decreased Mn-SOD activity.

The ultrastructural changes in the cornea show that Mn is necessary to maintain its structure. Because Mn is essential for the metalloenzyme related to the synthesis of protein, Mn deficiency may induce morphologic changes in corneal epithelial cells probably due to disturbed protein synthesis. Mn deficiency may decrease glycosaminoglycan (GAG) synthesis (Leach and Lilburn, 1978). GAG is important for the synthesis of proteoglycans, which are a main part of corneal stromal collagen (Smolin and Thoft, 1994). Mn deficiency may disturb actin formation in the microvilli and decrease tonofibrils in the cytoplasm. Thus manganese appears to be related to the cellular formation of actin filaments and fibrils in the cornea through protein metabolism. Microvilli and microplicae in the corneal epithelial cells have cores of actin filaments (Gipson and Anderson, 1977), which may allow some movement of the surface projections. Microvilli play an important role in mucin and tear film spread over the surface of the cornea. These changes may lead to a disappearance of the tear film on the corneal surface, which may result in serious damage to the defense mechanisms protecting the corneal surface from infection (Fawcett and Bloom, 1986). That may be the reason for the secretions seen around the eyelids of Mn-deficient rats. In the current experiment, Descemet's membrane was thinner in Mn-deficient rats than in the control group and of less uniform electron density. Microcracks were also noted between the endothelium and Descemet's membrane. Descemet's membrane is composed of type IV collagen, laminin and fibronectin. Mn is related to collagen metabolism, laminin, and fibronectin, which function in the adhesion of endothelial cells to Descemet's membrane (Gospodarowicz, Greenburg, Viodavsky et al, 1979; Waring Bourne, Edeilhausen et al, 1982). Although the corneal architecture might be weakened by Mn deficiency, the tight junctions in the corneal endothelium are intact and show no separation between the cells. The microcracks may be induced by Mn deficiency. Microcracks are not artifacts, as evidenced by their disappearance in recovery experiments.

Ultrastructurally the fibers appear to have uniform diameter, and there is little variation in their size at different depths in the central cornea of the normal rat. The whole corneal stroma in Mn-deficient rats is very thin, and the collagen fibers show a significant difference in diameter and irregular arrangement. The recovery of the corneal stroma is obvious: it becomes thicker, and collagen fibers increase in diameter. Keratocytes in the corneal stroma of Mn-deficient rats are higher in number and not damaged. Thus these keratocytes may be activated by Mn supplementation to produce collagen fibers. The increased number of keratocytes in the stroma of Mn-deficient rats might be the result of a concentration of cells in the thinned stroma. A striking feature of the endothelium in Mn-deficient rats is the presence of many small pit-like structures located on the endothelial surface, seen in both TEM and SEM examinations. Most of them are located near a neighboring cell. SEM shows pentagonal instead of hexagonal endothelial cells in Mn-deficient rats. It is well known that Descemet's membrane is synthesized by the endothelium and that endothelial cells are not self-renewing. As they decrease in number, their shape changes. The findings in the epithelium, Descemet's membrane, and endothelium in Mn-deficient rats and the high content of Mn in the normal cornea suggest that, although the role of Mn in living organisms has not yet been clarified, the cornea needs Mn for the maintenance of the cell structure.

IV. The Retina

Results

Electron Microscopic Findings

Slight retinal changes appeared in rats fed a Mn-deficient diet for 12 months, but definite changes occurred starting at 18 months.

In rats on a Mn-deficient diet for 12 months, photoreceptor outer segments decreased in number at some sites and disappeared at some sites (Fig. 6.4.1). Photoreceptor cell nuclei were still present in seven or eight layers. In rats fed a Mn-deficient diet for 18 months, the photoreceptor cells disappeared completely, and the inner nuclear layer nuclei came into direct contact with the retinal pigment epithelium (Fig. 6.4.2). The inner nuclear layer nuclei were mainly Müller and bipolar cell nuclei (Fif. 6.4.3A,3B), but some horizontal cell and amacrine cell nuclei remained. Outer plexiform layer components were occasionally found between the inner nuclear layer and the retinal pigment epithelium. The retinal pigment epithelium lost lamellar structures but contained secondary lysosomes and lipofusin granules (Fig. 6.4.2, 3A, 3B). Mitochondria increased significantly in the retinal pigment epithelium (Fig. 6.4.3A, 3B) and photoreceptor inner segment (Table 6.4.1). Microvili were elongated and were in contact with the inner nuclear layer. However, inner nuclear layer nuclei were still present in three or four layers (Fig. 6.4.3A, 4A).

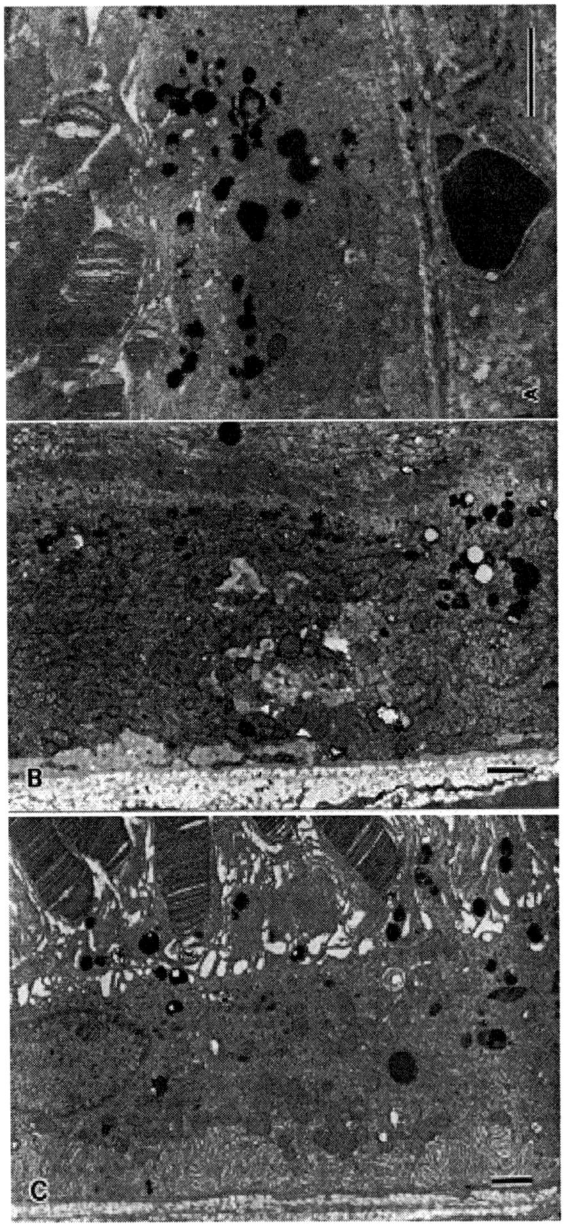

Figure 6.4.1. TEM micrographs of the retina of a rat fed a Mn-deficient diet for 12 months. The retinal pigment epithelium contains many round mitochondria with slightly destroyed cristae. Many secondary lysosomes are also seen (A). Photoreceptor outer segment discs are decreased at some site (A) and lost at some site. Round mitochondria are increased (B). C shows photoreceptor outer segment and the retinal pigment epithelium of a 12-months-old control rat. Bar: 1μm (A-C).

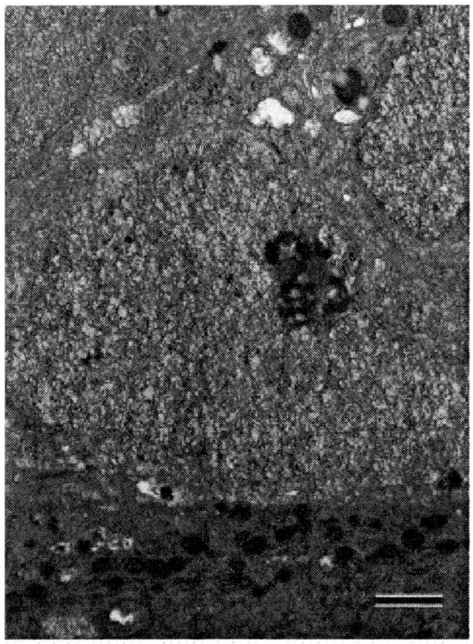

Figure 6.4.2. TEM micrograph of the retina of a rat fed a Mn-deficient diet for 18 months. Photoreceptor outer and inner segments and nuclei have disappeared completely. The retinal pigment epithelium is in direct contact with a nucleus of the inner nuclear layer. The retinal pigment epithelium contains many mitochondria and secondary lysosomes. Bar: 1µm.

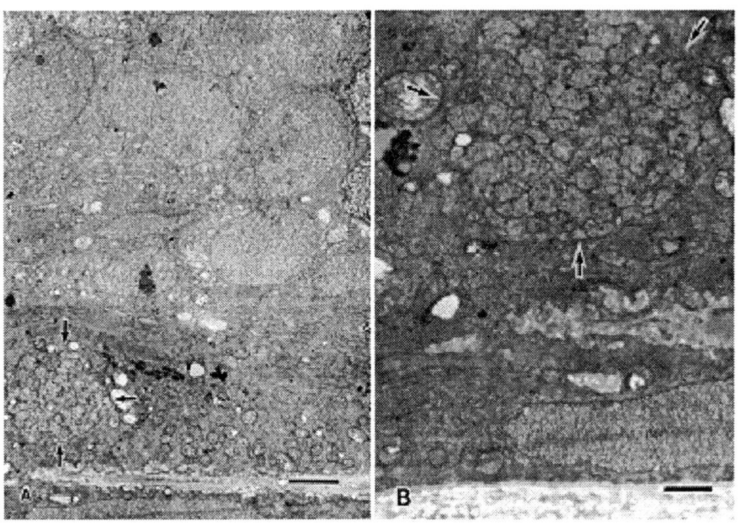

Figure 6.4.3. In a rat on Mn-deficient diet for 30 months, a cluster of unknown cell processes invades the retinal pigment epithelium (A). The retinal pigment epithelium has many round mitochondria and has lost basal infoldings and microvilli. Next to the retinal pigment epithelium are processes (arrows) and cells that have oval nuclei with dense bodies and much cytoplasm. The nuclei have homogeneous chromatin with low density. A higher magnification of the part indicated by the arrow shows a cluster of cell processes (arrows) (B). Bar: 5µm (A), 1µm (B).

Table 6.4.1. Number of mitochondria in the retinal pigment epithelium and the photoreceptor inner segment.

Pigment Epithelium	Examined field (N)	Mitochondria/ 10μm Baseline	P values (unpaired t-test)
12-month-old Mn-deficient rat	66	15.2±7.6	<0.0769
Equivalent age control rat	38	12.8±4.8	
18-month-old Mn-deficient rat	57	19.4±7.9	<0.0006
Equivalent age control rat	46	14.4±5.7	
30-month-old manganese deficient rat	54	33.3±40.7	<0.0001
Equivalent age control rat	46	12.0±4.1	
Inner segment			
12-month-old manganese deficient rat	96	18.3±7.3	<0.001
Equivalent age control rat	90	11.4±3.8	

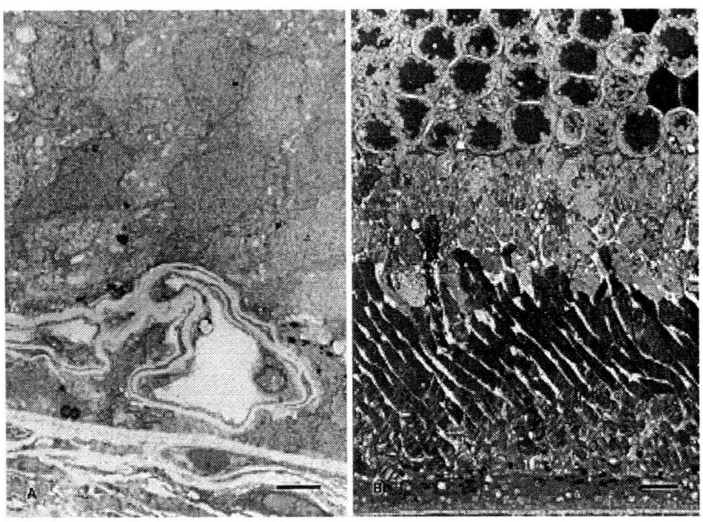

Figure 6.4.4. TEM micrographs of retinal pigment epithelium of a rat fed a Mn-deficient diet for 30 months (A) and an age-equivalent control rat (B). Two capillaries are seen in contact with the pigment epithelium. The capillary has an irregular lumen, many pinocytotic vesicles, and thick basement membranes (A). Microvilli of the retinal pigment epithelium have been lost, so the retinal pigment epithelium is in contact with many processes of several cells. Basal infoldings of the retinal pigment epithelium are few. Inner nuclear layer nuclei remain. B shows the photoreceptor outer segment and the retinal pigment epithelium of a 30-month-old control rat. Bar: 5μm (A, B).

In rats with Mn deficiency that lasted 30 months, retinal pigment epithelia with many mitochondria were in contact with cell processes and with cells resembling Müller cells with round nuclei, homogenously distributed chromatin, and much cytoplasm (Fig. 6.4.4, 6.4.6). Capillaries with thick basement membranes and the processes of some cells (Müller-like cells) frequently invaded the retinal pigment epithelium (Fig. 6.4.4A). The nerve fibers were decreased in number in the nerve fiber layer (Fig. 6.4.5A), while neurons in the inner plexiform layer lost synapses (Fig. 6.4.5B).

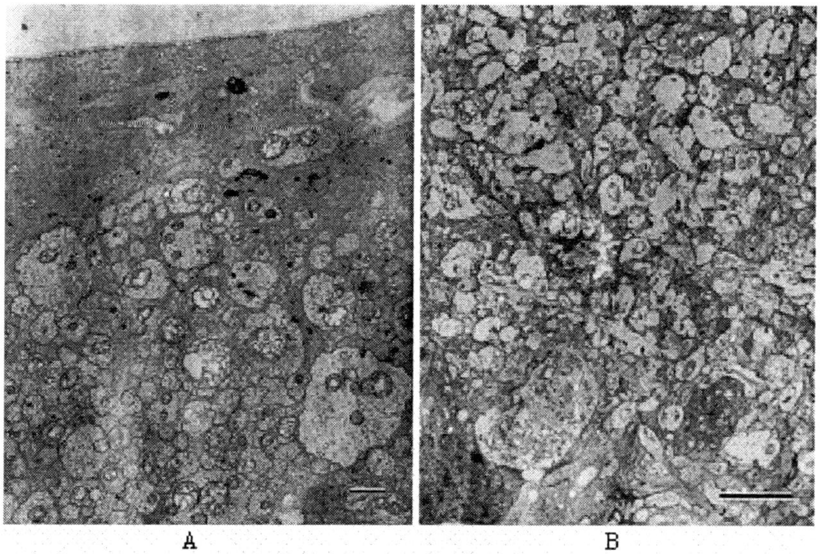

Figure 6.4.5. TEM micrographs of the retina from the internal limiting membrane to the inner plexiform layer of a rat fed a Mn-deficient diet for 30 months. Nerve fibers are decreased and ganglion cells disappear (A). Neurons in the inner plexform layer lose synapses (B). Bar: 1μm (A), 2μm (B).

In the choroid of 30-month-Mn-deficient rats, choriocapillaris was flat, but had normal-looking endothelial fenestration (Fig. 6.4.6). Choroidal vessels were prominently decreased behind choriocapillaris (Fig. 6.4.6).

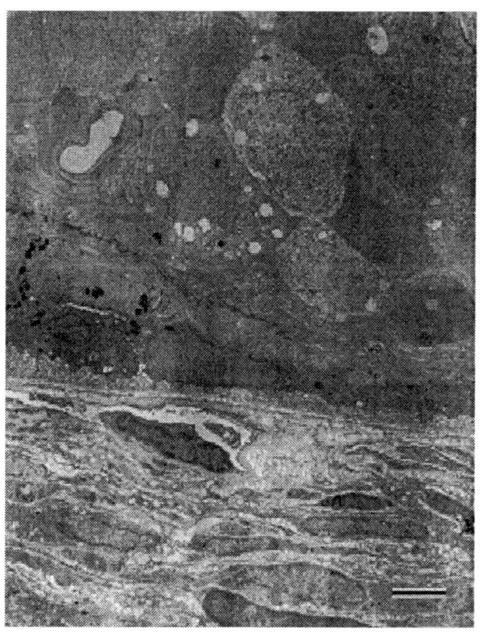

Figure 6.4.6. TEM micrograph of the retina and choroid of a rat fed a Mn-deficient diet for 30 months. The choroid shows a choriocapillaris with fenestrations, but no choroidal vessels behind it. The retinal pigment epithelium comes into contact with inner nuclear layer nuclei due to the disappearance of photoreceptor cells. Bar: 1μm.

Discussion

Serum Mn levels have been reported to decrease after prolonged depletion (Friedman, Freeland-Graves, Bales et al, 1987). However, in the current study, the serum Mn level fell rapidly in rats on a Mn-deficient diet, and retinal regions appeared late. The serum level of Mn declined to half the control level by 6 months on a Mn-deficient diet.

There have been few ultrastructural studies on Mn deficiency. Bell and Hurley (1973) demonstrated that Mn deficiency in mice results in changes in the integrity of their cell membranes, swollen and irregular endoplasmic reticulum and elongated stacked cristae of mitochondria in liver, heart and kidney cells. These findings, such as destruction of cell membrane structures and mitochondrial changes, are similar to those seen in the retina in the current study. A biochemical aberration caused by Mn deficiency is the diminished enzymatic activity of galactosyl transferase reactions related to chondroitin sulfate synthesis, which results in decreased polymerization (Leach and Muenster, 1962; Leach, Muenster and Wien et al, 1969; Leach 1971). In ocular tissues a Mn deficiency may result in decreased contact between photoreceptor outer segments and retinal pigment epithelium. This assumption is consistent with the role of Mn in mucopolysaccharide synthesis, because acid mucopolysaccharides are present between the photoreceptor outer segments and retinal pigment epithelium (Cohen, 1992). Another effect of Mn deficiency is a decrease of superoxide dismutase (SOD) activity. Two kinds of SOD are known: Cu·Zn SOD in the cytosol and Mn·SOD in the mitochondrial matrix. The function of SOD is thought to be associated in part with the protection of the cell from the toxic effects of free superoxide radicals (McCord, Keele, Fridvick et al, 1971). Mn·SOD would scavenge the O_2-generated by mitochondrial respiratory activity. If the activity of Mn·SOD is depressed by a dietary deficiency, changes of membrane structures may be the result of accumulation of O_2-radicals in the cell with consequent peroxidation of membrane components. Lipid peroxidation increases as Mn·SOD activity decreases (Zidenberg-Cherr, Keen, Lönnerdal et al, 1983). A Mn-deficient diet decreased Mn·SOD activity in the kidneys and hearts of Sprague-Dawley rats (Paynter, 1980). Photoreceptor outer segments are composed of lipid membrane accumulation, and photoreceptor inner segments contain many mitochondria. Thus, the disappearance of photoreceptor cells and mitochondrial membrane changes in the current study may be caused by depressed Mn-SOD activity, resulting in increased lipid peroxidation in biomembranes. In addition, protein metabolism may be disturbed. Lowered protein and glycogen metabolism may prevent the renewal of photoreceptor outer segment discs. Damage of the photoreceptor cells caused by Mn-deficiency is specific probably because of mitochondria-rich and membrane-rich special structures. The increase of mitochondria in the retinal pigment epithelium may be the result of compensation of mitochondrial dysfunction caused by Mn deficiency. Karyopyknosis of photoreceptor cell nuclei occur after 1 year of Mn deficiency and may be related to lowered DNA polymerase activity resulting from Mn deficiency. Mn is an important micronutrient in the maintenance of photoreceptor cells.

V. The Optic Nerve

Results

Light Microscopic Findings

In rats fed a Mn-deficient diet for 18 months, the diameter of the optic nerves was significantly shorter by light microscopy than that of control rats ($p<0.05$), but not significantly different than in the recovery group (Table 6.5.1). In both Mn-deficient and Mn-recovery rats, the number of myelinated axons was obviously decreased (Fig. 6.5.1) (Table 6.5.2).

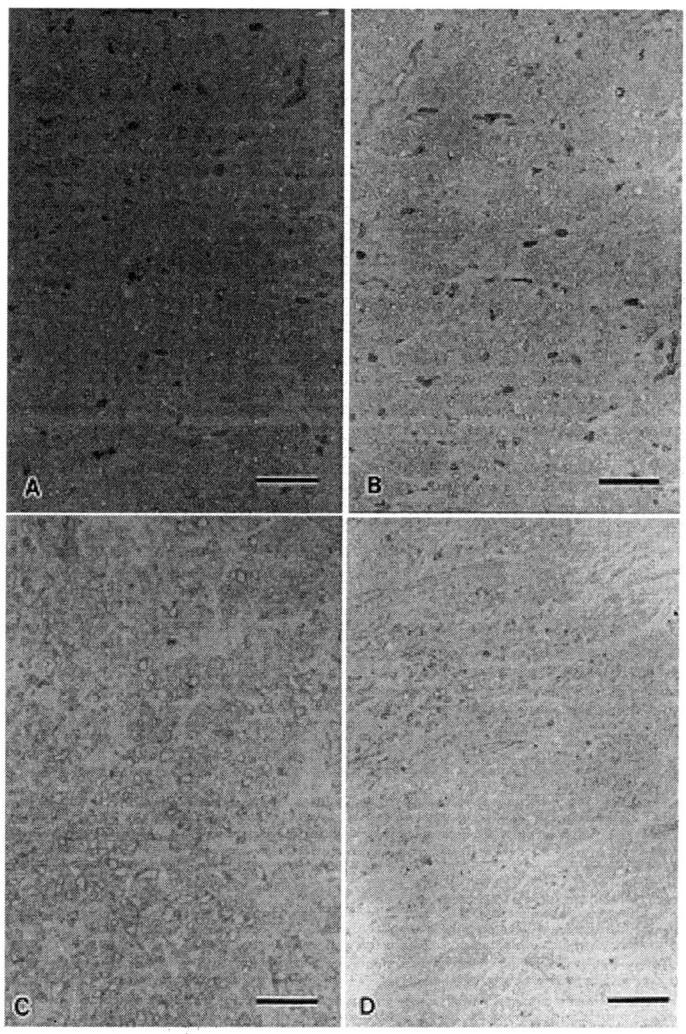

Figure 6.5.1. Light micrographs of transverse section of optic nerve 3 mm behind globe stained with toluidine blue. In a control rat (A) and a pair-fed control rat (B), myelinated nerve fibers are round, compactly arranged and appear normal. In Mn-deficient rat (C) and recovery (D) rats, the myelinated nerve fibers are irregular and loosely arranged. Compared with a control nerve, oligodendrocytes increase in number. Bar: 30μm (A-D).

Table 6.5.1. Diameter of optic nerves (μm).

Groups	Number of optic nerves counted	Diameter
Control	10	565±14
Recovery	12	578±11
Mn-deficiency	14	507±5.8

Diameter of optic nerves calculated in control, recovery and Mn-deficient rats in cross sections taken about 3 mm behind the eyeball. There are significant differences between the control and Mn-deficient group and between the recovery and Mn-deficient groups ($p<0.002$, $p<0.001$ respectively). There is no significant difference between the control and recovery groups ($p>0.25$).

Table 6.5.2. Number of myelinated axons in optic nerve (600μm²).

Groups	Number of fields examined	Number of myelinated axons
Control	185	156±23
Recovery	175	110±36
Mn-deficiency	197	136±34

The number of myelinated axons is significantly higher in the control group than in the recovery and Mn-deficient groups ($p<0.0001$) and the difference between the recovery and Mn-deficient groups is also significant ($p<0.01$).

Electron Microscopic Findings

Transmission electron microscopy (TEM) revealed significantly fewer myelinated axons in the optic nerves of rats fed a Mn-deficient diet for 18 months and recovery rats than in those of control rats (Table 6.5.2). The fiber density in myelinated axons in Mn-deficient and recovery rats was obviously decreased. Unmyelinated axons in the optic nerve were more numerous in the Mn-deficient and recovery rats than in the control rats, and oligodendrocytes with fine and evenly dispersed clumped chromatin were seen among the unmyelinated nerve fibers. Undeveloped myelin and unmyelinated axons were present (Fig.6.5.2). Degeneration of the myelinated axons was present: in the axoplasm there were osmiophilic substances, and the axoplasm and myelin sheath contained debris of cytoplasmic organelles. In transverse sections of Mn-deficient and recovery rats, the myelin sheaths of optic nerves were thin and undeveloped axons were frequently found (Fig. 6.5.3). The diameter of myelinated axons in the Mn-deficient and recovery rats was significantly shorter than that of those in the control rats (Table 6.5.3). Myelin sheath thickness and number of lamellae in Mn-deficient and recovery rats were significantly different from those of control rats (Tables 6.5.4, 5). In the number of myelinated axons, thickness of the myelin sheath and lamellar layers of myelinated fibers in optic nerves, the difference between the recovery and Mn-deficient rats was significant (Tables 6.5.4, 5). Large mitochondria were clumped, and some of the cristae disappeared from mitochondria in the myelinated axons of Mn-deficient rats (Fig. 6.5.4).

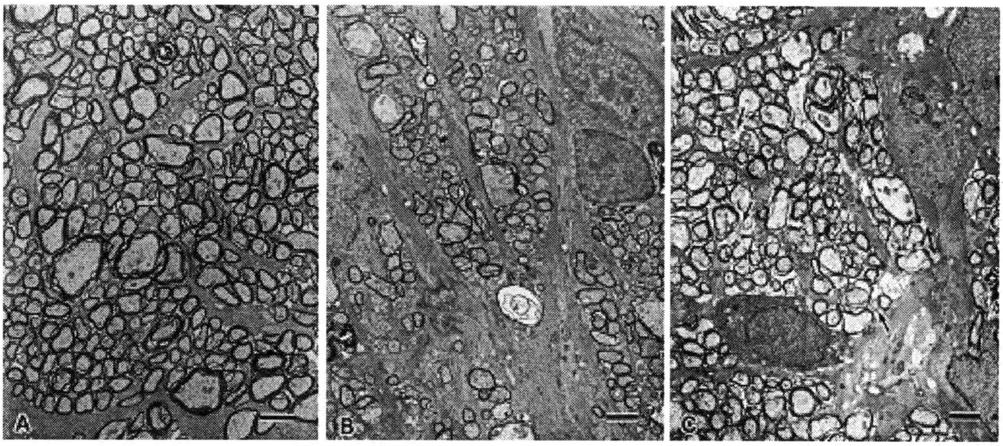

Figure 6.5.2. TEM micrographs of transverse sections of the optic nerves. In a control rat (A) myelin lamellae are compactly arranged. In a Mn-deficient rat (B), fewer axons and undeveloped myelin are seen. In a rat recovered from Mn deficiency (C), undeveloped myelin and unmyelinated axons (arrows) are present, and oligodendrocytes with finely clumped and dispersed chromatin and developed processes occupy the spaces between axons. Bar: 2μm (A-C).

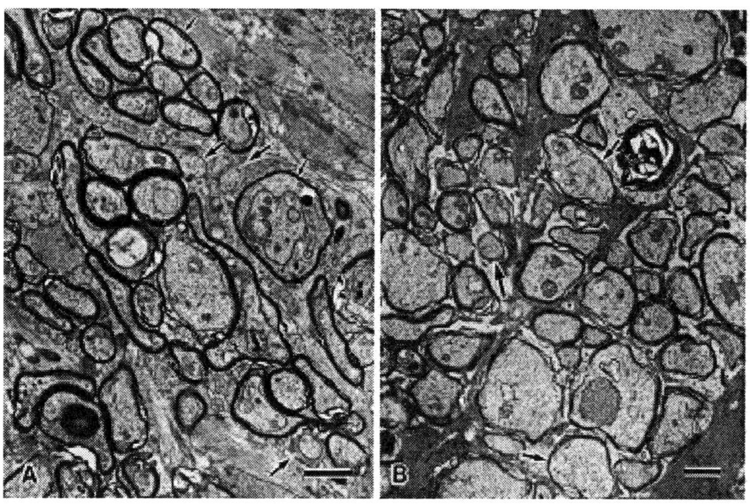

Figure 6.5.3. TEM micrographs of transverse sections of the optic nerves. In Mn-deficient (A) and Mn-recovery rats (B), the myelinated axons show degeneration (arrows), undeveloped myelin and unmyelinated axons (thickarrows). The number of lamellae is obviously decreased (thick arrows). Bar: 1μm (A, B).

Discussion

In human and animals the effects of Mn deficiency on the central nervous system (CNS) have been described on convulsion and ataxia in relation to L-dopa and manganese (Erway, Hurley and Fraser et al, 1966; Erway Hurley and Fraser et al, 1970; Dupont and Tanaka, 1985; Papavasilion, Millers and Cotzias, 1968; Cotzias Tang, Miller et al, 1972). To our knowledge, ours is the first report of ultrastructural changes in the CNS of Mn-deficient animals (Gong and Amemiya, 1996; Gong and Amemiya, 1999).

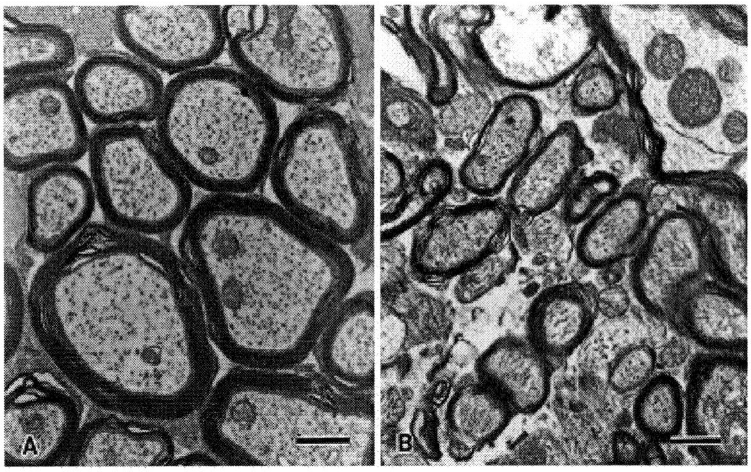

Figure 6.5.4. High magnification of TEM micrographs of transverse sections of the optic nerves. In a control rat (A), the myelin sheaths are thick, and the arrangement of myelin lamellae is regular. In a Mn-deficient rat (B), the mitochondria are abnormally large and some of the cristae have disappeared. The diameter of the axons varies. Bar: 500nm (A, B).

Table 6.5.3. Diameter of myelinated nerve fibers in optic nerves (μm).

Groups	Number of myelinated fibers counted	Diameter
Control	218	1.04±0.28
Recovery	224	0.67±0.23
Mn deficiency	246	0.74±0.22

The diameter of myelinated nerve fibers is significantly larger in the control group than in the recovery and Mn-deficient groups ($p<0.0001$), but the difference between the recovery and Mn-deficient groups is not significant ($p>0.05$).

Table 6.5.4. Thickness of myelin sheath in optic nerve (nm).

Groups	Number of myelin sheaths counted	Diameter
Control	238	148.4±54.8
Recovery	266	82.1±36
Mn deficiency	224	95.4±36.4

Myelin sheaths are significantly thicker in the control group than in the recovery and Mn-deficient groups ($p<0.0001$), and the difference between the recovery and Mn-deficient groups is also significant ($p<0.01$).

Table 6.5.5. Number of lamellar layers of myelinated fibers in optic nerve.

Groups	Number of myelinated fibers counted	Number of layers
Control	230	10.8±3.4
Recovery	243	5.9±2.0
Mn deficiency	272	6.9±2.7

The number of myelinated nerve fiber layers is significantly larger in the control group than in the recovery and Mn-deficient groups ($p<0.0001$), and the difference between the recovery and Mn-deficient groups is also significant ($p<0.002$).

The optic nerve contains 26.2µg/100g wet tissue and 101µg/100g dry tissue, which show one of the highest values in ocular tissue. The significant pathologic changes shown in this chapter fit in with the fact that there is a high content of manganese in the normal tissue, and there may be pathologic changes in Mn deficiency.

The diameter and the numbers of fibers and myelin lamellae of the optic nerves were significantly lower in the Mn-deficient rats than in the control rats. Even when the Mn-deficient rats were fed a usual diet, their optic nerves did not recover: the number of myelinated axons, the thickness of myelin sheaths and lamellar layers of myelinated fibers in optic nerves showed no significant differences between the Mn-deficient and the recovery rats. It appears that axons continue to degenerate after resumption of a normal diet. This means that when the CNS is destroyed it never recovers. One of the biochemical functions of manganese is its role in metalloenzymes such as manganese-superoxide dismutase (Mn-SOD) (Malecki, Huttner and Greger, 1994; Malecki and Greger, 1996; Utter, 1976; Wermer, Korc and Brannon, 1987). In the brain Mn-SOD activity was reported to be reduced by 50% in Mn-deficient mice (de Rosa, Keen, Leach et al, 1980), and it reached normal levels when these mice were fed a Mn-supplemented diet. Biochemical studies of myelin membranes exhibit a unique composition with >70% of dry weight consisting of lipids (Coetzee, Fujita, Dupree et al, 1996). Paynter (1980) has shown that Mn-deficient rats demonstrated a lower than normal activity of Mn-SOD in heart muscle, and the activity of the enzyme was correlated with the manganese concentration in the diet. SOD enzymes are thought to protect cells from the deleterious effects of superoxide free radicals (Malecki, Huttner and Greger, 1994). It is suggested that the changes in myelinated fibers produced by Mn deficiency are related to the role of this enzyme in lipid membrane stability (Davis, Ney and Greger, 1990; Leach and Lilburn, 1978; Malecki and Greger, 1996).

Mn deficiency also causes ultrastructural abnormalities of mitochondria (Bell and Hurley, 1973). Electron microscopy revealed elongation and reorientation of the cristae. It is possible that the changes in mitochondrial structure induced by Mn deficiency are related to the role of Mn-SOD in protecting cells (Malecki and Greger, 1996). Since Mn-SOD is located in the mitochondria, Mn deficiency may cause destruction or hypofunction of mitochondria, which induces an increase in the number of mitochondria to compensate for mitochondrial dysfunction (Gong and Amemiya, 1996). In the optic nerve, the mitochondria in myelinated nerve fibers showed morphologic changes in number and shape. These may be due to depressed Mn-SOD activity as a result of Mn deficiency, which increases lipid peroxidation in biomembranes.

Manganese as the preferred metal cofactor for a number of glycosyltransferases provides the clearest link between biochemical function and deficiency symptoms (Borello, De Leo and Galeotti, 1992). Glycosyltransferases are important in the biosynthesis of glycoprotein and glycosaminoglycans. Myelin is formed by oligodendrocytes in the CNS. Several proteins, especially myelin-associated glycoprotein (MAG), have been suggested or demonstrated to be involved in this neuroglia interaction and in the formation of myelin (Bartsch, Montag, Bartsch et al, 1995; Trapp, 1990). In the optic nerve, oligodendrocytes obviously increased in the Mn-deficient and recovery rats. It is reasonable to assume that because of the destruction in myelin, the oligodendrocytes are compensatorily increased. Rats in the second generation of Mn deficiency are affected by Mn deficiency from gestation through the postnatal period to adulthood. The development and maintenance of myelin may be affected by Mn deficiency and even if Mn is supplied to adult rats, destruction of the myelin structure may continue. Although the relationship of these observations to the fundamental biochemical functions of manganese is not clear, the role of manganese in optic nerve function may be related to the metabolism of the biogenic amines, to superoxide dismutase activity, to glycosyltransferase function, or, indeed, to all of these.

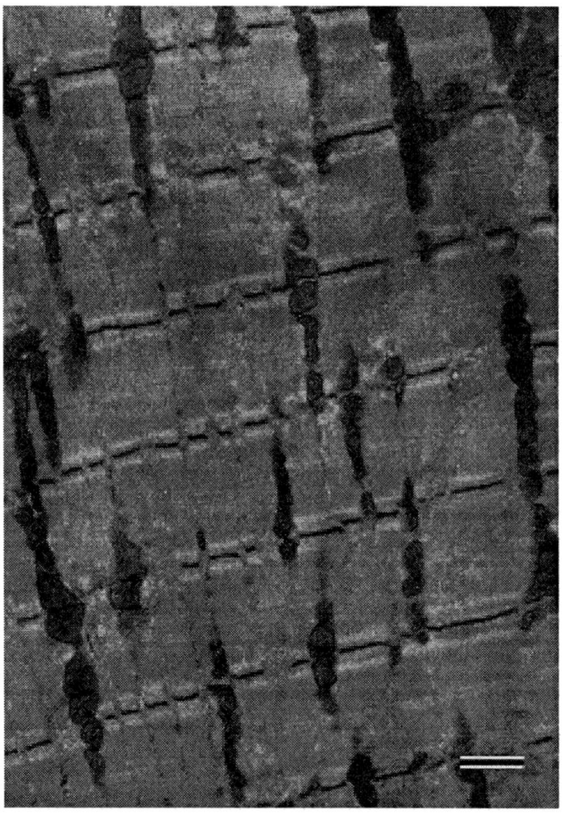

Figure 6.6.1. TEM micrographs of a rectus muscle of a rat fed a Mn-deficient diet for 30 months. The sarcoplasm contains almost normal nucleus and regularly arranged myofibrils with typical A-Z bands and long mitochondria with normal cristae. Bar: 2μm.

VI. Rectus Muscle

TEM Findings

In rectus muscle of 30-month-Mn-deficient rats, TEM showed normal features of the myocyte: regular arrangement of muscle fibers and A-Z bands and many normal mitochondria. No deposits of abnormal masses were seen in the sarcoplasm (Fig. 6.6.1).

Discussion

Mn deficiency induces neurological problems such as convulsion and ataxia, but no reports have been published on the rectus muscle disturbance. Mn deficiency causes ultrastructural changes of mitochondria (Bell and Hurley, 1973). Rectus muscle of Mn-deficient rats showed no abnormal mitochondria and ultrastructural changes in the current study. Thus rat rectus muscle may be unsusceptible to Mn deficiency.

References

Baly DL, Curry DL, Keen CL, Hurley LS. Dynamics of insulin and glucagon release in rats: Influence of dietary manganese. *Endocrinology*. 1985;116:1734-1740.

Bartsch U, Montay D, Bartsch S, Schachner M. Multiply myelinated axons in the optic nerve of mice deficient for the myelin-associated glycoprotein. *Glia*. 1995;14:115-122.

Bebndig A, Syensson B, Marklund SL, Karlsson K. Superoxide dismutase isoenzymes in the human eye. *Invest Ophthalmol Vis Sci*. 1998;39:471-475.

Bell LT, Hurley LS. Ultrastructural effects of manganese deficiency in liver, heart, kidney, and pancreas of mice. *Lab Invest*. 1973;29:723-736.

Bolze MS, Reeves RD, Lindbeck FE, Kemp SF, Elders MJ. Influence of manganese on growth, somatomedin and glycosaminoglycan metabolism. *J Nutr*. 1985;115:352-358.

Borg DC, Cotzias GC. Interaction of trace metals with phentothiazine drug derivatives. II.Formation. *Free Radic Biochem*. 1962:48:623-642.

Borrello S, De Leo ME, Galeotti T. Transcriptional regulation of Mn·SOD by manganese in the liver of manganese-deficient mice and during rat development. *Biochem Int*. 1992;28:595-601.

Coetzee T, Fujita N, Dupree J, Shi R, Bligh A, Suzuki K, Popko B. Myelination in the absence of galactocerebioside and sulfatide: normal structure with abnormal function and regional instability. *Cell*. 1996;86:209-219.

Cohen AL. The retina. In: Hart WM Jr, ed. *Adler's Physiology of the Eye*. 9th ed. St. Louis:Mosby Year Book;1992:592.

Comens P. Manganese depletion as an etiological factor in hydralazine disease. *Am J Med*. 1956;20:944-945.

Cotzias GC, Tang LC, Miller ST, Sladic-Simic D, Hurley LS. A mutation influencing the transportation of manganese, L-dopa, and L-triptophan. *Science*. 1972;176:410-412.

Davis CD, Ney DM, Greger JL. Manganese, iron and lipid interactions in rats. *J Nutr.* 1990;120:507-513.

de Rosa G, Keen CL, Leach RM, Hurley LS. Regulation of superoxide dismutase activity by dietary manganese. *J Nutr.* 1980;110:795-804.

Dupont CL, Tanaka Y. Blood manganese levels in children with convulsive disorder. *Biochem Med.* 1985;33:246-255.

Erway L, Hurley LS, Fraser AS. Neurological defect: manganese in phenocopy and prevention of a genetic abnormality of inner ear. *Science.* 1966;152:1766-1768.

Erway L, Hurley L.S, Fraser AS. Congenital ataxia and otolith defects due to manganese deficiency in mice. *J Nutr.* 1970;100:643-654.

Everson GJ, Shrader RE. Abnormal glucose tolerance in manganese-deficient guinea pigs. *J Nutr.* 1968;94:89-94.

Fawcett DW, Bloom W. *A Textbook of Histology.* Philadelphia:Saunders;1986:59.

Flessel CP. Metals as mutagenic initiators of cancer. In: Kharasch N, ed. *Trace Metals in Health and Diseases.* New York:Raven Press; 1979:109-115.

Friedman BJ, Freeland-Graves JH, Bales CW et al. Manganese balance and clinical observations in young men fed a manganese-deficient diet. *J Nutr.* 1987;117:133-143.

Gipson IK, Anderson RA. Actin filaments in normal and migrating corneal epithelial cells. *Invest Ophthalmol Vis Sci.* 1977;16:161-166.

Gong H, Amemiya T. Ultrastructure of retina of manganese deficient rats. *Invest Ophthalmol Vis Sci.* 1996;37:1967-1974.

Gong H, Amemiya T. Optic nerve changes in manganese-deficient rats. *Exp Eye Res.* 1999;68:313-320.

Gospodarowicz D, Greenburg G, Viodaosky I, Alvarado J, Johnson LK. The identification and localization of fibronectin in cultured corneal endothelial cells: cell surface polarity and physiological implications. *Exp Eye Res.* 1979;29:485-509.

Hurley LS. The roles of trace elements in foetal and neonatal development. *Philos Trans R Soc Lond B Biol Sci.* 1981;294:145-152.

Hurley LS, Keen CL and Baly DL. Manganese deficiency and toxicity: Effect on carbohydrate metabolism in the rat. *Neurotoxicology.* 1984;5:97-104.

Kemmer AR, Elvehjem CA, Hart EB. Studies on the relation of manganese to the nutrition of the mouse. *J Biol Chem.* 1931;92:623-630.

Klyce SD, Beuerman RW. Structure and function of the cornea. In: Kaufman HE, ed. *The Cornea.* Melbourne:Churchill Livingstone;1988:3-20.

Leach RM Jr, Muenster A-M. Studies on the role of manganese in bone formation: I. Effect upon the mucopolysaccharide content of chick bone. *J Nutr.* 1962;78:51-56.

Leach RM Jr, Muenster A-M, Wien EM. Studies on the role of manganese in bone formation: II. Effect upon chondroitin sulfate synthesis in chick epiphyseal cartilage. *Arch Biochem Biophys.* 1969;133:22-28.

Leach RM Jr. Role of manganese in mucopolysaccharide metabolism . *Fed Proc.* 1971;30:991-994.

Leach RM Jr, Lilburn MS. Manganese metabolism and its function. *World Rev Nutr Diet.* 1978;32:123-134.

Malecki EA, Huttner DL, Greger JL.. Manganese status, gut endogenous losses of manganese, and antioxidant enzyme activity in rats fed varying levels of manganese and fat. *Trace Element Res*. 1994;42:17-29.

Maleck EA, Greger JL. Manganese protects against heart mitochondrial lipid peroxidation in rats fed high levels of polyunsaturated fatty acids. *J Nutr*. 1996;126:27-33.

McCord JM, Keele BB, Fridovick I. An enzyme-based theory of obligate anaerobiosis: The physiological function of superoxide dismutase. *Proc Natl Acad Sci USA*. 1971;68:1024-1027.

Mehta R, Reilly JJ. Manganese levels in a jaundiced long-term total parenteral nutrition patient: Polentiation of haloperidol toxicity: Case report and literature review. *J Parenteral Enteral Nutr*. 1990;14:428-430.

Norose N, Arai K. Manganese deficiency due to long-term total parenteral nutrition infant. *Jpn Parenteral Enteral Nutr*. 1987;9:978-981.

Orent ER, McCollum EV. Effect of deprivation of manganese in the rat. *J Biol Chem*. 1931;92:651-678.

Papavasiliou PS, Millers ST, Cotzias GC. Functional interactions between biogenic amines, 3',5'-cyclic AMP and manganese. *Nature* 1968;220:74-75.

Paynter DI. Changes in activity of the manganese superoxide dismutase enzyme in tissues of the rat with changes in dietary manganese. *J Nutr*. 1980;110:437-447.

Rubenstein AH, Levin NW, Eliott GA. Manganese-induced hypoglycaemia. *Lancet*. 1962;2:1348-1351.

Shils ME, McCollum FV. Further studies on the symptoms of manganese deficiency in the rat and mouse. *J Nutr*. 1943;26:1-19.

Smolin G, Thoft RA. Anatomy of the conjunctiva, cornea, and limbus. In: Smolin G, Thoft RA, ed. *The Cornea*. 3rd ed. New York:Little Brown;1994:7-30.

Tauber FW, Krause AC. The role of iron, copper, zinc and manganese in the metabolism of the ocular tissues, with special reference to the lens. *Am J Ophthalmol*. 1943;26:260-266.

Trapp BD. Myelin-associated glycoprotein location and potential functions. *Ann NY Acad Sci*. 1990;605:29-43.

Utter MF. The biochemistry of manganese. *Med Clins N Am*. 1976;60:713-727.

Waring GD, Bourne WM, Edeilhauser H, Kenyon KR. The corneal endothelium: normal and pathologic structure and function. *Ophthalmology*. 1982;89:531-590.

Werner L, Korc M, Brannon PM. Effects of manganese deficiency and dietary composition on rat pancreatic enzyme content. *J Nutr*. 1987;117:2079-2085.

Wedler FC, Denman RB, Roby WG. Glutamine synthetase from ovine brain is a manganese (II) enzyme. *Biochemistry*. 1982;21:6389-6396.

Zidenberg-Cherr S, Keen CL, Lönnerdal B, Hurley LS. Superoxide dismutase activity and lipid peroxidation in the rat: Developmental correlations affected by manganese deficiency. *J Nutr*. 1983;113:2498-2504.

Chapter 7

ALUMINUM
ALUMINUM INTOXICATION

I. SIGNIFICANCE

Aluminum (Al) is one of the most abundant elements in nature. But because of the absence of Al in the living cell, Al is doubtful to be an essential trace element.

Al is clinically well known to be toxic to the CNS (central nervous system), skeletal system, and hematopoietic system in humans. Exposure to Al is common by oral intake, inhalation, transdermal introduction, or via potential administration through hemodialysis. Thus Al content in animals and humans is increased with age. There have been many neurological and pathological studies of potential Al toxicity (Wilhelm, Jager and Ohnesorge1990; Yokel and McNamara, 2001). The injection of Al compounds into animal brains has been found to produce neurofibrillary degeneration in the CNS similar to that observed in Alzheimer's disease (Crapper, Quittkat, Krishman et al, 1980; De Boni, Scott and Crapper, 1974). The retina and optic nerve are derivatives of the forebrain: consequently their morphology and physiology are very much like that of the brain (Hogan, Alvarado and Weddell, 1971). Since it has an affinity for the CNS, Al may be deposited in ocular tissue. However, that possibility has not been studied in the context of the above-mentioned neurological disorders.

Now that it is very difficult to examine Al-deficient effects in ocular tissue because of a possibility of almost no presence of Al in the living cell, the effect of excessive Al on ocular tissue is described in this book.

II. AL EXCESSIVE EXPERIMENT

Material and Methods

Normal 4-week-old Wistar Kyoto rats were divided randomly into Al-treated and control groups. The Al toxicosis group was injected in with 0.3ml of 4% aluminum chloride ($AlCl_3$) every day for up to 16 weeks. The rats were killed (at least 5 rats in each group) on the first day of the 8th, 12th, and 16th weeks after the start of administration of $AlCl_3$. The posterior pole of the retina of rats treated with Al was examined on the day following the last injection. Eyes were enucleated under pentobarbital sodium (Dainabor, USA) anesthesia, and blood was simultaneously drawn from the aorta 8, 12, and 16 weeks after the start of the experiment. The measurement of serum aluminum levels was performed by an atomic absorption spectrophotometer. Age-equivalent normal Wistar Kyoto rats were used as controls and were treated with physiological sodium solution instead of aluminum chloride.

Clinical Features of the Al-Excessive Animal

The serum Al level increased with the dose of Al administration; in the controls it was always less than 10μg/l, the limit of sensitivity (Table 7.2.1). The difference between Al treated and control groups was significant ($p<0.001$) (Table 7.2.1). Al-treated rats showed no abnormal changes in weight gain or body hair, but the entire body of rats treated for 16 weeks showed severe torsive activity.

Table 7.2.1. Rat Serum Aluminum Levels.

Time treated	Serum aluminum levels (μg/l)		
	8 weeks	12 weeks	16 weeks
Rats treated with $AlCl_3$	54.0 ±8.1*	60.3±4.6*	245.2±35.1*
Control rats	undetected	undetected	undetected

Note. Values are mean ±SD. Treated rats, n=5; control rats, n=10
* P<0.001(Student's t-test significant difference).

III. THE CORNEA

Results

Light Microscopic Findings

In the cornea of Al excess rats, light microscopy showed normal features: the normal thick epithelial layer, regularly arranged stromal lamellae, normal thick Descemet's membrane and one layer endothelium.

Electron Microscopic Findings

In the cornea of rats administrated with $AlCl_3$ for 16 weeks, electron microscopic examination showed no abnormalities. The most superficial epithelial cells kept many microvilli and microplicae, and epithelial cells had many fibrils, ribosomes, mitochondria and well-developed intercellular junctions (Fig. 7.3.1). The stroma consisted of regularly arranged collagen fibers and normal keratocytes. Descemet's, membrane was normal in thickness and endothelial cells were arranged in one sheet (Fig. 7.3.2).

Energy dispersive X-ray analyzer showed no Al deposits in any components of the cornea.

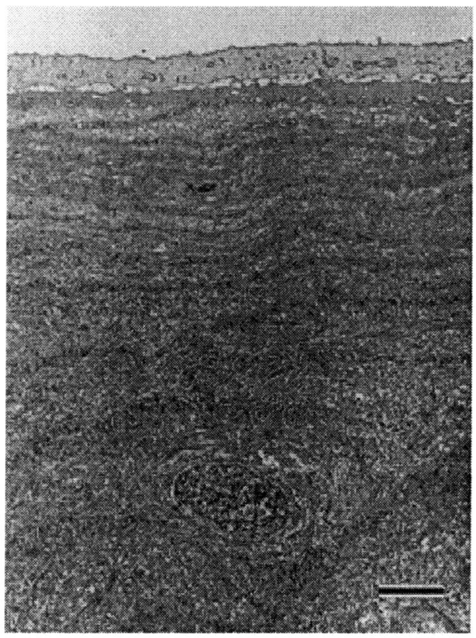

Figure 7.3.1. Electron micrograph of the cornea of a rat treated with $AlCl_3$ for 16 weeks. The epithelium shows no abnormalities. Bar: 2μm.

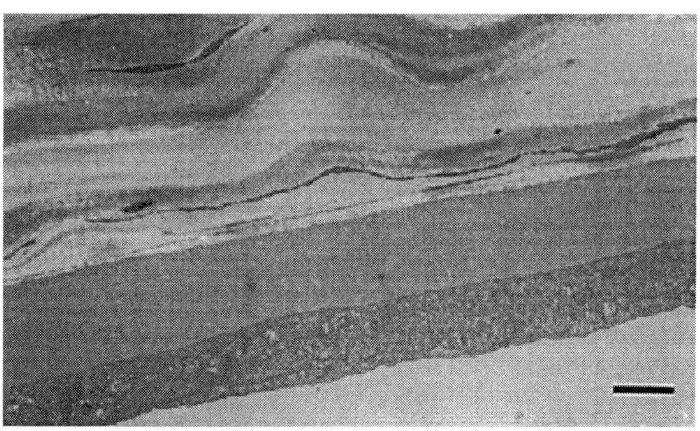

Figure 7.3.2. Electron micrograph of the cornea of a rat treated with $AlCl_3$ for 16 weeks. The stroma and endothelium show no abnormal findings. Bar: 2μm.

Discussion

It is unknown whether Al is present at birth in humans or if it animals and is essential. However, Al increases in the body with age. Ocular tissue consists of a combination of the CNS, muscles, connective tissues, adipose tissues, pigment tissues, epithelial and endothelial tissues, vascular tissue, etc. That is, almost all kinds of tissues are involved in the eye and orbit. Al has an affinity for the retina and is toxic to it. In rats with all intoxication directed to the retina, the cornea showed neither morphological changes nor Al accumulation. Since the cornea consists of epithelial and endothelial cells and collagenous tissues, the current results suggest that Al has scarce affinity for the connective tissue and is non-toxic to the cornea.

Table 7.4.1. Numbers of nuclei in outer nuclear layer at the posterior pole in control and treated rats.

Rat	Time treated		
	8 weeks	12 weeks	16 weeks
Control	27.2 ±1.92	27.0±1.87	26.2±1.7*
Treated	25.2 ±0.3	26.8±2.78	0*

Note. Values are mean ±SD. Nuclei were counted in a 30×30μm area.
Control and treated rats, n=20
*P<0.0001(Student's t-test significant difference).

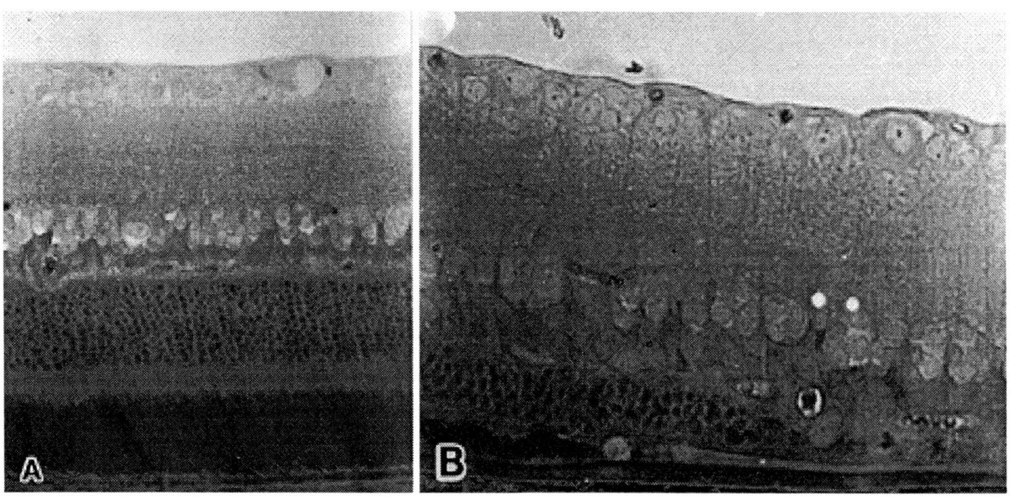

Figure 7.4.1. Light micrograph of retinas of rats. (A) Retina of a control rat; (B) retina of a rat treated with $AlCl_3$ for 16 weeks, showing two-thirds that of the control rat retina in thickness. Original magnification. × 400.

IV. THE RETINA

Results

Light and Electron Microscopic Findings

In rats treated with $AlCl_3$ for 8 and 12 weeks, the photoreceptor cell nuclei did not decrease (Table 7.4.1A), but Müller cells in the outer nuclear layer were vacuolated and some have disappeared altogether (Fig. 7.4.2). However, the retina of rats treated for 16 weeks showed two-thirds that of the control rat retina in thickness (Fig. 7.4.1B). The energy dispersive X ray analyzer (EDXA) failed to detect Al in any of the intracytoplasmic organelles, including lysosomes, mitochondria, dense bodies, nucleus, photoreceptor outer segment discs, and abnormal granules suspected of containing Al-related substances.

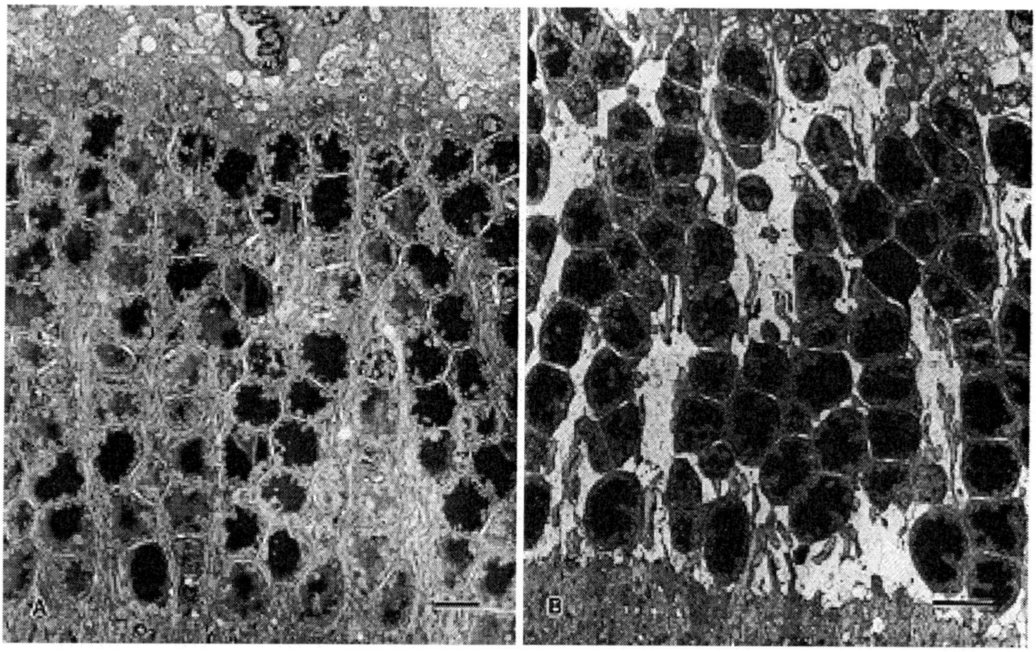

Figure 7.4.2. Electron micrographs of the outer nuclear layer of a retina of a control rat (A) and that of a rat treated with $AlCl_3$ for 8 weeks (B). The number of photoreceptor nuclei has not decreased, however, some Müller cells have lost their cytoplasmic components. Bar: 2μm (A), 5μm (B).

Rats treated with $AlCl_3$ for 16 weeks showed prominent pathologic changes, i.e., a thin retinal pigment epithelium (RPE) and disappearance of the outer and inner segments and nuclei of photoreceptors (Fig. 7.4.3). The retina between the RPE and the inner nuclear layer (INL) was almost completely destroyed and contained unidentifiable cells that had no cytoplasmic membrane; debris of intracytoplasmic organelles and dense irregular granules are also observed. Pyknotic nuclei were seen in unidentified cells in the inner nuclear layer, but no apoptotic nuclei. The granules were also seen in dendrite and/or neurons in the inner and outer plexiform layers due to the damaged retinal structure. Very dense irregular granules were seen in the nuclei and the cytoplasm of unidentified cells between the inner nuclear layer and the RPE (Fig. 7.4.4). These granules appeared in intracytoplasmic debris, in the nucleus, in the cytoplasmic matrix (Fig. 7.4.5), and in the RPE. The RPE cells were dark and contained numerous granules (Fig. 7.4.3A).

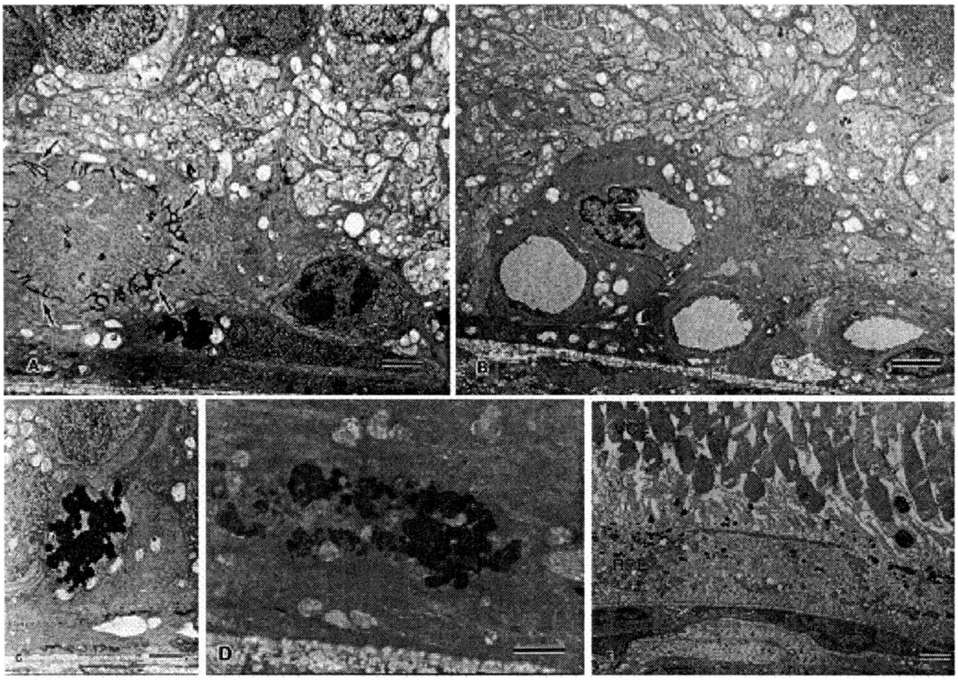

Figure 7.4.3. Electron micrographs of the retinas of a rat treated with $AlCl_3$ for 16 weeks. The retina shows a thin retinal pigment epithelium (RPE) and loss of the photoreceptor outer and inner segments and nuclei (A, B, C). Dense and irregular granules (arrows) are deposited in the cytoplasm of the cells and in neurons and /or dendrites between the RPE and the INL (inner nuclear layer) (A, B, C). The RPE also contains dense and irregular granules (A, B, D). (E) The retinal structure from the RPE to the visual cell layer (VCL) of a control rat. Bar: 2μm (A-D), 1μm (E).

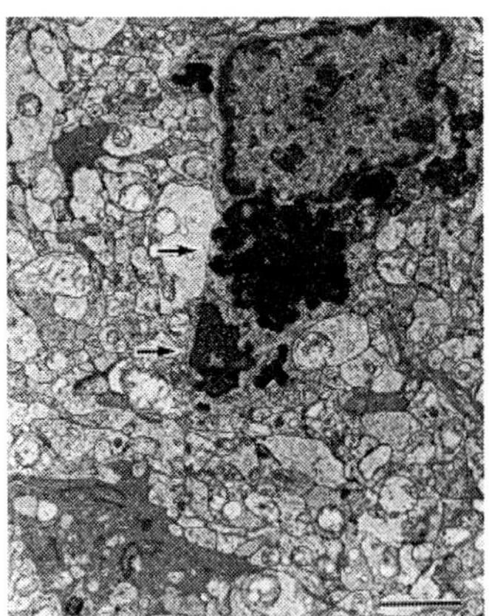

Figure 7.4.4. Electron micrographs of rat retinas treated with $AlCl_3$ for 16 weeks. Very dense, irregular granules (arrows) are seen in cytoplasm of an unidentified cell and around the nuclei in the INL (inner nuclear layer) or IPL (inner plexiform layer). Bar: 2μm.

EDXA detected Al at the dense irregular granules in the unidentified cells between the inner nuclear layers and in the RPE cells (Fig. 7.4.6), between the RPE and neurons and dendrites in the inner plexiform layer, and in the outer plexiform layer as well.

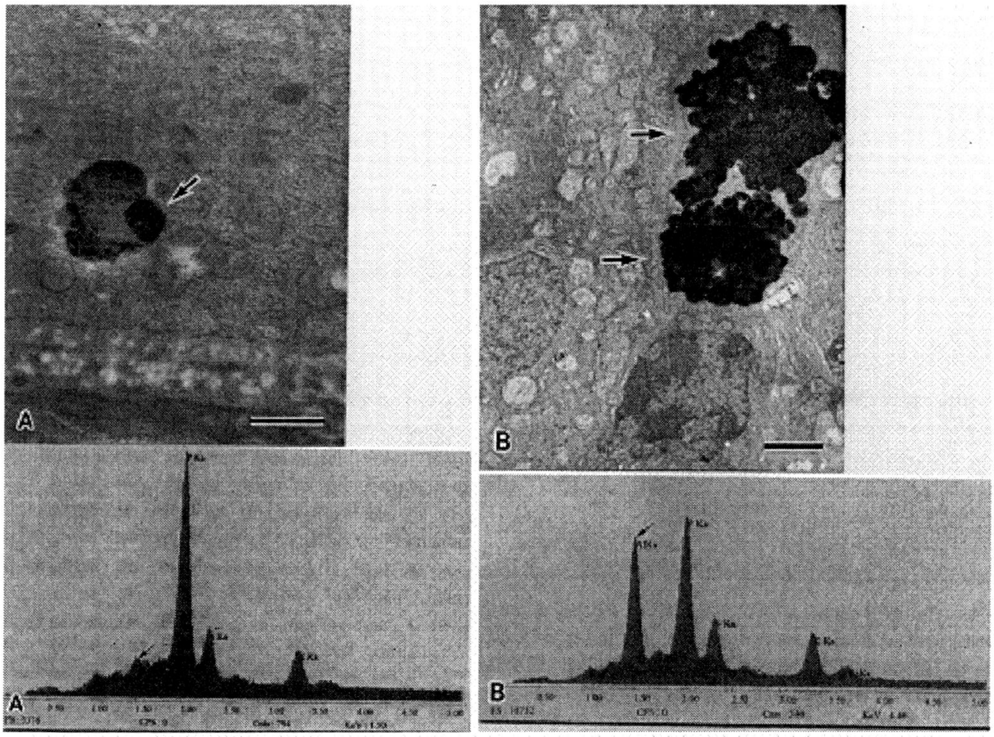

Figure 7.4.5. Electron micrographs of the retinas of a rat treated with $AlCl_3$ for 16 weeks. The RPE contains several clumps (arrow) of dense granules in the cytoplasm (A). Several clumps (arrow) of dense granules are seen in unidentified cells near the INL nuclei (N) (B). EDXA analysis reveals that the dense bodies (thick arrow) contain no Al (thin arrow) in the control rats. Bar: 0.5μm (A), 2μm (B).

Discussion

The current study showed a high concentration of Al in the serum of rats injected intraperitoneally with 5 or more mg Al/kg daily for 8-16 weeks, and EDXA showed Al in their degenerated retinas.

Experimental Al intoxication has certain silent characteristics; namely, it is hard to induce Al intoxication by specific doses and therefore it takes a long time to induce Al intoxication. In addition, Al intoxication occurs suddenly after long-term administration of Al, and the effect of Al exposure might be indirect rather than direct, due to Al accumulation (Swegert, Dave and Katyare et al, 1999). There have been no reports of abnormal retinal function due to Al intoxication. In the current study, Lu et al (2002) used $AlCl_3$ and the dose was determined according to that used in previous reports (Ebina, Okada, Hamazaki et al, 1984; Uemura, 1984). The rats that were administrated 0.3ml of 4% $AlCl_3$ daily first showed retinal changes at the 8th week of the experiment, and they showed very slight changes at the

12th week. Prominent changes in the retina (severe degeneration and the disappearance of photoreceptor cells) were first observed at the 16th week, Al was also detected by EDXA in dense granules in the inner nuclear layer nuclei, inner plexiform layer, dendrites and/or neurons of the outer plexiform layer. These progressing changes correlate with the serum Al level.

Thus, long-term exposure with a large quantity of Al may be necessary for Al intoxication. The total dose of Al administered during the current experiment is unusually high, and such excessive amounts of Al do not enter the human body. In fact, Al intoxication occurs in hemodialysis patients after long-term hemodialysis (Lin, Kou and Leu, 1996). Although Al was first demonstrated in the retina of rats treated with $AlCl_3$ for 16 weeks, there is a possibility that the retina already contained excessive Al in the rats that were treated for 8 or 12 weeks, since the threshold sensitivity of EDXA is too low to detect the element in the cytoplasm without deposits of Al. Rats treated for 16 weeks showed retinal degeneration with deposits of Al in the retina. In addition, cell nuclei were pyknotic but not apoptotic. These findings suggest that Al may combine with chromatin in the nuclei and in neurons and/or dendrites of the outer and inner plexiform layers. Histochemical and subcellular fragmentation studies on intracellular binding sites of Al show that Al concentration specifically increases in the large euchromatic neocortical neuronal chromatins (De Boni, Scott and Crapper, 1974; Lukiw, Krishman, Wong et al, 1992; Lukiw, Kruck and McLachlan, 1987; McLachlan, 1986; Wen and Wisniewski, 1985). Experimental aluminum encephalopathy (EAE) shows that Al lactate or Al chloride injected into an Al-susceptible animal induces a rapid accumulation of Al in the nuclear structure of the glia and large neurons (Crapper, Quittkat and Krishman et al, 1980; Crapper-McLachlan and De Boni, 1980; Wen and Wisniewski, 1985). In EAE neuronal tissue, a high concentration of Al is found in glial or neuronal lysosomes (Schuumans-Stekhaven, Renkawek, Otte-Holler et al, 1990). The photoreceptor cells are assumed to be the most sensitive to Al toxicity, because they were the most severely damaged. In hemodialysis patients, high Al levels have been observed in the periosteum and epiphyseal cartilage. Certain brain lesions such as Alzheimer amyloid structures and other encephalopathies contain Al and are related to Al deposition. Similarly, in the current experiments, the Al deposits were found not only in the nucleus but also in the cytoplasmic matrix.

V. THE OPTIC NERVE

Results

TEM Findings

The optic nerve of rats treated with $AlCl_3$ for 16 weeks showed decreased myelinated nerve fibers, irregular myelin lamellae and a thin myelin sheath (Fig. 7.5.1A). Glial cell proliferation was prominent (Fig. 7.5.1A), but in some sites glial cells scarcely invaded among myelinated axons (Fig. 7.5.1B). The axoplasmal membrane was detached from the myelin sheath (Fig. 7.5.1A,B). Any deposition was found in the optic nerve.

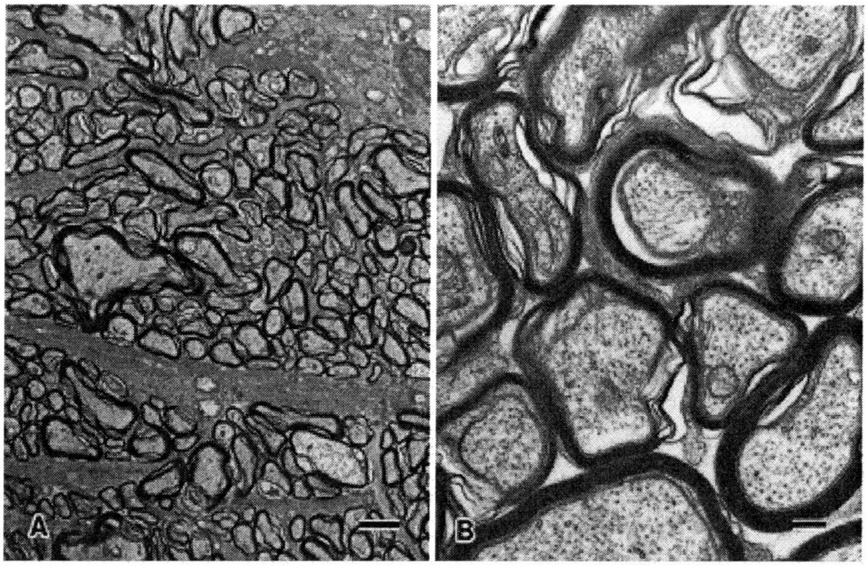

Figure 7.5.1. Electron micrographs of the transverse section of the optic nerve in a rat treated with $AlCl_3$ for 16 weeks. Myelinated nerve fibers are decreased and myelin lamellae are irregularly arranged and thin. Glial cell proliferate (A). Higher magnification of myelinated axons (B). Scarce glial cells are present among axons. Axoplasmal membrane is detached from myelin sheath. Bar: 2μm (A), 200nm (B).

Discussion

Although the rat retina demonstrated severe changes with a rapid accumulation of Al after a long-term administration with a large amount of Al, the cornea showed neither accumulation of Al nor ultrastructural alterations and the optic nerve had moderate changes without dense deposition containing Al. The ultrastructural changes are less severe in comparison with those in deficiencies of vitamins A (Chapter 8), E (Chapter 9) and C (Chapter 12) and trace elements Mg (Chapter 1), Zn (Chapter 2), Cu (Chapter 3) and Mn (Chapter 6). Thus the optic nerve damages may be due to secondary degeneration following retinal degeneration. It has been reported that Al lactate or Al chloride injected into an Al-susceptible animal induces a rapid accumulation of Al in the nuclear structure of the glia and large neurons (Crapper, Quittkat, Krishnan et al, 1980; Crapper-McLachlan and De Boni, 1980; Wen and Wisniewski, 1985). However, glial cells in the optic nerve of rats treated with $AlCl_3$ contained no Al-containing deposits and had no degeneration.

References

Crapper DR, Quittkat S, Krishman SS, Dalton AJ, De Boni U. Intranuclear aluminum content in Alzheimer's disease dialysis encephalopathy, and experimental aluminum encephalopathy, and experimental aluminum encephalopathy. *Acta Neuropathol (Berl)*. 1980;50:19-24.

Crapper-McLachlan DR, De Boni U. Aluminium in human brain disease. *Neuro-toxicology.* 1980;1:3-16.

De Boni U, Scott JW, Crapper DR. Intracellular aluminium binding; a histochemical study. *Histochemistry.* 1974;40:31-37.

Ebina Y, Okada S, Hamazaki S, Midorikawa O. Liver, kidney, and central nervous system toxicity of aluminium given intraperitoneally to rats: A multiple dose sub-chronic study using aluminium nitrilotriacetate. *Toxicol Appl Pharmacol.* 1984; 75: 211-218.

Hogan MJ, Alvarado JA, Weddell JE. Retina. In Hogan MJ, Alvarado JA, Weddell JE, ed. *Histology of the Human Eye.* Philadelphia:Saunders;1971:393-522.

Lin JL, Kou MT, Leu ML. Effect of long-term low-dose aluminium-containing agents on hemoglobin synthesis in patients with chronic renal insufficiency. *Nephron.* 1996; 74:33-38.

Lu ZY, Gong H, Amemiya. Alminum chloride induces retinal changes in the rat. *Toxicol Sci.* 2002;66:253-260.

Lukiw WJ, Krishman B, Wong L, Kruck TP, Bergeron C, Crapper Mclachlan DR. Nuclear compartmentalization of aluminium in Alzheimer's disease (AD). *Neurobiol. Aging.* 1992;13:115-121.

Lukiw WJ, Kruck TP, McLachlan DR. Alterations in human linker histone-DNA binding in the presence of aluminium salts in vitro and in Alzheimer's disease. *Neurotoxicology.* 1987;8:291-301.

McLachlan DR. Aluminium and Alzheimer's disease. *Neurobiol Aging.* 1986;7:525-532.

Schuumans-Stekhoven JH, Renkawek K, Otte-Holler I, Stols A. Exogenous aluminium accumulates in the lysosomes of cultured rat cortical neurons. *Neurosci Lett.* 1990;119:71-74.

Swegert CV, Dave KR, Katyare SS. Effect of aluminium-induced Alzheimer-like condition on oxidative energy metabolism in rat liver, brain, and heart mitochondria. *Mech Aging Dev.* 1999;112:27-42.

Uemura E. Intranuclear aluminium accumulation in chronic animals with experimental neurofibrillary changes. *Exp Neurol.* 1984;85:10-18.

Wen GY, Wisniewski HM. Histochemical localization of aluminium in the rabbit CNS. *Acta Neuropathol (Berl).* 1985;68:175-184.

Wilhelm M, Jager DE, Ohnesorge FK. Aluminium toxicokinetics. *Pharmacol Toxicol.* 1990;66:4-9.

Yokel RA, McNamara PJ. Aluminium toxicokinetics: An updated minireview. *Pharmacol Toxicol.* 2001;88:159-167.

Chapter 8

VITAMIN A

PART I. VITAMIN A DEFICIENCY

Significance

Since ancient Egypt and Greece, the curative value of liver containing vitamin A has been recognized for night blindness and the effect on growth. In the 1920s and 1930s, the chemical structure of vitamin A was determined as an all-trans-retinol and retinoic acid was found to be a growth effect (Arens and van Dorp, 1946;Ross, 1999). In the 1950s vitamin A was shown to be the essential visual pigment of the photoreceptor cells (Wald, 1958, 1968). The discovery of retinol-binding protein (RBP) and its significance accelerate the elucidation of vitamin A function occurred in the 1960s and 1970s. After the 1980s retinoid receptor research rapidly developed and two main subfamilies of nuclear retinoid receptors (RAR and RXR) are recognized (Chambon, 1996;Ross, 1999). Vitamin A has four main functions: vision, cellular differentiation, development, and immunity.

Vitamin A deficiency has been known to result in xerophthalmia, keratomalacia, and blindness (Carter-Dowson, Tanaka, Kuwabara et al, 1980; Van Horn, Schutten and Hyndriuk, 1980). Previous studies have shown that vitamin A deficiency causes various changes in the conjunctiva and cornea (Carter-Dowson, Tanaka, Kuwabara et al, 1980; Kobayashi, Tsubota, Takamiya et al, 1997; Pfister and Renner, 1978; Pirie, 1978; Shams, Hanrinen, Chaves et al, 1993; Van Horn, Schutten and Hyndiuk et al, 1980). In other words, vitamin A is essential for the proper differentiation and maintenance of mucosal epithelium and its absence causes a loss of goblet cells and keratinizing metaplasia of the epithelium (Anderson, Richard and Rock, 1993; Hatchel, Ubels, Stekiel et al, 1985; Sullivan, McCulley and Dohlman, 1973).

Vitamin A Deficiency Experiment

Materials and Methods

Normal male infant Wistar Kyoto rats from normal mothers were weaned 20 days after birth and divided into two groups: rats fed a vitamin A deficient diet and control rats fed a usual diet with vitamin A 8.80IU/g and vitamin E 0.091mg/g. The vitamin A deficient solid diet was commercially prepared and obtained from Nippon Clea (Tokyo, Japan) (Reeves, Nielsen and Fahey, 1993). This diet contains less than 0.01mg of retinal per 100g diet and all other nutrients. Distilled and deionized water was provided freely to both groups. All the rats were killed at 13 weeks of age.

Clinical Features of Vitamin A Deficient Animal

Body weight: At 13 weeks of age the body weight of vitamin A deficient rats (207.7±32.0g, n=11) was significantly lower than that of control rats (410±11.5g, n=5) ($p=0.0372$).

Serum vitamin A: At 13 weeks of age the serum vitamin A level was 25.6±18.4ng/ml (n=11) in the vitamin A deficient rats and 526.8±54.6ng/ml (n=5) ($p<0.0001$).

The Conjunctiva and Cornea

Light Microscopic Findings

The conjunctiva: The conjunctiva of the vitamin A deficient rats showed severe keratinization and lack of goblet cells (Fig. 13.1.1A), while control rats had numerous goblet cells and no keratinization.

The cornea: The corneas of the vitamin A deficient rats showed severe keratinization. Some abnormal vessels were seen in the anterior stroma, and the basal cells had lost their columnar appearance (Fig. 13.1.2A). The control corneas had the columnar features of basal epithelial cells and no keratinization.

Scanning (SEM) and Transmission (TEM) Electron Microscopic Findings

The conjunctiva: SEM showed severe keratinization, many dark cells and a lack of goblet cells at the conjunctival surface in the vitamin A deficient rats (Fig. 8.3.1). In contrast, the conjunctiva of the control rats had many more densely arranged goblet cells (Fig. 8.3.2) and microplicae than that of the vitamin A deficient rats. The difference between the control and vitamin A deficient rat conjunctivae were statistically significant: 80.8±11.2 goblet cells per standard field in control rats and 5.0±8.3 in vitamin A deficient rats ($p<0.0001$).

TEM showed many keratohyalin granules, an absence of goblet cells and a loss of microvilli in vitamin A deficient conjunctivae (Fig. 8.3.3). On the other hand, control conjunctivae had many goblet cells rich in secretory granules (Fig. 13.3.3A). Hemidesmosomes decreased in number in the basal cells and fine granular clusters were accumulated in concavity of infolded basement membrane (Fig. 8.3.4).

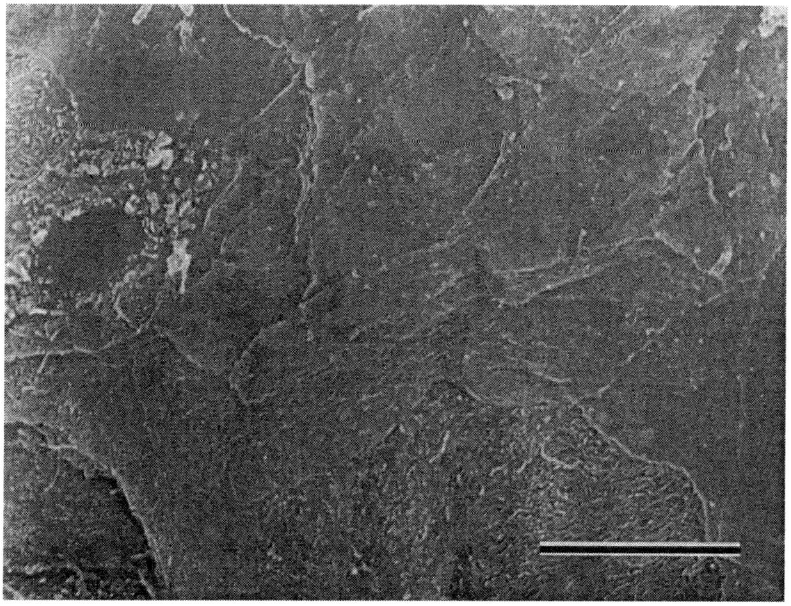

Figure 8.3.1. SEM micrograph of the conjunctival epithelium of a vitamin A deficient rat. The conjunctiva demonstrates severe keratinization, but no microvilli and goblet cells. Bar: 10μm.

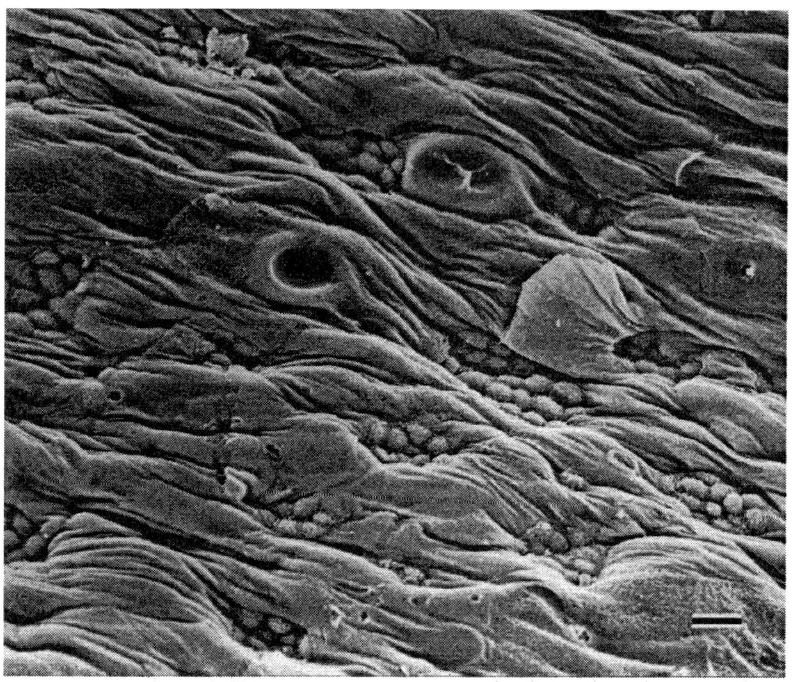

Figure 8.3.2. SEM micrograph of the conjunctival epithelium of a control rat. The conjunctiva has many goblet cells and microvilli. Bar: 10μm.

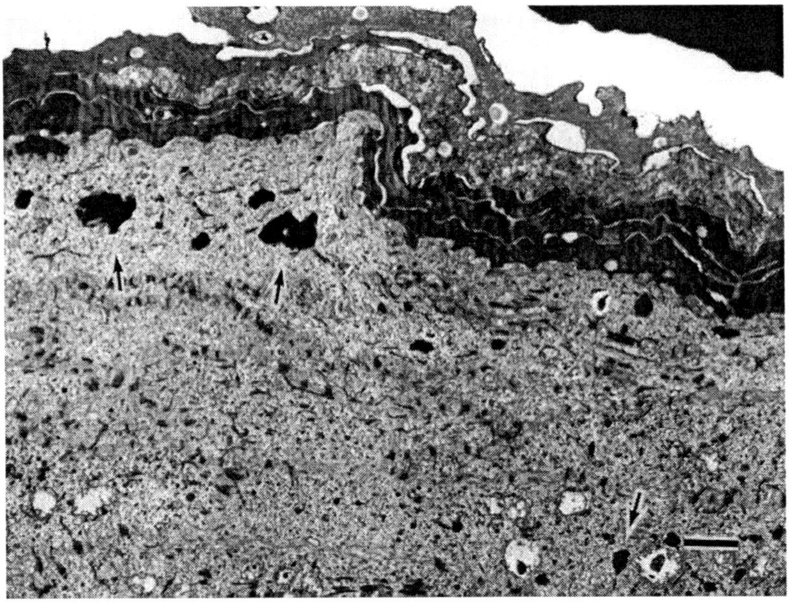

Figure 8.3.3. TEM micrographs of the conjunctiva. In a vitamin A deficient rat, the most superficial epithelial cells lose microvilli and show severe keratinization. Epithelial cells contain many keratohyalin granules. They are present in the deep epithelium as well as the superficial layer. Bar: 2μm (A).

The cornea: SEM revealed that the vitamin A deficient rat corneas had many more dark cells than the control rat corneas. At high magnification, vitamin A deficient rat corneas showed very few microvilli and a rough and uneven surface (Fig. 8.3.5. Control corneas had many microvilli and microplicae on the surface (Fig. 13.3.2A). In SEM micrographs of corneas, the ratio of light cells/light cells plus dark cells of vitamin A deficient rat corneas was significantly lower than that of control rat corneas ($p=0.0003$). The epithelial cells of vitamin A deficient rat corneas were smaller than those of control rat corneas because vitamin A deficient rat corneas had more epithelial cells per $600\mu m^2$ field on SEM micrographs than did control rat corneas ($p=0.0001$).

TEM showed that corneas in vitamin A deficient rats showed significant epithelial keratinization including keratohyalin granules and loss of microvilli (Fig. 8.3.6A). Vitamin A deficient rat corneas had 0.78 ± 0.77 microvilli per/μm standard field, compared with 2.83 ± 0.52 ($p<0.0001$) in control rat corneas. Hemidesmosomes in the cornea decreased in number.

The corneal stroma of vitamin A deficient rats had macrophage-like cells containing many cellular debris and multiple nuclei (Fig. 8.3.7).

The control rat cornea had many microvilli and no keratinization in the epithelium (Fig. 8.3.6B), and many hemidesmosomes and an intact basement membrane.

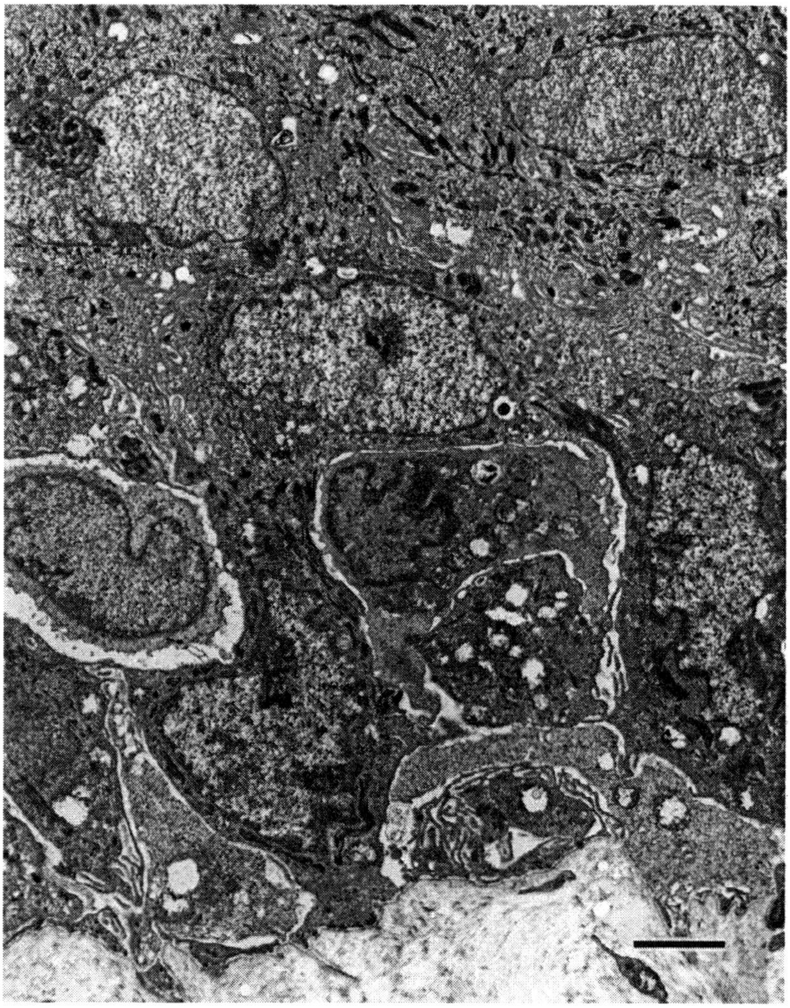

Figure 8.3.4. TEM micrograph of the conjunctiva in a vitamin A deficient rat. The basal cells in the epithelium lose hemidesmosomes, and clusters of fine granular masses are accumulated in concavity of infolded basement membrane. Bar: 1μm.

The conjunctiva of the upper eyelids of rats fed a vitamin A deficient diet for 4 months was examined with electron microscopy and energy dispersive X-ray analyzer. Compared with normal controls (Oba, Gong, Amemiya et al, 2001), vitamin A deficient rats had about the same amounts of Na, P, S, K and Fe in their goblet cells, but more Cl, Mg and Ca (Oba, Gong, Amemiya, 1998).

Discussion

Our study confirms that vitamin A deficiency causes keratinization and a decrease and loss of microvilli and microplicae in the most superficial epithelial cells of the conjunctiva and cornea. Beta-carotene and other carotenoids have antioxidant functions such as the quenching of singlet oxygen and other electronically excited molecules that are produced by photoexcitation or chemoexcitation reactions. Thus vitamin A is one of the major fat-soluble antioxidants, which carry an important role of non-enzymatic antioxidant defense. Antioxidant functions include lowered DNA damage, diminished lipid peroxidation, and inhibition of transformation in vitro. In addition to its action as an antioxidant, vitamin A accelerates the development of the epithelium, prevents keratinization of the epithelium, and supplies fatty acids which combine with vitamin A. Vitamin A may stimulate the synthesis of glycoconjugates that may appear on the cell surface or be secreted as basement membrane components (Hatchell and Sommer, 1984; Ubels et Edelhauser and Austin, 1983).

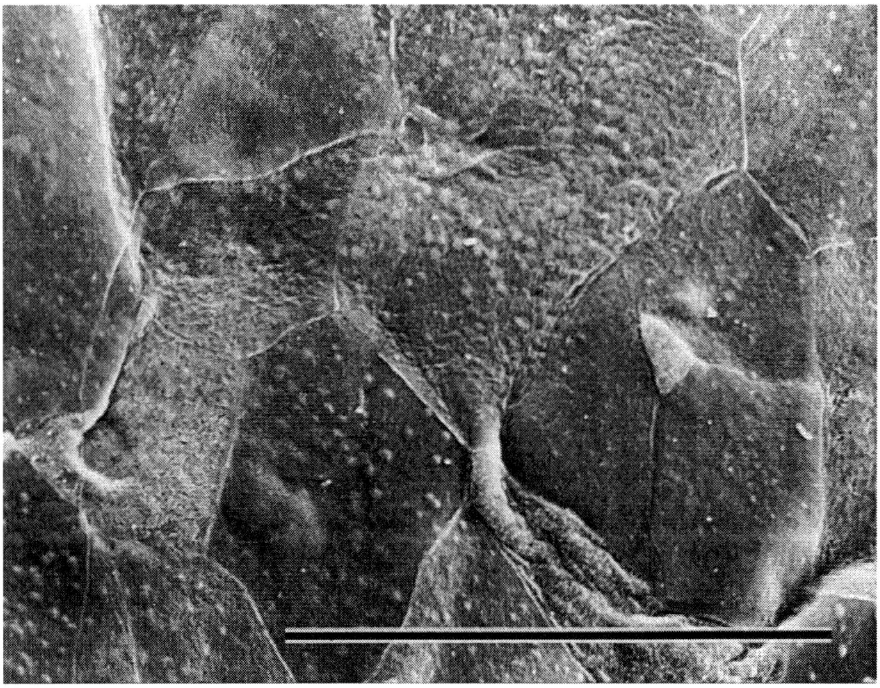

Figure 8.3.5. SEM micrograph of the corneal surface. A. A vitamin A deficient rat shows few microvilli in the most superficial epithelium. Bar:10μm (A).

The cells in the conjunctival and corneal epithelium have several cellular retinoid-depending proteins and nuclear retinoid receptors which depend upon retinoic acid. The structure integrity of the cornea, an avascular tissue, depends upon vitamin A delivered via tear fluid. The lacrimal gland can synthesize and secrete PBP, which may be important in solubilizing the retinol in tears (Lee, Ubels and Soprano, 1992). These conjunctival and corneal changes may be due to a lack of retinoic acid.

Acitretin, a synthetic retinoid, which is an analogue of retinoic acid and is used in dermatology for treatment, normalizes hyperproliferative states and induces differentiation of basal cells in the dermis toward a less keratinized, more epithelial phenotype (Orfanos, Zouboulis, Almond-Roesler et al, 1997). Thus retinoid deficiency induces keratinization in the conjunctiva and cornea. In the current experiment conjunctival and corneal keratinization disappeared by administration of vitamin A after its deficiency. Bitot's spots, formy-appearing deposits of cells and bacteria in the outer quadrant of the eye occur in vitamin A deficiency. Vitamin A is known for a long time to have a function for resistance to infection.

Vitamin A is concerned with cell-mediated immunity and antibody-mediated responses, and vitamin A deficiency induces poor resistance to infection which is related to bacterial infection in Bitot's spots. Vitamin A, as retinoic acid, maintains normal differentiation of the conjunctival and corneal epithelial cells preventing keratinization.

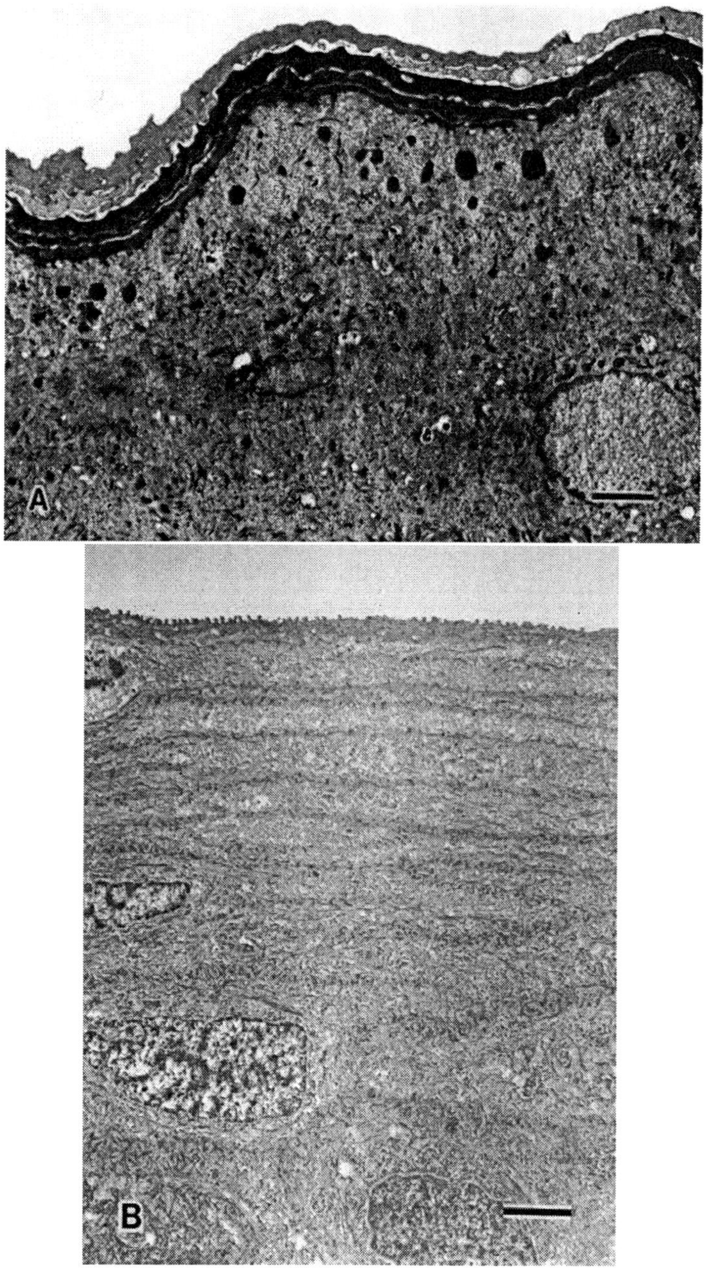

Figure 8.3.6. TEM micrographs of the corneal epithelium. A. In a vitamin A deficient rat, the corneal surface shows keratinization and epithelial cells contain many keratohyalin granules in deep layers as well as superficial layers. B. The epithelial cells of a control rat have many microvilli and no keratinization. Bar: 2μm (A, B).

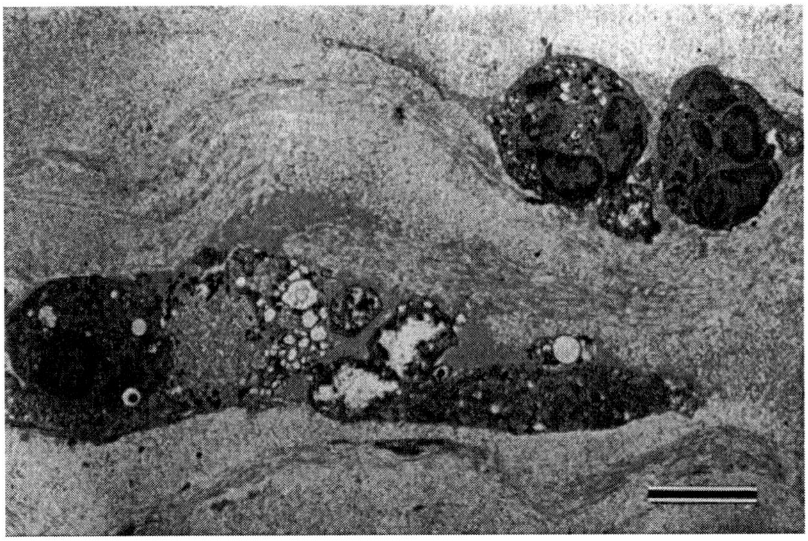

Figure 8.3.7. TEM micrograph of the corneal stroma of a vitamin A deficient rat. The stroma shows macrophage-like cells which contain multiple nuclei and many cellular debris. Bar: 4μm.

In vitamin A deficient rats, the basal cells in the epithelium have been reported to lose hemidesmosomes to induce microseparation of the plasma membrane (Sommer, 1983). This change is assumed to be the finding that vitamin A deficiency weakens the cellular attachment related to laminin. The same changes were seen in the current study and the conjunctiva showed disappearance of hemidesmosomes, but the basement membrane remained. Hemidesmosomes in the conjunctiva may be more sensitive to vitamin A deficiency than those in the cornea.

Changes of cell membranes in degeneration permit Ca to intrude into cells from the extracellular fluid. The analytical results suggest that the relationship between Ca and Mg is disturbed in vitamin A deficiency so that the function of goblet cells is abnormal (Oba, Gong , Amemiya et al, 1998; Oba, Gong, Amemiya et al, 2001)

The Effect of Vitamin A Deficiency on Retinal Development

Materials and Methods

Female Wistar Kyoto rats were fed a vitamin A deficient diet supplemented with retinoic acid for two or three months starting about 25 days after birth. Then they were mated with male Wistar Kyoto rats fed a usual diet. Subsequently, female rats were placed on a vitamin A deficient diet.

Animals were separated into four groups as follows:

1. Developing rats from vitamin A deficient rats were killed on the 7th, 12th, 14th or 18th day and 21st day after birth.
2. Developing rats from vitamin A deficient rats were injected intraabdominally with 1,250 IU of vitamin A on the first postnatal day, and killed on the 7th or 12th day after birth.

3. Developing rats from vitamin A deficient rats were injected intraabdominally with 1,250 IU of vitamin A on the 7th day after birth and killed on the 12th day.
4. Male and female rats fed a usual diet were mated, and developing rats from these rats were killed on the 7th or the 12th day after birth.

Clinical Features of the Fetus and Neonate

About eighty per cent of litters from vitamin A deficient mother rats were dead within 4 days after birth, even if they were given vitamin A on the first postnatal day. The rest of rats survived and developed. Fig. 8.4.1 shows the growth of the animals. There was little difference in body weight until the 12th postnatal day between the control and vitamin A deficient groups. However, vitamin A deficient rats began to show retarded growth after the 12th postnatal day.

Results

Light Microscopic Findings

By light microscopy, the 12-day-old control rat retina seemed to have almost complete retinal layers. The photoreceptor inner segments were identified. The outer segment layer of photoreceptor cells was seen in spite of its thinness. The retina of 12-day-old vitamin A deficient rats showed prominent undifferentiation. The inner segment layer of photoreceptor cells was identified to be thin. The photoreceptor outer segments could hardly be seen.

Electron Microscopic Findings

By electron microscopy, the rats of the control group were seen to have a lamellar structure like photoreceptor outer segments between the young photoreceptor cells and the retinal pigment epithelium (RPE) on the 7th day after birth. On the 12th day the photoreceptor outer segments developed rather well. Cilia extended from the photoreceptor inner segments which contained many polysomes and mitochondria.

In the retinas of the 12-day-old rats in vitamin A deficiency, the distinct photoreceptor outer segments could not be found between the photoreceptor inner segments and the RPE (Fig. 8.4.2). Very rarely, however, a few lamellae were found to be continuous with the cilium extending from the basal body in the distal part of the inner segment (Fig. 8.4.3). The photoreceptor inner segments were opposed to the RPE. The photoreceptor inner segments contained polysomes, mitochondria and centrioles. The RPE appeared normal, but thin. The retina of 14-day-old vitamin A deficient rats showed development of photoreceptor outer segments (Fig. 8.4.4). They were not as many as those in the 14-day-old normal rats, but showed irregular arrangement of the discs (Fig. 8.4.4). The photoreceptor outer segments of 18-day-old rats with vitamin A deficiency showed degeneration, but inner segments were rather well developed. The RPE cells contained many lipid-like droplets (Fig. 8.4.5).

In the retina of 21-day-old vitamin A deficient rats, which survived longest after birth, dark cells were seen in the RPE and inner segments, and outer segments were degenerated (Fig. 8.4.6).

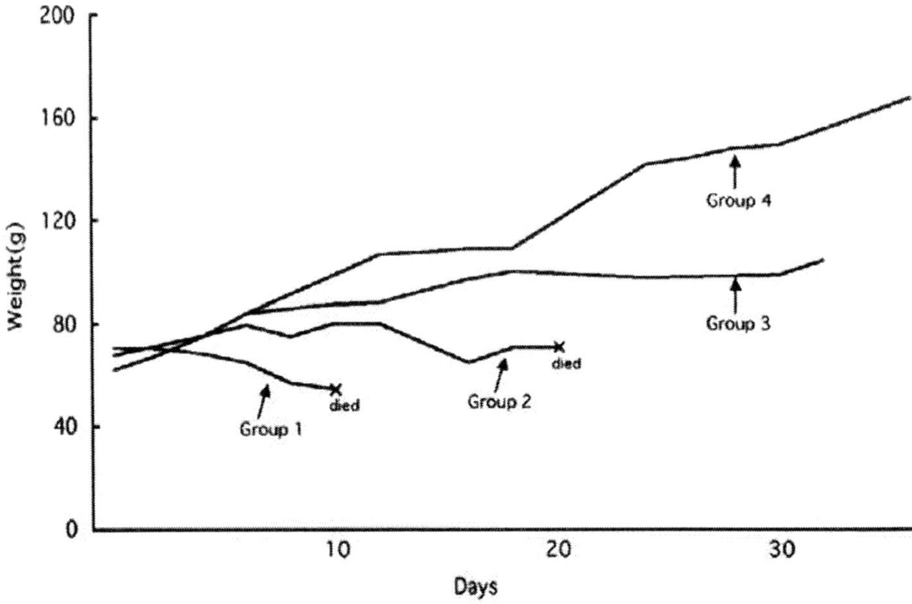

Figure 8.4.1. Growth of animals
Group 1: Control rats (10 rats).
Group 2: Rats raised by vitamin A deficient mother rats (16 rats).
Group 3: Rats injected with vitamin A on the 7th postnatal day (4 rats).
Group 4: Rats injected with vitamin A on the 1st postnatal day (1 rat).
2)-4) rats from vitamin A deficient mother rats (16 rats).

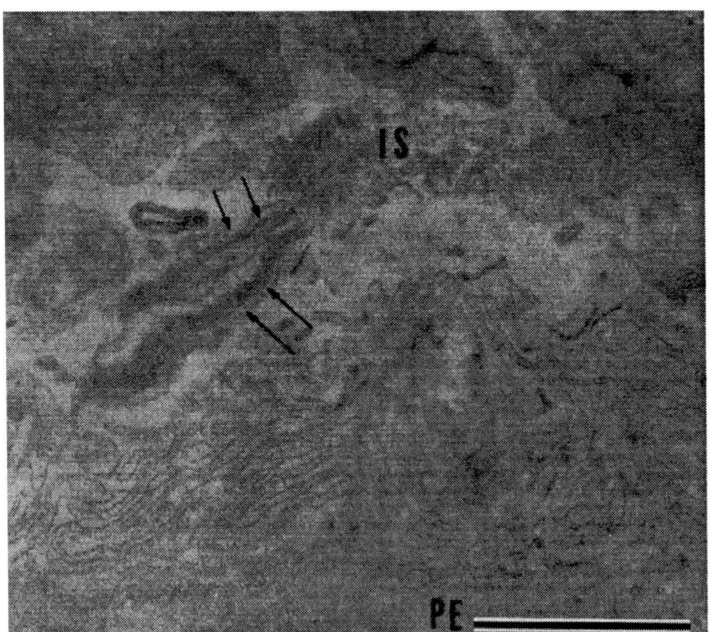

Figure 8.4.2. Electron micrograph of a 12-day-old rat in vitamin A deficiency. A few lamellar membranous structures (arrows) are seen between the RPE (PE) and the photoreceptor inner segments (IS). Bar: 3μm.

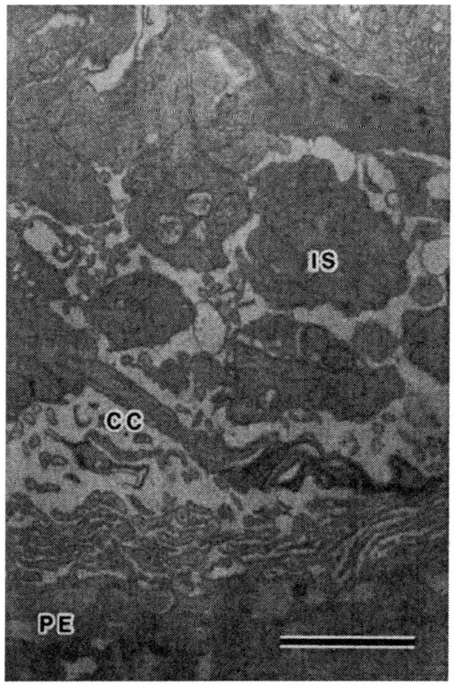

Figure 8.4.3. Electron micrograph of the retina of a 12-day-old rat in vitamin A deficiency. Poorly developed lamellar membranous structures (arrows) are very scarcely seen to be continuous with a connecting cilium (CC) extending from the basal body in the distal portion of the inner segment (IS). It contains many mitochondria. PE:RPE. Bar: 1μm.

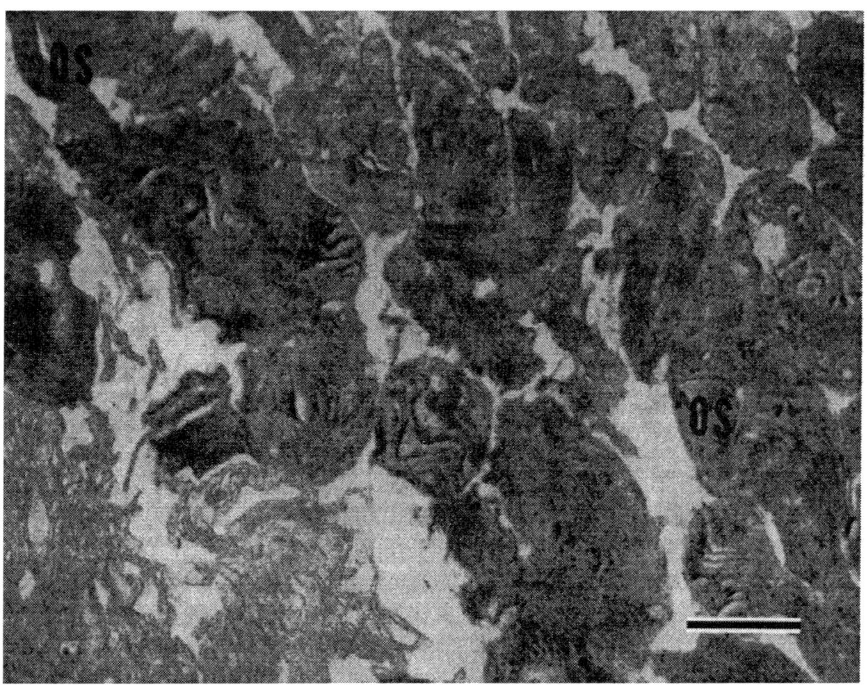

Figure 8.4.4. Electron micrograph of outer segments of a 14-day-old rat in vitamin A deficiency. There are many outer segments with irregularly arranged discs. Bar: 1μm.

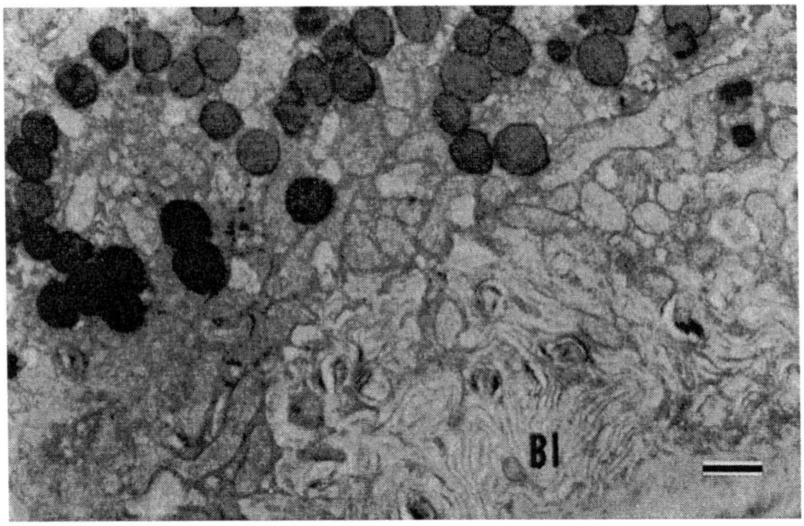

Figure 8.4.5. Electron micrograph of the RPE of a 18-day-old rat in vitamin A deficiency. The RPE has many lipid-like droplets and well-developed basal infoldings. Bar: 1μm.

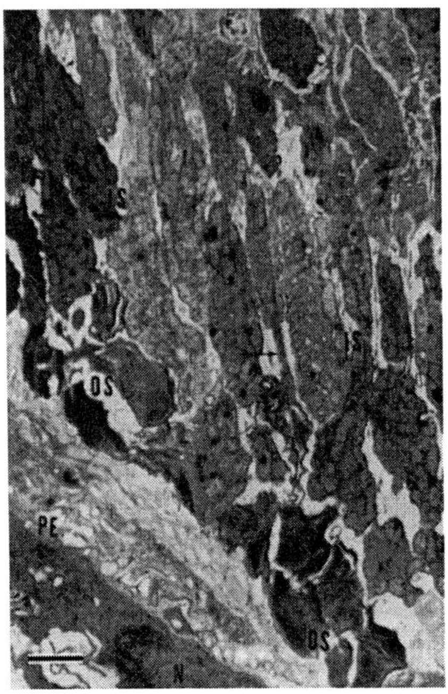

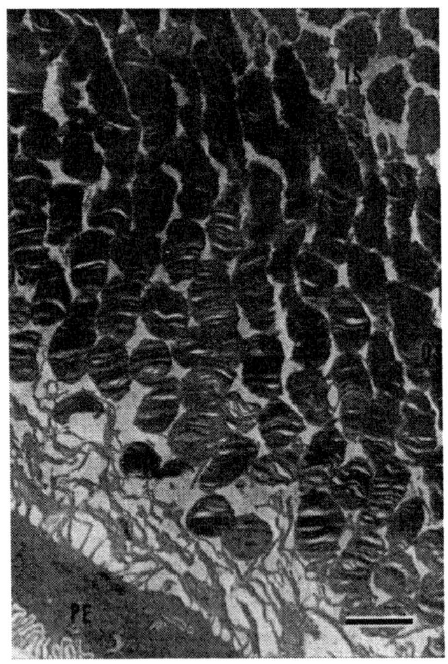

Figure 8.4.6. Electron micrograph of the retina of a 21-day-old rat in vitamin A deficiency. The inner segments and RPE cells are dark. The outer segments are scarce and their discs are irregularly arranged. IS: Inner segment, OS: Outer segment, PE: Pigment epithelium. Bar: 1μm.

Figure 8.4.7. Electron micrograph of the RPE (PE) and outer segments (OS) of a 43-day-old rat injected with vitamin A on the 7th postnatal day born from vitamin A deficient mother rat. There are many outer segments with regularly arranged discs. The RPE looks intact despite high basal infoldings. IS: Inner segment. Bar: 2μm.

In the retina of 43-day-old rats fed a usual diet after the 21st postnatal day following being weaned by a vitamin A deficient mother, many outer segments were present (Fig. 8.4.7) and the RPE cells contained lyosomes and phagocytized lamellar structures (Fig. 8.4.8).

In the retina of developing rats from the vitamin A deficient mother, injected with vitamin A on the first or 7th postnatal day, the lamellar structure like photoreceptor outer segments was found between the photoreceptor inner segments and the RPE on the 12th day after birth. There was little difference in morphology between the recovery and control groups.

The retina of vitamin A deficient mother rats showed moderate degeneration of the photoreceptor outer segments.

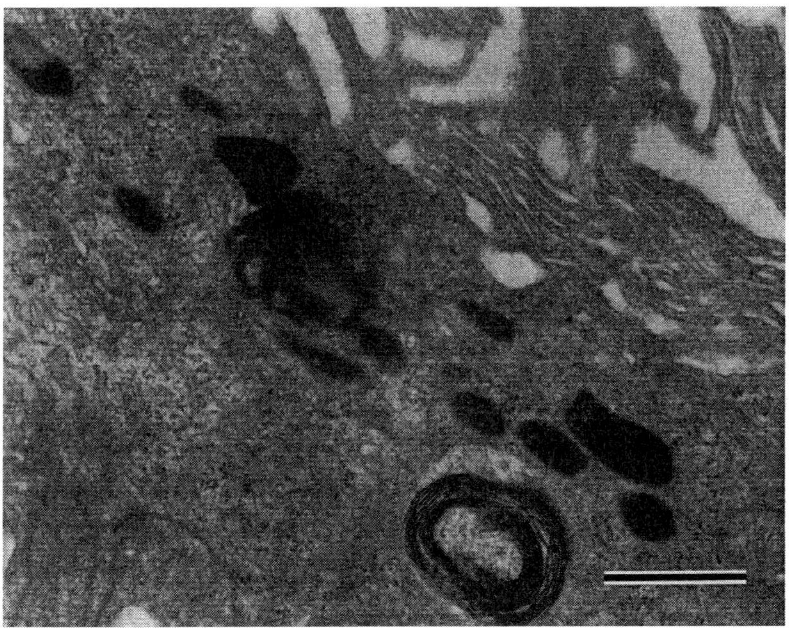

Figure 8.4.8. Electron micrograph showing phagocytized lamellar structure and secondary lysosomes in the RPE of a 43-day-old rat fed a usual diet after 21st postnatal day following being raised by a vitamin A deficient mother. Bar: 1µm.

Discussion

Both vitamin A deficiency and excess cause a failure of embryonic development and congenital malformations. Retinoic acid may induce undifferentiated stem cells to cease proliferation and to assume a differentiated, mature phenotype (Strickland and Mahdavi, 1978;Ross, 1999).

It is well-known that vitamin A deficient pregnant animals resorb their embryos or fetuses, or produce the offsprings with congenital malformations (Warkany and Schraffenberger, 1946; Wilson, Roth and Warkany, 1953). The eye is the organ most frequently involved. If the discussion is limited on ocular abnormalities, the litters from vitamin A deficient mother rat demonstrate postlenticular fibroplasias, incomplete closure of the choroidal fissure (coloboma), eversion and abnormal folding of the nervous layer of the retina, and less frequent defects involving the lids and lens.

Judging from the experiments (Amemiya, 1976, 1977a, b; Warkany and Schraffenberger, 1946; Wilson, Roth and Warkany, 1953), seventy-five or eighty per cent of the litters from the mother rat with vitamin A deficiency have some abnormalities and die within 4 days after birth. The rest of litters survive after the 4th postnatal day even if they are raised by a vitamin A deficient mother rat. It is unknown what has happened to these surviving litters. Major focus on the fate of the litters from the mother rat with vitamin A deficiency has been concentrated here to development of the retina without retinal dysplasia, especially to the development of the photoreceptor outer segments.

In the regions that form the eyes, specific isoforms of retinal dehydrogenase, which mediates retinoic acid biosynthesis, are expressed at appropriate times during development in tissue that will differentiate into the ventral and dorsal portions of the eye (McCaffery and Drager, 1995;Ross, 1999). Mice lacking cellular retinol-binding protein (CRBP) happen to appear normal at birth (Morriss-Kay and Sokolva, 1996;Ross, 1999).

Judging from the light and electron microscopic findings, the maturity of the photoreceptor outer segments of the 12-day-old rats with vitamin A deficiency seemed to be about equivalent to that of the 7- or 8-day-old control rats, although there was little difference in body weight between vitamin A deficient and control groups until the 12th postnatal day. The development of photoreceptor outer segments of vitamin A deficient mother rats was apparently retarded. On the other hand, when litters from vitamin A deficient mother rats were given vitamin A at birth or on the 7th day after birth, surviving developing rats demonstrated nearly normal development of the photoreceptor outer segments. These results may suggest that, if newborn rats from a vitamin A deficient mother have no severe anomalies leading to death, the retinal cells develop gradually according to the amount of vitamin A supplied from moderately vitamin A deficient mother rat. In addition, it means that a suitable supplementation of vitamin A can lead to the correct retinal development in vitamin A deficient litters. Vitamin A deficient rats in the current study had apparent photoreceptor outer segments after the 14th postnatal day. They were normal in size, but not as many as normal ones. This indicates that, as far as vitamin A is supplied to the developing rats from moderately vitamin A deficient mother even if it is a small amount, photoreceptor outer segments can develop and increase in number according to the amount of vitamin A.

The Retina

Vitamin A-Deficient Experiment

Materials and Methods

The animals used were female Wistar Kyoto rats obtained from the Pure Line Animal Center of Kyoto University.

Rats were divided into three groups as follows:

Group 1 was fed a vitamin A deficient diet starting 25 to 30 days after birth.

(a) Rats killed in the 3rd or 4th month of the experiment showing slight or moderate symptoms of vitamin A deficiency.
(b) Rats killed in the 6th or 7th month of the experiment showing symptoms of severe vitamin A deficiency.
(c) Rats killed after 2 or 16 daily injections of 5,000 I.U. of vitamin A following 6 months on the vitamin A deficient diet.
(d) Rats killed about 6 months on a usual diet following 6 months on a vitamin A deficient diet.

Group 2 was fed a vitamin A deficient diet and received daily injections of 20 mμ of retinoic acid starting 25 to 30 days after birth. Rats were killed after about 4 months.

Group 3: control rats were fed a usual diet from 90 to 360 days after birth.

Cytochemistry of alcohol dehydrogenase activity: The rat retina was incubated in the medium (Amemiya, 1967) without fixation and observed with an electron microscope. Alcohol dehydrogenase activity was demonstrated as TNBT (tetranitroblue tetrazolium) - formazan aggregates.

Clinical features of vitamin A deficient animal

The rats in group 1 began to show mild symptoms of vitamin A deficiency about 2 months after being fed the vitamin A deficient diet only: they showed retarded growth (Fig. 8.5.1) and slight roughening of the fur. From 3 to 4 months after being fed the vitamin A deficient diet only, the rats showed moderate roughening of the fur and ceased to gain weight (Fig. 8.5.1), and sometimes showed light inflammation of the conjunctiva. At the end of 5 or 6 months on the vitamin A deficient diet, the rats in group 1 showed marked loss of weight (Fig. 8.5.1), dirty fur or marked roughening of the fur, inflammation of the conjunctiva, tremors of all limbs, and corneal opacity or corneal ulcer. Many of them died.

The rats in group 2 did not show roughening of the fur, inflammation of the conjunctiva, or corneal opacity until at least 130 days after being fed the vitamin A deficient diet and injected with vitamin A acid, but their growth was slightly stunted compared with that of the control group (Fig. 8.5.1).

The rats recovered from vitamin A deficiency: They gained weight rapidly (Fig.8.5.1), and the luster of the fur reappeared. Inflammation of the conjunctiva and corneal opacity disappeared.

Results

Electron Microscopic Findings

Group 1. a. In rats killed 3 months on the vitamin A deficient diet, most of the photoreceptor outer segments looked normal and the RPE had lamellar structures. In rats fed the vitamin A deficient diet for 4 months, the outer segment discs were decreased in number and degenerated (Fig. 8.5.2), and immature outer segments appeared frequently (Fig. 8.5.3). The outer segment discs broke into vesicles. The RPE scarcely contained lamellar structures. Alcohol dehydrogenase activity, as evidenced by TNBT-formazan, decreased slightly or moderately in the RPE, especially in the endoplasmic reticulum, but remained normal in the inner segment.

b. The electron micrographs of the retinas of rats that were fed the vitamin A deficient diet for 5 months showed an extremely decreased number of outer segments and destruction of mitochondria in the RPE. Alcohol dehydrogenase activity disappeared in the RPE (Fig. 8.5.4), but remained normal or decreased slightly in the discs of the outer segments.

In rats fed the vitamin A deficient-diet for 7 months, the RPE showed severe destruction of mitochondria, vacuolation of the endoplasmic reticulum and absence of lamellar structures (Fig. 8.5.5), but ribosomes remained. The outer segments disappeared (Fig. 8.5.5). In the inner segments mitochondria were severely destroyed and vacuolated, and the endoplasmic reticulum was dilated. The terminal processes of Müller's fibers were vacuolated (Fig. 8.5.5).

c. In rats treated with 5,000 I.U. of vitamin A for 16 days after about 6 months on the vitamin A deficient diet, the RPE and inner segments showed reconstruction of mitochondria and gradual closing of the endoplasmic reticulum. The outer segments showed various stages of regeneration (Fig. 8.5.6), and disappearance of disc vesiculation and elongation of cilia. Alcohol dehydrogenase activity reappeared in normal amounts and sites or increased in the RPE and inner segments, especially in the endoplasmic reticulum.

d. The retinas of rats fed a usual diet for 6 months following 6 months on the vitamin A deficient diet showed the photoreceptor cells morphologically completely recovered from the destruction, normally repaired RPE, and recovery of alcohol dehydrogenase activity in the pigment epithelium and inner segments.

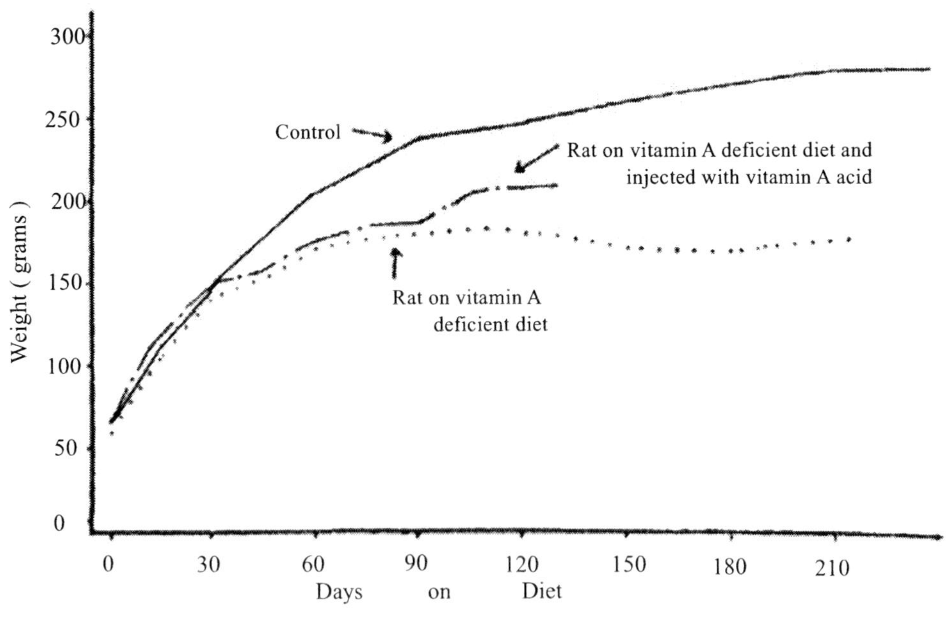

Figure 8.5.1. Growth of animals

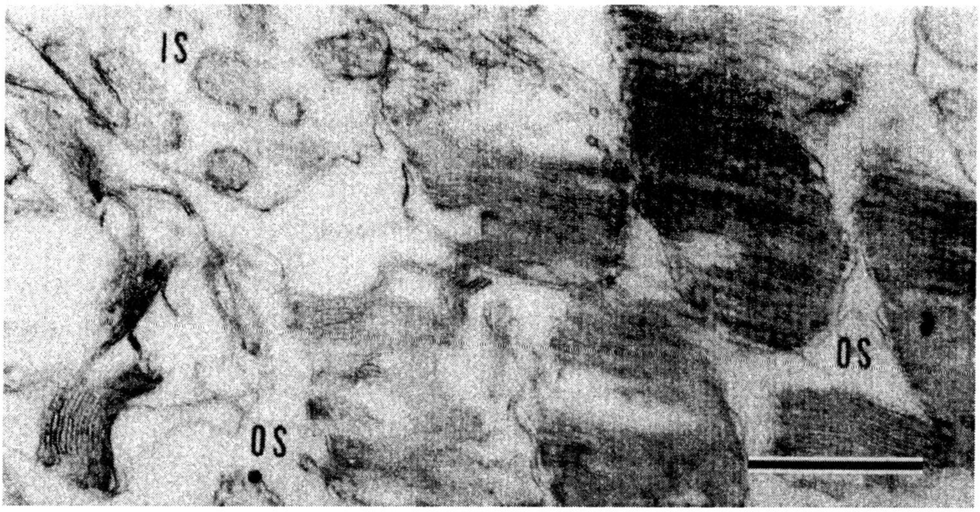

Figure 8.5.2. Electron micrograph of the retina of a rat fed a vitamin A deficient diet for 4 months. The outer segment discs show a decrease and slight degeneration. Bar: 1μm.

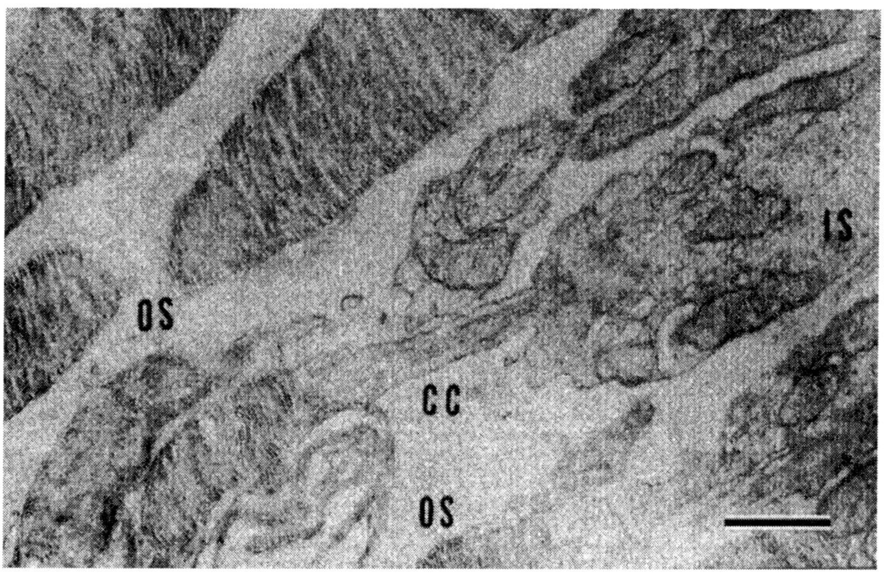

Figure 8.5.3. In the retina of a rat fed a vitamin A deficient diet for 4 months, an immature outer segment is seen. Bar: 1μm.

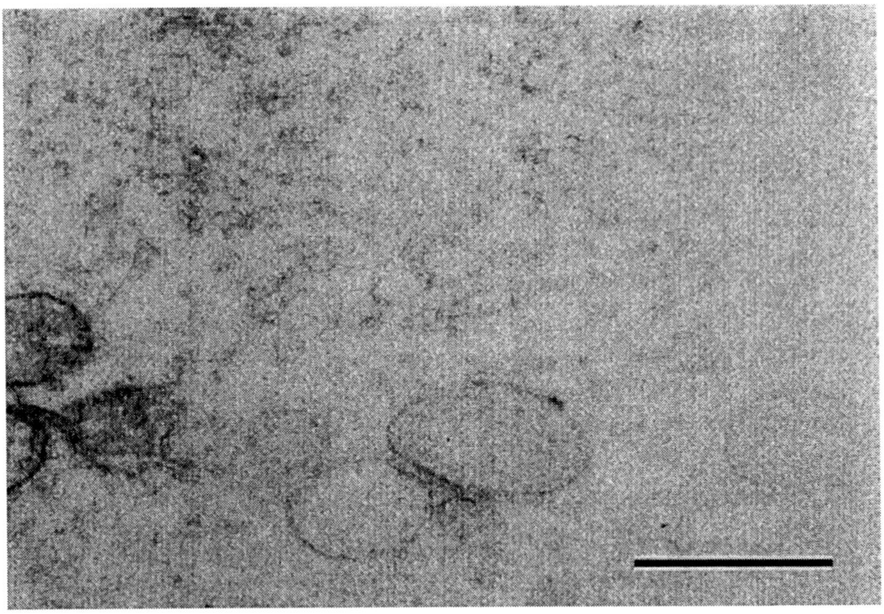

Figure 8.5.4. Electron micrograph of alcohol dehydrogenase activity in the photoreceptor outer segment of a rat fed a vitamin A deficient diet for 5 months. Alcohol dehydrogenase activity as evidenced by deposits of TNBT-formazan is not seen on the disc membranes. Bar: 1μm.

Group 2. There was not much difference in the kind and severity of degeneration at the equivalent stages between the retinas of rats on the vitamin A-free diet and those on the vitamin A deficient diet and injected with vitamin A acid.

Group 3. The electron micrographs of the retina of rats fed the usual diet showed no abnormal findings.

Discussion

Vitamin A as 11-cs-retinol plays a role for vision in the retina in transduction of light into the neural signals necessary for vision. The essential light-absorbing unit is composed of opsin, 11-cis-retinal bound to a protein, which is involved in the photoreceptor outer segment. In retinoid metabolism in vision, all-trans-retinal to retinol happens in the photoreceptor outer segment and its movement is processed across the photoreceptor space to the RPE cells by interphotorecepter retinoid-binding protein (IRBP) and a protein is present in the photoreceptor space. In the RPE cells, all-trans-retinol is esterified through a lecithin:retinol acyltransferase-mediated reaction, providing a local storage pool of retinyl ester that, when needed, is hydrolyzed and isomerized to form 11-cis-retinol (Ross, 1999).

The studies on the retina in vitamin A deficiency are those by Dowling and Wald (1960) and Dowling and Gibbons (1961) excel the others in a few respects. The first is that they used a vitamin A free diet supplemented with retinoic acid which allows rats to grow normally, but cannot enter into the visual cycle (Dowling and Wald, 1960). The second is that they discussed the electron microscopic findings in relation to the ERG findings in rats with hypovitaminosis A; the third is that histological and cytological changes in the retina of rats with vitamin A deficiency were studied and discussed on the basis of detailed measurements of the biochemical composition of the outer segments. Rats fed a vitamin A deficient diet grew less than those fed a vitamin A deficient diet and injected with retinoic acid. The former had dirty or rough fur, while the latter appeared normal. The ERG findings suggested, however, that the rats in both groups were night-blind (Dowling and Wald, 1960; Dowling and Gibbons, 1961). Not much difference in morphology could be detected by electron microscopy between rats on the vitamin A deficient diet and those with vitamin A acid supplementation. Thus retinoic acid maintains the growth of the rats, but the morphological findings in the retinas of rats with vitamin A deficiency are not affected by vitamin A acid.

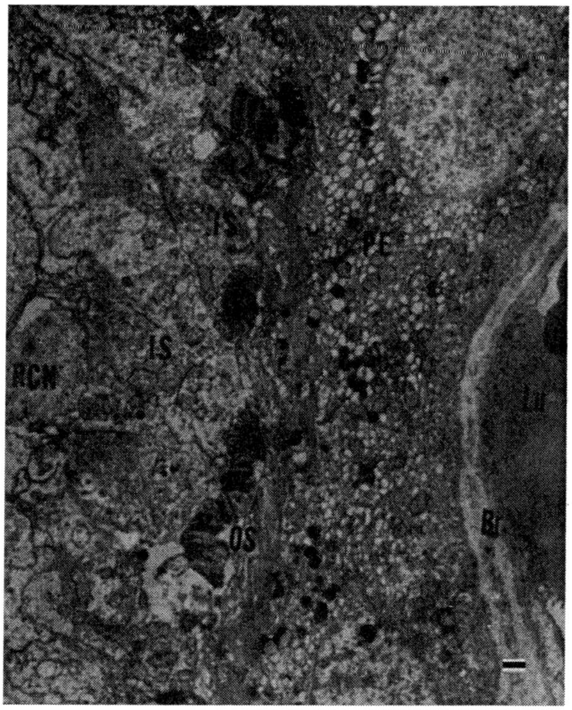

Figure 8.5.5. Electron micrograph of the retina of a rat fed a vitamin A deficient diet for 7 months. The inner segments (IS) are in contact with the RPE (PE) due to disappearance of the outer segments (OS). Only remnants of lamellar structures remain. The endoplasmic reticulum of the RPE is vacuolated and Müller's fibers show destruction in the terminal processes and among photoreceptor cell nuclei (RCN). El: Elastic zone, BM: Basement membrane, Br: Bruch's membrane, Lu: Lumen of the choriocapillary. Bar: 1 μm.

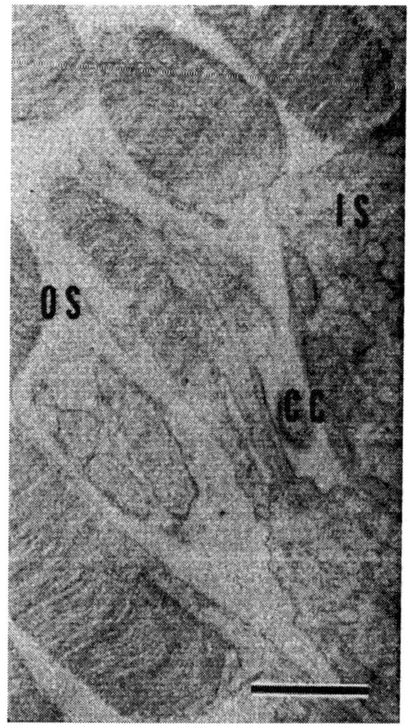

Figure 8.5.6. Electron micrograph of the retina of a rat treated with 5,000 I.U. of vitamin A for 16 days after about 6 months on the vitamin A deficient diet. An outer segment show a stage of regeneration. Bar: 1μm

The activity of alcohol dehydrogenase, which disappeared in the endoplasmic matrices of the RPE and inner segments and on the outer segment discs in 5 months of the deficient experiment (Amemiya, 1967a,c). This stage corresponded to the time of a lower or absent alcohol dehydrogenase requirement as the vitamin A stored in the RPE decreases or disappears. It is suggested that alcohol dehydrogenase remains in the outer and inner segments, allowing the physiological action of the scant amount of vitamin A left in the photoreceptor cells to continue until vitamin A deficiency is extreme. Alcohol dehydrogenase in the inner segments may lie in the endoplasmic reticulum near the outer segments, providing for more efficient utilization of working supplies of vitamin A and meeting the urgent need of vitamin A by the outer segments. These speculations are supported by the fact that alcohol dehydrogenase activity reappeared and returned to normal in the RPE and photoreceptor cells after recovery from vitamin A deficiency. The degeneration in vitamin A deficiency began in the RPE and then extended to the outer segments, while the inner segments remained rather normal in the later stages, and that regeneration during recovery from the deficiency also began in the RPE, because the RPE is related to the structural and functional maintenance of the outer segments (Bernstein, 1961; Wald, 1958). The elongated cilia began to protrude from occasional inner segments of the retina of rats treated with intraperitoneal injections of 5,000 I.U. of vitamin A for 2 days after vitamin A injection and those cilia contained vesicular materials and much alcohol dehydrogenase activity. It is well-known that the outer segments gradually differentiate at the distal end of the inner segments after the development of mitochondria and the Golgi complex in the inner segments (De Robertis, 1956; Samorajski, Keefe and Ordy, 1965). The mode of regeneration of the outer segments in recovery from vitamin A deficiency was similar to normal morphogenesis.

The Optic Nerve

Results

TEM Findings

After 4 months on a vitamin A deficient diet, rats showed that the postlaminar part of the optic nerve had a decreased amount of myelinated axons, irregularly arranged myelin lamellae, thinned myelin sheaths and proliferated glial cells (Fig. 8.6.1a). Axons contained vacuoles, destructed mitochondria and high density masses which looked like lipid debris or degenerated myelin lamellae. Neurotubules and neurofilaments were decreased (Fig. 8.6.1b). On the other hand, the optic nerve of control rats had many myelinated axons containing many neurotubulus and neurofilaments (Fig. 6.5.1A).

Discussion

Vitamin A is a fat soluble vitamin. Histochemical examination for the fat constitution in the retina showed that the retina of vitamin A deficient rats is stained weakly by all the staining methods examined (Amemiya, 1967b). On the other hand, the retina of rats with excess vitamin A is intensely stained: the specific finding is intense staining in the photoreceptor inner segment of vitamin A excessive rats despite of the fact of intense staining in the photoreceptor outer segment in normal rats and weak staining in vitamin A deficient rats (Amemiya, 1967b). There may be no evidence showing that vitamin A itself is related to the lipid metabolism. However, the reduction of fatty acids such as palmitic acid, stearic acid and oleic acid containing vitamin A may induce lipid degeneration of myelinated axons due to vitamin A deficiency. Vitamin A has an antioxidant action. Carotenoids, such as β-carotene, lycopene and some oxycarotenoids exert antioxidant functions in lipid phases by quenching $^1O_2$ or free radicals (Sies, Stahl and Sundquist, 1992). Thus vitamin A deficiency also has a possibility that myelin lamellae are broken by peroxidation of lipid membrane. Another possibility is that myelin degeneration may be secondary to retrograde degeneration of axons initiated by the decrease of retinal nerve fibers following to loss of photoreceptor cells due to vitamin A deficiency. Retinoids have been implicated in the development of the central nervous system (Morris-Kay and Sokolova, 1996). Thus vitamin A deficiency might disturb optic nerve development.

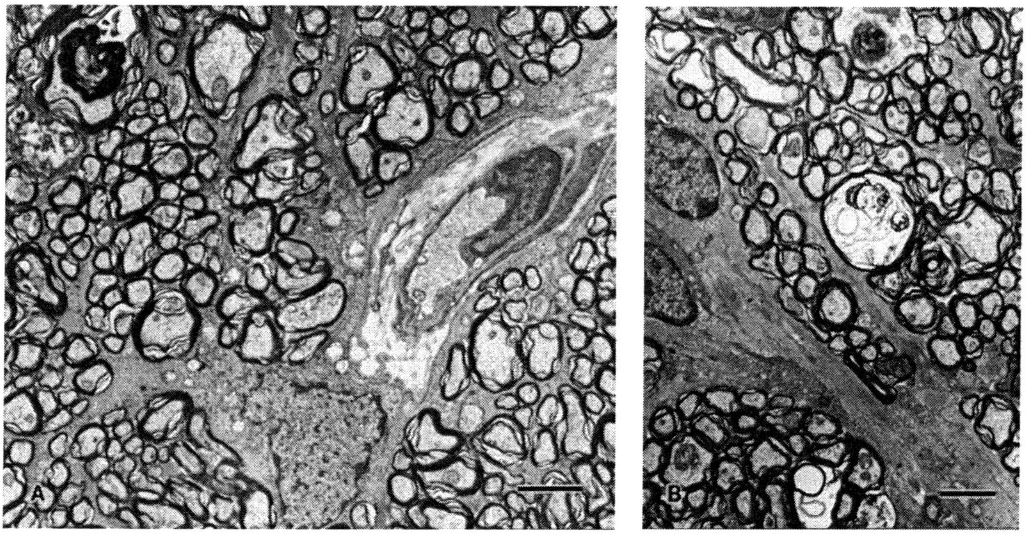

Figure 8.6.1. Electron micrographs of the optic nerve of a vitamin A deficient rat. The myelin sheath becomes thin and irregularly deformed. Glial proliferation is seen (A). Some axons show decrease or loss of microtubulus and neurofilaments, destructed mitochondria and cellular debris. Glial proliferation is seen (B). Bar: 2μm (A), 1μm (B).

PART 2. VITAMIN A EXCESS

I. Significance

Hypervitaminosis occurs due to acute or chronic overconsumption of preformed vitamin A (not carotenoids). Signs of toxicity are associated with chronic consumption of doses in excess of 10 times the RDA resulting from food faddism, e.g. excessive consumption of liver, or self-medication with high-dose vitamin A preparation (Ross, 1999). Signs and symptoms of retinoid toxicity are usually dose-dependent and are headache, vomiting, alopecia, dryness of mucous membranes, desquamation, bone and joint pain, liver disturbance, hemorrhage and coma. Ocular signs and symptoms include itching, particularly around the eye, conjunctivitis, blurred vision, double vision and papilledema.

In chronic hypervitaminosis A, holo-RBP in the plasma is not elevated, while retinyl esters are often increased markedly (Smith and Goodman, 1976). Retinyl esters can react more randomly with the membranes of cells than the physiologically sequestered retinol bound in holo-RBR. Thus circulating retinyl esters, by disrupting membrane functions, may well be a major toxic form of vitamin A (Olson, 1988). That is, hypervitaminosis A and vitamin A toxicity may be caused by steps that retinoids first break membranes of cells, insert into, then expand and destabilize membranes. Physiologic conditions or disease that enhance the plasma levels of lipoprotein-bound retinyl ester, therefore, may well increase the risk of vitamin A toxicity (Olson, 1988). The excessive dietary intake of carotenoids does not induce hypervitaminosis A, but induces hypercarotenosis which is rather benign. The long-term large daily therapeutic doses of some carotenoids can induce retinopathies (Olson, 1988).

Vitamin A and other carotenoids easily produce various kinds of malformations such as craniofacial anomalies, congenital heart disease, kidney defects, thymic abnormalities and central nervous system disorders. Synergistic actions between vitamin A and other teratogens including alcohol and drugs possibly induce malformation at nonteratogenic doses of each (Olson, 1988). The sclera of the eye is clear in hypercarotenosis unlike jaundice (Olson, 1988).

II. Vitamin A Excess Experiment

Materials and Methods

Female Wistar Kyoto rats were used. The animals were divided into six groups as follows:

Group 1 received 30,000 I.U. of vitamin A intraperitoneally each day for 8 days starting 25 to 30 days after birth.

Group 2 was injected intraperitoneally for 16 days with 10,000 I.U. of vitamin A daily starting 25 to 30 days after birth.

Group 3 was injected intraperitoneally for 30 days with 5,000 I.U. of vitamin A daily starting 25 to 30 days after birth.

Group 4 received intraperitoneal injections for 150 days of 500 I.U. of vitamin A daily after birth

Group 5 was fed a vitamin A deficient diet for 90 days starting 25 to 30 days after birth.

Group 6: control rats were fed the usual diet from 90 to 120 days after birth.

Clinical features of vitamin A excess animals

The rats injected daily with 30,000 I.U. or with 10,000 I.U. of vitamin A lost weight rapidly and died within 18 days. They showed inflammation of the conjunctiva, pseudoexophthalmos, paralysis of the limbs, and loss of hair starting a few days before death. The rats injected daily with less than 5,000 I.U. of vitamin A could survive more than 2 months, but their growth was stunted (Fig. 8.7.1.1). The above-mentioned signs of hypervitaminosis A appeared later.

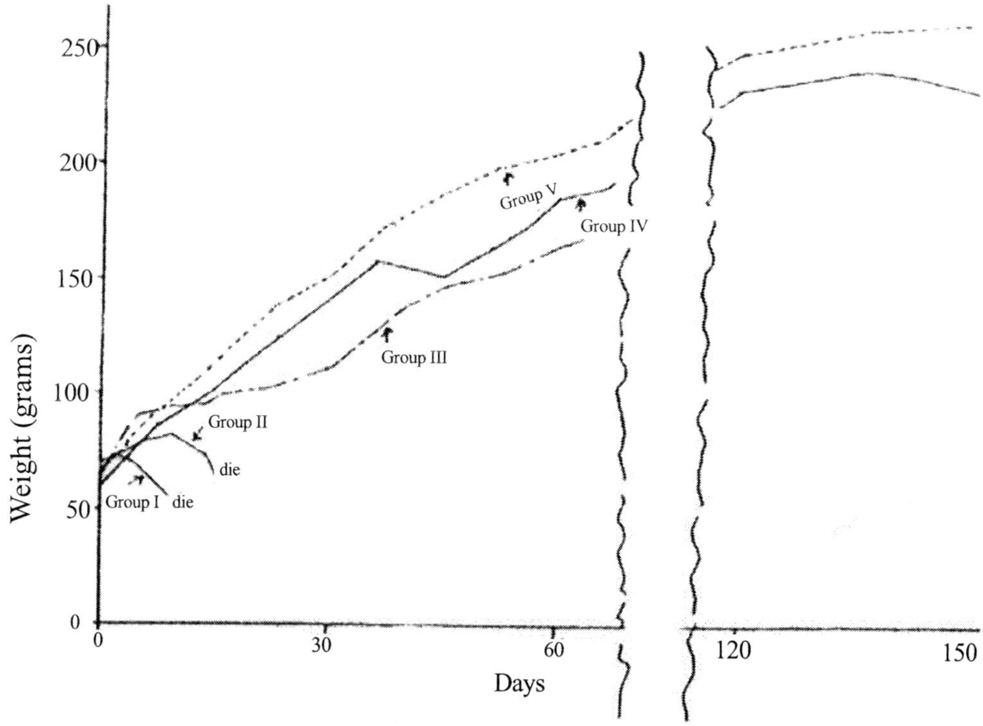

Figure 8.7.1.1. Growth of animals.

III. The Retina

Results

Histochemical Findings

The results obtained by the various histochemical staining methods and the lipid profiles in the retinas of each group are shown in Tables 8.7.2.1-4.

Sudan black B stained blue-black between the nuclei of the outer and inner nuclear layers, but not the nuclei.

Nile blue sulfate showed metachromasia between the nuclei of the outer and inner nuclear layers, that is, nile blue sulfate stained pink between the nuclei of the outer and inner nuclear layers. The nuclei of the outer and inner nuclear layers stained blue intensely or moderately with nile blue sulfate, but this staining of the nuclei does not mean the presence of fat, judging from the results of other stainings.

Table 8.7.1 The results of staining for lipids in retinas of normal, vitamin A excess and deficient rats

Retina	Staining methods / Groups	Sudan black B	Nile blue	Osmium tetroxide (primary blackening)	Okamoto et al's methods for cholesterin using: conc.sulphuric aciod	Okamoto et al's methods for cholesterin using: sulphuric acid-iodine tincture	Okamoto et al's method for fatty acid	Schultz's method for cholesterol	Okamoto et al's method for phosphatide (general, primary and secondary differential demonstrations)
Pigment epithelium	Normal	black (±)	blue (±)	brown (+)	(-)	(-)	(-)	(-)	royal purple (±)
	Hyper vitaminosis A	black (±)	blue (±)	dark brown - brown	(-)	(-)	(-)	(-)	royal purple (±)
	Hypovitaminosis A	black (±)	blue (±)	brown (±)	(-)	(-)	(-)	(-)	royal purple (±)
Outer segment	Normal	black (+++)	blue (++)	brown (+—++)	(-)	(-)	(-)	(-)	royal purple (+++)
	Hypervitaminosis A	black(++—+++)	blue (+—++)	dark brown—brown	(-)	(-)	(-)	(-)	royal purple (++—+)**
	Hypovitamiinosis A	black (++)	blue (+)	brown (+)	(-)	(-)	(-)	(-)	royal purple (+)
Inner segment	Normal	black (++)	blue (+)	brown (+—++)	(-)	(-)	(-)	(-)	royal purple (++)
	Hypervitaminosis A	black(+—++)	blue (+)	brown (+—++)	(-)	(-)	(-)	(-)	royal purple (+++—++)
	Hypovitaminosis A	black (+)	blue (±)	brown (±—+)	(-)	(-)	(-)	(-)	royal purple (+)
Outer nuclear layer	Normal	black* (±)	blue** (+++), pink*	dark brown***	(-)	(-)	(-)	(-)	(-)
	Hypervitaminosis A	black* (±)	blue** (+++), pink*	dark brown***	(-)	(-)	(-)	(-)	(-)
	Hypovitaminosis A	black* (±)	blue** (++), pink*	brown (++)***	(-)	(-)	(-)	(-)	(-)
Outer plexiform layer	Normal	black (++)	(-)	brown (+—++)	(-)	(-)	(-)	(-)	royal purple (++—+++)
	Hypervitaminosis A	black(+—++)	(-)	brown (+—++)	(-)	(-)	(-)	(-)	royal purple (++—+)
	Hypovitaminosis A	black (+)	(-)	brown (+)	(-)	(-)	(-)	(-)	royal purple (+)

Table 8.7.1 The results of staining for lipids in retinas of normal, vitamin A excess and deficient rats (continued)

Retina	Staining methods / Groups	Sudan black B	Nile blue	Osmium tetroxide (primary blackening)	Okamoto et al's methods for cholesterin using		Okamoto et al's method for fatty acid	Schultz's method for cholesterol	Okamoto et al's method for phosphatide (general, primary and secondary differential demonstrations)
					conc.sulphuric aciod	sulphuric acid-iodine tincture			
Inner nuclear layer	Normal	black* (±)	blue** (++), pink*	dark brown***	(-)	(-)	(-)	(-)	(-)
	Hypervitaminosis A	black* (±)	blue** (+—++), pink*	dark brown***	(-)	(-)	(-)	(-)	(-)
	Hypovitaminosis A	black* (±)	blue** (+), pink*	brown (+)	(-)	(-)	(-)	(-)	(-)
Inner plexiform layer	Normal	black (++)	(-)	brown (+)	(-)	(-)	(-)	(-)	royal purple (+)
	Hypervitaminosis A	black(+—++)	(-)	brown (+)	(-)	(-)	(-)	(-)	royal purple (+—++)
	Hypovitaminosis A	black (+)	(-)	brown (±)	(-)	(-)	(-)	(-)	royal purple (+)
Ganglion cell layer	Normal	black (+)	blue (±)	dark brown	(-)	(-)	(-)	(-)	(±)
	Hypervitaminosis A	black (+)	blue (±)	dark brown—brown	(-)	(-)	(-)	(-)	(±)
	Hypovitaminosis A	black (+)	blue (±)	brown (- - ±)	(-)	(-)	(-)	(-)	(±)

The designations refer to the intensity of staining where: - is unstained; ± is questionable and faint; + is weak; ++ is moderate; +++ is intense.
*, *** Sudan black B and osmium tetroxide stained the fibers between the nuclei of the outer and inner nuclear layers.
**, * With nile blue sulfate, the nuclei stained blue, and the fibers between the nuclei stained pink.
** See text.

Table 8.7.2 Lipid profiles of retinas

Retina	Experimental Conditions	Fat Constitution
Pigment epithelium	Normal	Phosphatide (S. & L.) (+), Fatty acid (+)
	Hypervitaminosis A	Phosphatide (S. & L.) (+), Fatty acid (+)
	Hypovitaminosis A	Phosphatide (S. & L.) (±), Fatty acid (±)
Outer segment	Normal	Phosphatide (S. & L.) (+++), Fatty acid (++)
	Hypervitaminosis A	Phosphatide (S. & L.) (+—++), Fatty acid (+—++)
	Hypovitaminosis A	Phosphatide (S. & L.) (+), Fatty acid (+)
Inner segment	Normal	Phosphatide (S. & L.) (++), Fatty acid (+)
	Hypervitaminosis A	Phosphatide (S. & L.) (++—+++), Fatty acid (+—++)
	Hypovitaminosis A	Phosphatide (S. & L.) (+), Fatty acid (±)
Outer nuclear layer	Normal	Neutral fat (+)
	Hypervitaminosis A	Neutral fat (+)
	Hypovitaminosis A	Neutral fat (±—+)
Outer plexiform layer	Normal	Phosphatide (S. & L.) (++—+++)
	Hypervitaminosis A	Phosphatide (S. & L.) (+—++)
	Hypovitaminosis A	Phosphatide (S. & L.) (+)
Inner nuclear layer	Normal	Neutral fat (+)
	Hypervitaminosis A	Neutral fat (+)
	Hypovitaminosis A	Neutral fat (- —±)
Inner plexiform layer	Normal	Phosphatide (S. & L.) (+)
	Hypervitaminosis A	Phosphatide (S. & L.) (+—++)
	Hypovitaminosis A	Phosphatide (S. & L.) (+)
Ganglion cell layer	Normal	Fatty acid (+), Phosphatide (±)
	Hypervitaminosis A	Fatty acid (+), Phosphatide (±)
	Hypovitaminosis A	Fatty acid (±), Phosphatide (±)

The designations refer to the intensity of staining where: ± is questionable and faint; + is weak; ++ is moderate; +++ is intense.

S. is sphingomyelin; L. is lecithin.

Table 8.7.3 Results of staining for lipids in normal retinas

Retina	Staining methods / Authors	Sudan III	Nile blue sulfate	Neutral rot	Osmium tetroxide	Smith-Dietrich	Ciaccio	Fischler	Colodetz	Double refraction
Pigment epithelium	Sugita	Yellowish red (±)	blue	pink (±)			(+)	(+)	(-)	
	Maki	Yellowish red	blue (±)	pink (±)	dark brown	(+)	(+)	dark purple	(-)	(-)
	Majima	Yellowish red	blue	pink (±)	black	(±)	(+)	(+)	(-)	(-)
Outer segment	Sugita	Yellowish red (±)	blue	pink (±)		purple	(+)	(+)	(-)	(+)
	Maki	Yellowish red	blue	pink (±)	dark brown	blue black	bright orange	(+)	(-)	(-)
	Majima	Yellowish red	blue	pink (+)	black	(±) (+)	(+)	(+)	(-)	(+)
Inner segment	Sugita	Yellowish red (±)	blue (±)	pink (±)		Purple (±)	(+)	(-)	(-)	(-)
	Maki	Yellowish red (±)	blue	pink (±)	grey	blue black	bluish yrllow	(-)	(-)	(-)
	Majima	Yellowish red (±)	blue (±)	pink (±)	grey	(+)	(+)	(±)	(-)	(-)
Outer nuclear layer	Sugita	Yellowish red (±)	blue	pink		purple	(+)		(-)	(-)
	Maki	Yellowish red — (-)	blue(±)	pink (±)	grey	blue black	yellowish blue (±)	(-)	(-)	(-)
Outer plexiform layer	Sugita			pink (±)		purple	(+)		(-)	(-)
	Maki	Yellowish red	blue pink (±)	(-)	grey	blue black	(±)	(-)	(-)	(-)
Inner nuclear layer	Sugita		blue	pink		(+)	(+)	(-)	(-)	(-)
	Maki	Yellowish red — (-)	blue (±)	pink	grey	blue black	yellowish blue (±)	(-)	(-)	(-)
Inner plexiform layer	Sugita	Yellowish red (±)	(-)	pink (±)		(-)	(-)	(-)	(-)	(-)
	Maki	Yellowish red	blue pink (±)	(-)	grey	blue black	bluish yellow	(-)	(-)	(-)
Ganglion cell layer	Sugita	Yellowish red (±)	blue (±)	pink (±)		(+)	(+)	(-)	(-)	(+)
	Maki	Yellowish red — (-)	blue (±)	pink	grey	blue black	yellowish blue (±)	(-)	(-)	(-)
Nerve fiber layer	Sugita	Yellowish red (±)	blue (±)	pink (±)		(+)	(+)	(-)	(-)	(-)
	Maki	Yellowish red	blue pink (±)	(±)	grey	blue black	bluish yellow	(-)	(-)	(-)

Materials: Sugita; albino mouse, albino rat, albino rabbit, guinea pig, and monkey.
Maki; frog., Majima; frog.

The designations: - is unstained or negative; ± is weak; + is stained or positive.

Table 8.7.4 Lipid profiles in retinas examined histochemically

Authors	Sugita	Maki	Oguchi	Majima	Yamamoto
Animals / Retina	albino mouse, albino rat, albino rabbit, guinea pig, monkey	frog	frog	frog	chicken
Pigment epithelium	cephalin, soaps, fatty acid	cephalin, soaps, fatty acid		cephalin, soaps, fatty acid	
Outer segment	sphingomyelin, cephalin, fatty acid, cerebroside	neutral fat, cephalin, soaps, fatty acid	cholesterin, cephalin, soaps	cephalin, soaps, fatty acid	phospholipid
Inner segment	cephalin	cephalin	lipoid	cephalin	phospholipid
Outer nuclear layer	—	cephalin			
Outer plexiform layer	—	cholesterin, glyceryl esters			phospholipid
Inner nuclear layer	cephalin	cephalin			
Inner plexiform layer	—	cholesterin, glyceryl esters			phospholipid
Ganglion cell layer	sphingomyelin, cerebroside, cephalin	cephalin			phospholipid
Nerve fiber layer	cephalin	cephalin, cholesterin, glyceryl esters			

The method by Okamoto et al for general phosphatide demonstrated intense staining of the photoreceptor outer segment and outer plexiform layer in the control rat retina, moderate staining of the photoreceptor inner segment, and faint staining of the pigment epithelium and inner plexiform layer (Fig. 8.7.2.1). The outer and inner nuclear layers contained no phosphatide. The primary and secondary demonstrations of differential methods for phosphatide by the same workers showed the presence of lecithin and sphingomyelin in the same layers as in those demonstrated by the general method. That is, there was not much difference in intensity of staining in each layer of the control rat retina among the general and differential demonstrations, but the intensity of staining in the secondary differential demonstration was greater than in the primary. In some retinas of rats receiving intraperitoneal injections of 500 I.U. of vitamin A for 150 days or 30,000 I.U. for 8 days, the method of Okamoto et al for phosphatide demonstrated intense staining of the photoreceptor inner segment and moderate to faint staining of the outer segment (Fig. 8.7.2.2).

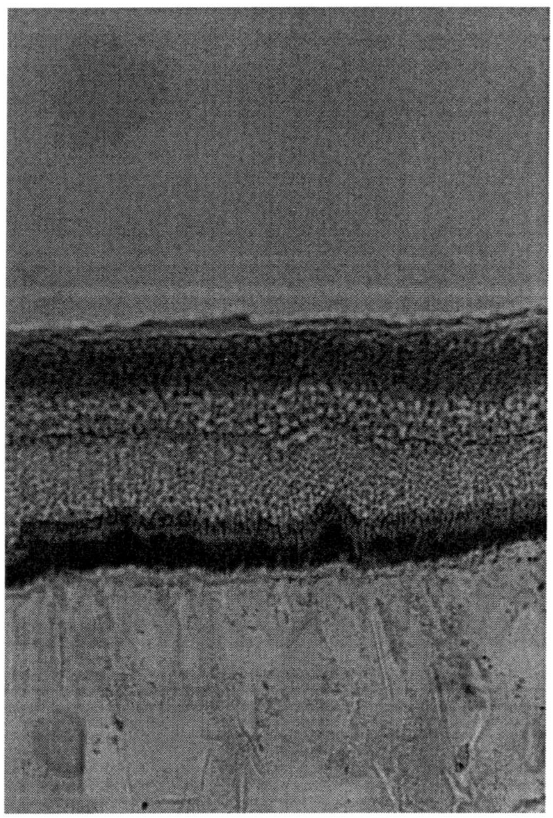

Figure 8.7.2.1. Light micrograph of the retinas stained by Okamoto et al's method for general phosphatide. The photoreceptor outer segment layer shows intense staining in a control rat retina. × 200.

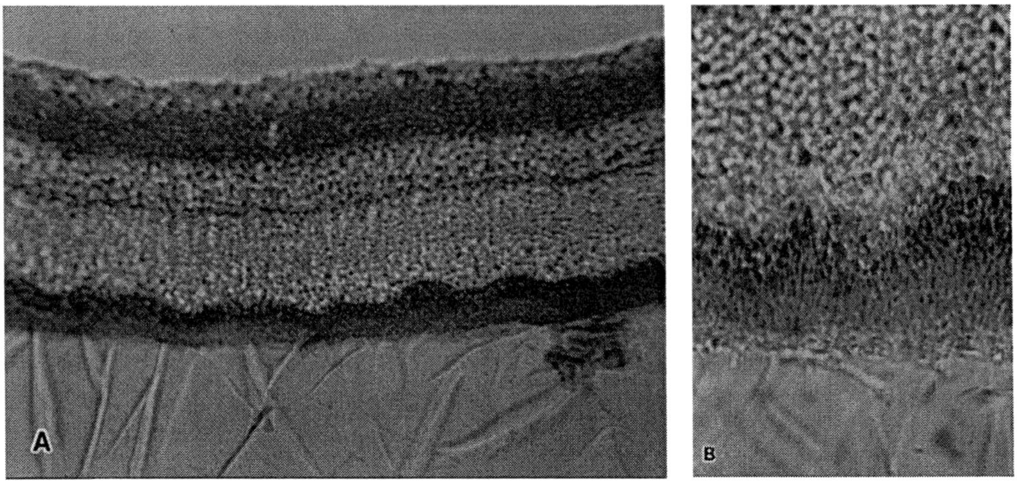

Figure 8.7.2.2. Light micrographs of the retina of a vitamin A excess rat. Okamoto et al's staining method for lecithin and sphingomyelin shows intense staining in the inner segment layer(A,B) A: × 200, B: × 400.

The retinas of rats with vitamin A deficiency showed low stainability in all of the fat staining methods, suggesting low lipid concentration. But no changes were observed in the fat constitution in each layer of the retina.

Schultz's method for cholesterol did not demonstrate the presences of cholesterol in the retinas of control rats or those with hypo- or hyper-vitaminosis A.

The methods for cholesterin by Okamoto et al using conc. sulphuric acid or sulphuric acid-iodine tincture failed to demonstrate cholesterin in any of the rat retinas.

Electron microscopic findings

Group 1: In rats intraperitoneally injected with 30,000 I.U. of vitamin A daily starting 25 to 30 days after birth, the RPE showed slightly higher electron density of the cytoplasmic membrane and many lipid droplets, and ribosomes were increased in the inner segments (Fig.8.7.2.3). Mitochondria were swollen and destroyed in the RPE and the inner segments.

Group 2: In rats intraperitoneally injected with 10,000 I.U. of vitamin A daily starting 25 to 30 days after birth, many lipid droplets and ribosomes appeared in the RPE (Fig. 8.7.2.4). In the outer segments their fine structure appeared to remain normal. In the RPE and the inner segments mitochondria were swollen and destroyed.

Group 3: In rats killed after 30 days of intraperitoneal injections with 5,000 I.U. of vitamin A, the RPE epithelium had many ribosomes and lipid droplets, which were different in shape and electron density from those in group 2 (Fig. 8.7.2.5). In rats killed 70 days after stopping the injections of 5,000 I.U. of vitamin A for 30 days, no difference in electron micrographs could be noted in the RPE or in the photoreceptor cells, compared with those of rats injected intraperitoneally for 30 days with 5,000 I.U. of vitamin A.

Group 4: In rats injected intraperitoneally for 150 days with 500 I.U. of vitamin A starting 25 to 30 days after birth, the RPE showed increased ribosomes. The photoreceptor cell outer segments showed no abnormalities. Mitochondria were swollen and destructed in the RPE and the inner segments.

Group 5: Control rats showed no abnormal changes in the RPE and the photoreceptor cells.

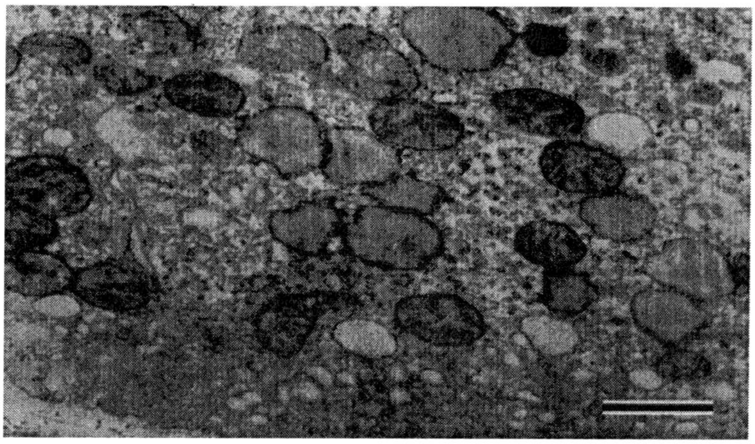

Figure 8.7.2.3. Electron micrograph of the RPE of the retina of a rat with intraperitoneal injection of 30,000 I.U. of vitamin A for 8 days. Many lipid droplets and ribosomes appear in the RPE, which shows increased electron density. Bar: 1μm.

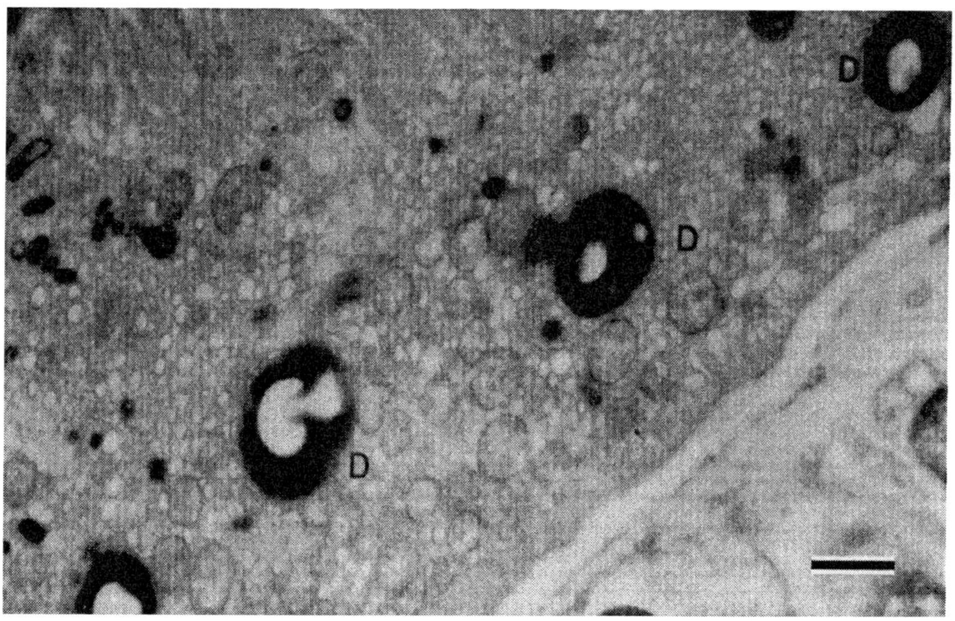

Figure 8.7.2.4. Electron micrograph of the RPE of the retina of a rat killed after 16 days of intraperitoneal injections with 10,000 I.U. of vitamin A (group 2). The RPE shows increased electron density and many lipid droplets (D). Bar: 1μm

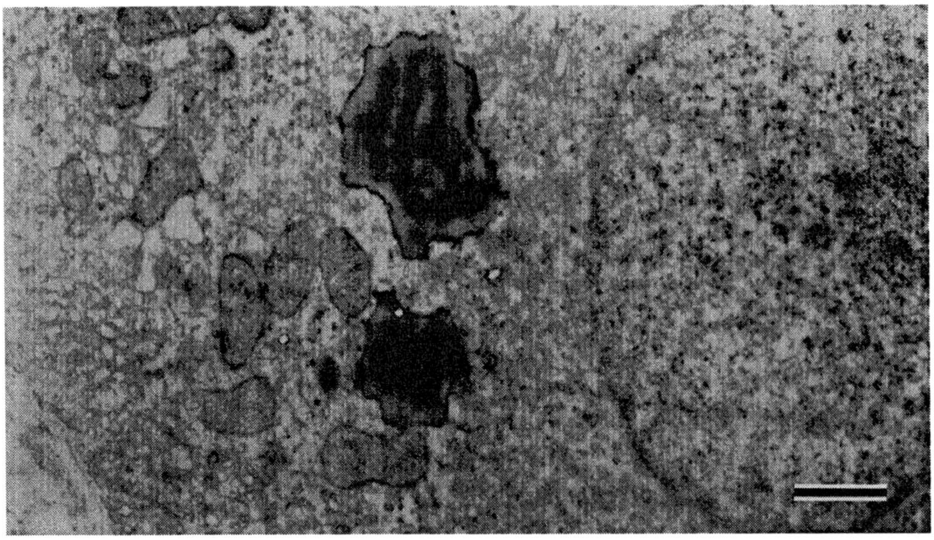

Figure 8.7.2.5. Electron micrograph of the RPE of the retina of a rat killed after 30 days of intraperitoneal injections with 5,000 I.U. of vitamin A (Group 3a). The RPE has lipid droplets, which are different in shape and electron density from those observed in Figs 8.7.2, 3,4. Bar: 1μm.

Alcohol dehydrogenase cytochemistry

Alcohol dehydrogenase activity, as evidenced by deposits of TNBT-formazan, was scarce in the RPE in all hypervitaminosis A groups (Amemiya, 1967), and there was not much difference in the enzymatic activity of the alcohol dehydrogenase system in the RPE between the control and recovering groups (Fig. 8.7.2.6).

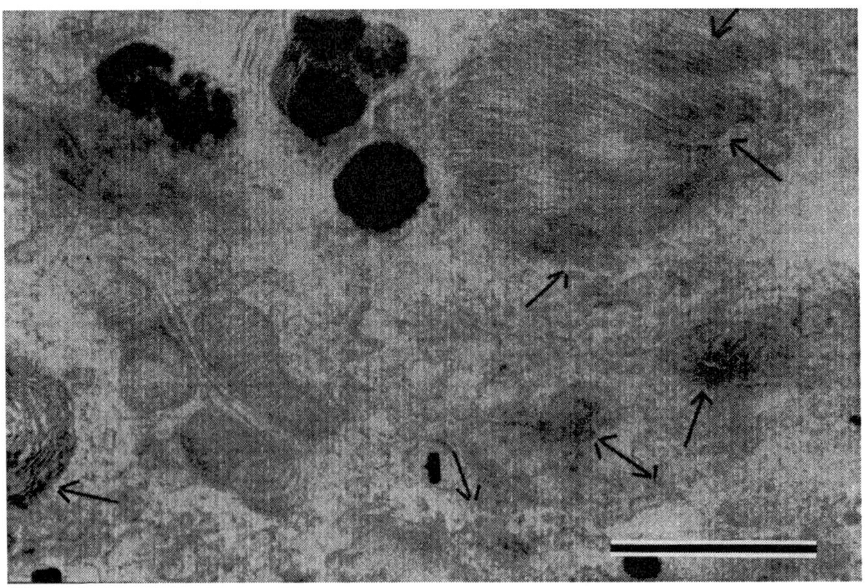

Figure 8.7.2.6. Aggregates of TNBT-formazan (arrows) in the preparation incubated in the medium for alcohol dehydrogenase are mainly in the endoplasmic reticulum, especially in the cytoplasmic matrix adjacent to mitochondria, and less frequently of the outer and inner limiting membranes of mitochondria and cristae mitochondriales. Bar: 1μm.

In the retinal photoreceptor cells of rats receiving intraperitoneal injections of 30,000 I.U. of vitamin A for 8 days or 10,000 I.U. for 16 days, alcohol dehydrogenase activity, as evidenced by deposits of TNBT-formazan, was in the same location as in the control group, and no considerable difference in amount was noted between the control and vitamin A excess groups (Fig. 8.7.2.7). But in the rats killed on the 30th day of daily injection with 5,000 I.U. of vitamin A, enzymatic activity of the alcoholic dehydrogenase system as aggregates of TNBT-formazan could not be found in the endoplasmic reticulum or in or on mitochondrial profiles of the inner segments (Fig. 8.7.2.8). In the photoreceptor cells on the 70th day after recovering from vitamin A excess, enzymatic activity of the alcohol dehydrogenase system as deposits of TNBT-formazan reappeared in the same location as in the control group (Fig. 8.7.9), and no difference in amounts was noted between the control and recovering groups.

Discussion

According to Moore (1964), the continuation of overdosing causes vitamin A to spill over into the kidney, lungs, adrenal cortices and probably into the retina, and when the absorptive power of the liver is completely overwhelmed, frozen sections clearly demonstrate the accumulation of large masses of lipids, presumably mostly vitamin A, around the Kupffer cells of the liver.

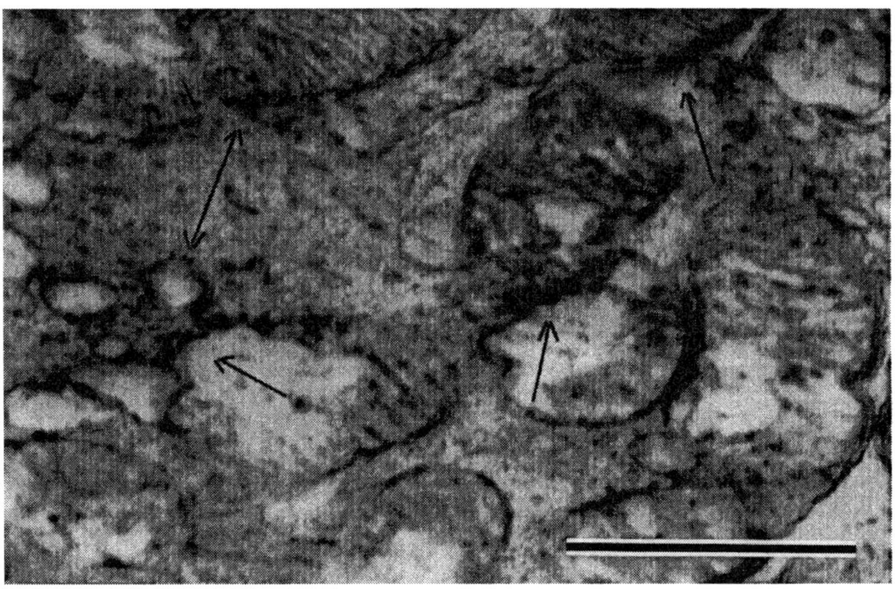

Figure 8.7.2.7. Electron micrograph shows the activity of alcohol dehydrogenase, as evidenced by deposits of TNBT-formazan (arrows) in the RPE of a rat recovered from vitamin A deficiency. Aggregates of TNBT-formazan reappear in the same location as in the control group, and there is not much difference in amount between the normal and recovering groups. Bar: 0.5μm.

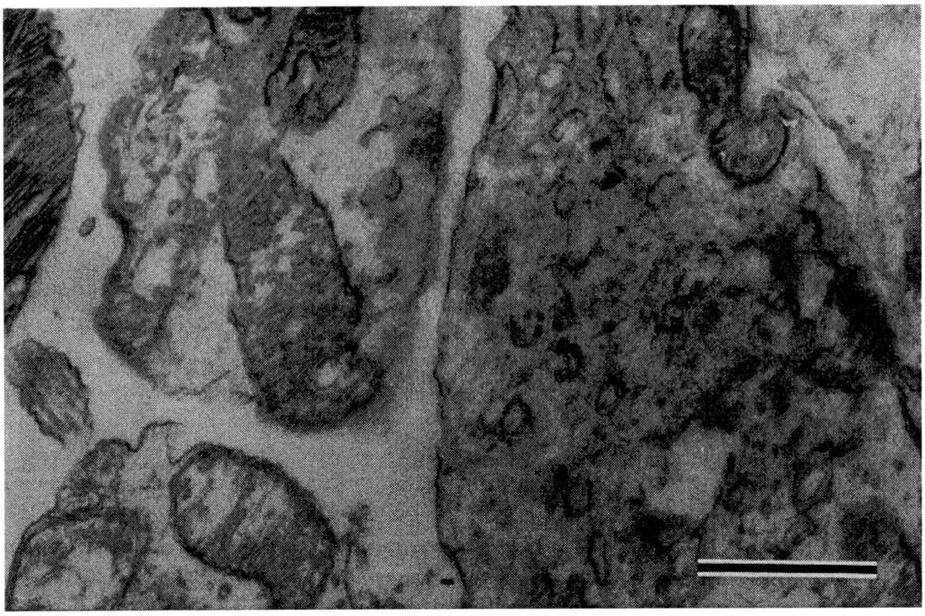

Figure 8.7.2.8. Electron micrograph of the enzymatic activity of alcohol dehydrogenase in the inner segment of the retina of a rat killed on the 30th day of daily injection with 5,000 I.U of vitamin A. Alcohol dehydrogenase activity as aggregates of TNBT-formazan cannot be found in the endoplasmic reticulum or in or on mitochondrial profiles of the inner segment. Bar: 1μm.

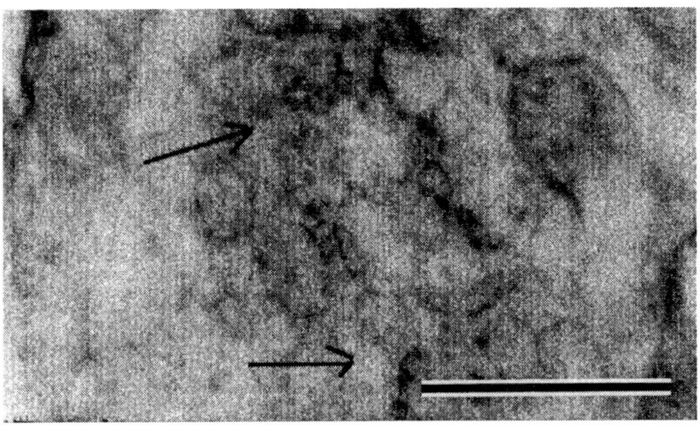

Figure 8.7.2.9. Electron micrograph of alcohol dehydrogenase activity in the inner segment of the retina of a rat on 70th day after recovering from vitamin A excess. Alcohol dehydrogenase activity as deposits of TNBT-formazan (arrows) reappears in the same location as in the control group, and no difference in amount is noted between the control and recovering groups. Bar: 1μm.

Lipids comprise about 20% of the dry weight of the retina; the nerve fiber layer contains 34%, the photoreceptors 22-25% and the outer nuclear layer 12% (Lowry, Roberts and Lewis, 1956). Phospholipids constitute the major class of lipids, about 65-75% of the total, followed by cholesterol (10-12%), diglycerides, triglycerides, free fatty acids (5-7% each), and sphingolipids (2%) (Fliesler and Schroepfer, 1982; Bazan, Reddy, Redmond et al, 1985).

Phosphatidyl-choline (PC) and phosphatidylethanolamine (PE) account for about 80% of the total phospholipids (Anderson, Maude and Zimmerman, 1975).

The major saturated fatty acids in the retina are palmitic (16:0) and stearic (18:0). Palmitic acid is high in PC, stearic acid in PE and PS (phosphatidylserine) (Bergman, 1991). Histochemistry can demonstrate phospholipids, but not individual fatty acids. On the other hand, the retina has the highest content of unsaturated fatty acids in the body; in most species over 50% of these fatty acids are unsaturated, and about 60% of these are polyunsaturated (Bergman, 1991).

Krause (1935) showed that the cattle retina was characterized by its very high proportion of lecithin and its overall high content of phospholipids. The current histochemical data showed that the principal phospholipids in the retina are sphingomyelin and lecithin. The presence of sphingomyelin and lecithin in the retina, especially in the outer segment, should be emphasized in respect to their high contents and specific changes in the fat constitution of the retina in hypervitaminosis A.

The lipid profile of the retina in hypervitaminosis A in the current study was similar to that of the control retina except for a few changes. In some rats injected daily with 30,000 I.U. of vitamin A for 8 days or 500 I.U. for 150 days, phosphatide increased in the inner segment while it decreased strikingly in the outer segment, but in other cases various staining techniques showed no remarkable difference between vitamin A excess and control rats.

Many of the changes in hypervitaminosis A can be explained on the hypothesis that vitamin A penetrates lipoprotein membranes and that membranes containing an excess of the vitamin exhibit increased permeability or decreased stability (Smith and Goodmar, 1976; Olson, 1988).

Electron micrographs of the retina of rats with vitamin A excess showed many lipid droplets, increased ribosomes and slight destruction of the mitochondrial structure in the retinal pigment epithelium, and increased ribosomes and destructed mitochondria. The photoreceptor outer segment showed no abnormalities except higher electron density of discs. Higher electron density in photoreceptor cell outer segment discs of rats with vitamin A excess may be due to the lipids combined with vitamin A, i.e. for the most part, palmitic acid. Many studies (Lucy, Luscombe and Dingle, 1963) have shown that penetration of the lipoprotein membrane of isolated mitochondria from the liver induces the most rapid mitochondrial swelling by vitamin A and mitochondria from the spleen and the brain are the least affected by vitamin A and that these results reflect differences in the lipoprotein membranes of mitochondria of various tissues and hence a difference in the ability of vitamin A to penetrate these membranes. There was no action of vitamin A on mitochondria isolated from cattle retina and further it was noted that the swelling in retinal mitochondria induced by thyroxine and calcium was less than that in liver mitochondria under similar conditions.

The appearance of many droplets and increased electron density in the retinal pigment epithelium and the outer segment discs appear to be in harmony with the results of histochemical demonstrations of fatty constitution in the retina of rats with vitamin A excess.

Lucy et al (1963) have described the possibility and the fact that the absence of vitamin A in hypovitaminosis A as well as its excess in hypervitaminosis A leads to distortion of the mitochondrial structure (Sheldon and Zetterqvist, 1955). The current experiments confirmed these facts and possibilities with the electron microscope.

In rats injected intraperitoneally with 30,000 I.U. of vitamin A for 8 days or 10,000 I.U. for 16 days, alcohol dehydrogenase activity decreased or disappeared in the pigment epithelium, but appeared to remain normal in photoreceptor cells. In rats injected intraperitoneally for 30 days with 5,000 I.U. of vitamin A, alcohol dehydrogenase activity disappeared in both the retinal pigment epithelium and photoreceptor cells. These facts suggest that the pigment epithelium is affected more readily than the photoreceptor cells and that the rats injected daily with more than 10,000 I.U. of vitamin A die before severe damage can appear in the retina. If vitamin A were permitted to accumulate by the excessive intake of vitamin A, it would not only distort the mitochondrial structure, but also inhibit the neighboring enzymes, and thereby act as a toxic agent in the retina.

The disappearance and reappearance of alcohol dehydrogenase activity in the retinal pigment epithelium and photoreceptor cells of rats with vitamin A excess are not inconsistent with the ERG findings reported by Dowling and Gibbons (1961): a diminution of a- and b-waves and disappearance of c- wave.

REFERENCES

Amemiya T. Alcohol dehydrogenase system in the pigment epithelium of the rat retina --- normal, hypo- and hypervitaminosis A. *Acta Soc Ophthalmol Jpn.* 1967a;71:2115-2123.

Amemiya T. Histochemical examination of retinas of rats with vitamin A excess and deficiency. Report 2. Effect of vitamin A on the fat constitution in the retina. *Acta Soc Ophthalmol Jpn.* 1967b;71:2203-2211.

Amemiya T. Cytochemical and electron microscopic examination of the retina of rats with hypervitaminosis A. *Acta Soc Ophthalmol Jpn.* 1967c;71:2236-2251.

Amemiya T. Cytochemical and electron microscopic examination of the retina of rats with hypovitaminosis A. *Acta Soc Ophthalmol Jpn.* 1968;72:1074-1099.

Amemiya T. Postnatal development of photoreceptor outer segments of vitamin A deficient rats. In *22nd International Congress of Ophthalmology Concilium.* 1976;2:171-179.

Amemiya T. Postnatal maldevelopment of the retina. *Biol Neonate.* 1977a;32:319-326.

Amemiya T. The effect of vitamin A deficiency during the fetal and early postnatal periods on development of the photoreceptor cells and the retinal pigment epithelium of the rat. *Acta Soc Ophthalmol Jpn.* 1977b;81:347-354.

Anderson RE, Maude MB, Zimmerman W. Lipids in ocular tissues. X. Lipid composition of subcellular fractions of bovine retina. *Vision Res.* 1975;15:1087-1090.

Anderson JA, Richard NR, Rock ME. Requirement of human cornea. *Invest Ophthalmol Vis Sci.* 1993;34:3442-3449.

Arens JF, van Dorp DA. Synthesis of some compounds possessing vitamin A activity. *Nature.* 1946;157:190-191.

Bazan NG, Reddy TS, Redmond TM, Wiggert B, Chader GJ. Endogenous fatty acids are covalently and noncovalently bound to interphotoreceptor retinoid-bounding protein in the monkey retina. *J Biol Chem.* 1985;260:13677-13680.

Bergman ER. Biochemistry of the Eye. New York: Plenum; 1991:343-345.

Bernstein MH. Functional architecture of the retinal epithelium. In Smelser GK, ed. *The Structure of the Eye.* New York:Academic Press Inc;1961:139-150.

Carter-Dawson L, Tanaka M, Kuwabara T, Bieri JG. Early corneal changes in vitamin A-deficient rats. *Exp Eye Res.* 1980;30:261-268.

Chambon P. A decade of molecular biology of retinoic acid receptors. *FASEB.* 1996;10:940-954.

De Robertis E. Morphogenesis of the retinal rods; an electron microscope study. *J Biophys Biochem Cytol.* 1956;2(Suppl):209-218.

Dowling JE, Wald G. The biological function of vitamin A acid. Proc Natl Acad Sci USA. 1960;46:587-608.

Dowling JE, Gibbons IR. The effect of vitamin A deficiency on the fine structure of the eye. In: Smelser GK, ed. *The Structure of the eye.* New York:Academic Press Inc;1961:85-99.

Fliesler SJ, Schroepfer GJ Jr. Sterol composition of bovine retinal rod outer segment membranes and whole retinas. *Biochim Biophys Acta.* 1982;711:138-148.

Hatchell DU, Sommer A. Detection of ocular surface abnormalities in experimental vitamin A deficiency. *Arch Ophthalmol.* 1984;102:1389-1393.

Hatchell DU, Ubels JL, Stekiel, Hatchell MC. Corneal epithelial wound healing in normal and diabetic rabbits treated with tretionin. *Arch Ophthalmol.* 1985;103:98-100.

Huang AI, Tseng S, Kenyon KR. Changes of paracellular permeability of ocular surface epithelium by vitamin A deficiency. *Invest Ophthalmol Vis Sci.* 1991;32:633-639.

Kobayashi TK, Tsubota K, Takamura E, Sawa M, Ohashi Y, Usui M. Effect of retinol palmitate as a treatment for dry eye: a cytological evaluation. *Ophthalmologica.* 1997;211:358-361.

Krause AC. The lipids of the retina. *Acta Ophthalmol.* 1934;12:372-374

Lee S-Y, Ubels JL, Soprano DR. The lacrimal gland synthesizes retinal-binding protein. Exp Eye Res. 1992;55:163-171.

Lowry OH, Roberts NR, Lewis C. The quantitative histochemistry of the retina. *J. Biol Chem.* 1956;220:879-892.

Lucy JA, Luscombe M, Dingle JT. Studies on the mode of action of excess of vitamin A. 8. Mitochondrial swelling. *Biochem J.* 1963;89:419-425.

McCaffery P, Dräger UC. Retinoic acid synthesing enzymes in the embryonic and adult vertebrate In: Weiner H, Holmes RS, Wermuth B, ed. *Enzymology and molecular biology of carbonyl metabolism 5.* New York: Plenum Press;1995:173-183.

Moore T. Systemic action of vitamin A. *Exp Eye Res.* 1964;3:305-315.

Morriss-Kay GM, Sokolova N. Embryonic development and pattern formation. FASEB. 1996;10:961-968.

Oba K, Gong H, Amemiya T, Baba K. Role of trace elements in goblet cells in vitamin A deficient rats. *Biomed Res Trace Elements.* 1998;9:173-174.

Oba K, Gong H, Amemiya T, Baba K, Takaya K. Applying secondary ion mass spectrometry to the analysis of elements in goblet cells of conjunctiva. *J Electron Microsc.* 2001;50:325-332.

Olson JA. Vitamin A excess. In: Shils ME, Young VR, ed. *Modern Nutrition in Health and Disease.* 7th ed. Philadelphia:Lea & Febriger;1988:292-312.

Orfanos CE, Zoubaulis CC, Almond-Roes B, Geilen CC. Current use and future potential role of retinoids in dermatology. *Drugs.* 1997;53:358-388.

Pirie A. Effect of vitamin A deficiency on the cornea. *Trans Ophthalmol Soc* UK. 1978;98:357-360.

Pfister RP, Renner ME. The corneal and conjunctival surface in vitamin A deficiency. *Invest Ophthalmol Vis Sci.* 1978;17:874-883.

Reeves PG, Nielsen FH, Fahey GC Jr. AIN-93 purified diets for laboratory rodents: final report of the American Institute of Nutrition ad hoc writing committee on the reformulation of the AIN-76A rodent diet. *J Nutr.* 1993;123:1939-1951.

Ross AC. Vitamin A and retinoids. In: Shils ME, Olson JA, Shike M, Ross C, ed. *Modern Nutrition in Health and Disease.* 9th ed. Philadelphia: Lippincott Williams & Wilkins; 1999:305-327.

Samorajski T, Keefe JR, Ordy JM. Morphogenesis of photoreceptor and retinal ultrastructure in a sub-human primate. *Vision Res.* 1965;5:639-648.

Shams NBK, Hanninen LA, Chaves HV. Effect of vitamin A deficiency on the adhesion of rat corneal epithelium and the basement membrane complex. *Invest Ophthalmol Vis Sci.* 1993;34:2646-2654.

Sheldon H, Zetterqvist H. Experimental induced changes in mitochondrial morphology: vitamin A deficiency. *Exp Cell Res.* 1956;10:225-228.

Sies H, Stahl W, Sundquist AR. Antioxidant functions of vitamins: vitamin E and C, β-carotine, and other carotenoids. Ann NY Acad Sci. 1992;669:7-20.

Smith FR, Goodman DS. Vitamin A transport in human vitamin A toxicity. *N Engl J Med.* 1976;294:805-808.

Sommer A, Emran N, Tamba T. Vitamin A responsive punctative keratopathy in exerophthalmia. *Am J Ophthalmol.* 1979;87:330-333.

Sommer A, Emran N. Tear production in vitamin A responsive xerophthalmia. *Am J Ophthalmol.* 1982;93:84-87.

Sommer A, Green WR. Goblet cell response to vitamin A treatment for corneal exerophthalmia. *Am J Ophthalmol.* 1982;94:213-215.

Sommer A. Effect of vitamin A deficiency on the ocular surface. *Ophthalmology.* 1983;90:592-600.

Strickland S, Mahdavi V. The induction of differentiation in teratocarcinoma stem cells by retinoic acid. *Cell.* 1978;15:393-403

Sullivan WR, McCulley JP, Dohlman CH. Return of goblet cells after vitamin A therapy in xerosis of the conjunctiva. *Am J Ophthalmol.* 1973;75:720-725.

Ubels JL, Edelhauser HE, Austin KH. Healing of experimental corneal wounds treated with topically applied retinoids. *Am J Ophthalmol.* 1983;95:353-358.

Van Horn DL, Schutten WH, Hyndiuk RA. Xerophthalmia in vitamin A-deficient rabbits. Clinical and ultrastructural alterations in the cornea. *Invest Ophthalmol Vis Sci.* 1980;19:1067-1079.

Wald G. Photochemical aspects of visual excitation. Exp Cell Res. 1958;14(Suppl5):389-410.

Wald G. Molecular basis of visual excitation. *Science.* 1968;162:230-239.

Warkany J, Schraffenberger E. Congenital malformations induced in rats by maternal vitamin A deficiency. *Arch Ophthalmol.* 1946;35:150-169.

Wilson JG, Roth CB, Warkany J. An analysis of the syndrome of malformations induced by maternal vitamin A deficiency. Effects of restoration of vitamin A at various times during gestation. *Am J Anat*. 1953; 92:189-217

Chapter 9

VITAMIN E

I. SIGNIFICANCE

Vitamin E functions in vivo as a chain-breaking antioxidant that prevents propagation of free radical damage in biologic membranes (Tappel, 1962; Burton, Joyce and Ingold, 1983; Ingold, Webb, Witter et al, 1987). Vitamin E is a potent proxyl radical scavenger and especially protects polyunsaturated fatty acids within phospholipids of biologic membranes and in plasma lipoproteins (Burton, Joyce and Ingold, 1983). In addition to its antioxidant function, α -tocopherol shows structure-specific effects on several enzyme activities and membrane properties (Taube and Pacher, 1995).

Vitamin E deficiency occurs only rarely in humans and virtually never results from dietary deficiencies because of the almost ubiquitous distribution of tocopheroles in foods, especially oils and fats. Vitamin E deficiency does occur as a result of genetic abnormalities in α -tocopherol transfer protein (α TTP) and a result of various fat malabsorption syndromes. Genetic abnormalities in α TTP are involved in homozygous hypobetalipoproteinemia and abetalipoproteinemia. Fat malabsorption syndromes are involved in fat metabolism syndromes such as chronic cholestasis in children and adults, cystic fibrosis and pancreatic insufficiency, short bowel syndromes such as Crohn's disease, chronic steatorrhea and total parenteral nutrition.

In the ophthalmic field, retinitis pigmentosa is seen in vitamin E-deficient patients whose visual field and dark adaptation are occasionally improved with administration of vitamin A and E even though its effects are temporally. It is assumed that the antioxidant action of vitamin E prevents the oxidation of vitamin E. In systemic diseases inducing vitamin E deficiency such as chronic cholestasis (Alvarez, Landrieu, Laget et al, 1983) and short bowel syndromes (Howard, Ovesen, Satya-Multi et al, 1982) and abetalipoproteinemia (Müller, Lloyd, Bird, 1977), plasma levels of vitamin A and E are lowered accompanied with atypical retinitis pigmentosa.

Since Owens and Owens (1949) reported that premature retinopathy is improved with vitamin E administration because patients with premature retinopathy occasionally show low concentration of vitamin E in the blood. There have been many studies of vitamin E-related retinal diseases (Friedrichson, Kalbach, Buck et al, 1995; Fryer, 1993; Mares-Parlmen,

Bredy, Klein et al, 1995; Mojon, Bascocoinik, Haas et al, 1994; West, Vitale, Hallfrisch et al, 1994).

It is a great controversy whether cataract is prevented by vitamin E. According to the reports on clinical symptoms of patients with vitamin E deficiency due to various fat malabsorption syndromes, such patients have never been reported to have cataract. Thus, cataract may not be caused by vitamin E deficiency alone.

In animal experiments, vitamin E deficiency induces defects in various organs, such as sterility, encephalomalacia in chicks, degeneration and necrosis of cardiac and skeletal muscles, vascular lesions in rabbits and monkeys, hepatic necrosis, edema, yellow discoloration of body fat and anemia (Grant, 1961; Mahan, Jones, Cline et al, 1973; Obel, 1953; Schwarz and Folz, 1957; Van Vleet, Carlton and Olander, 1970; Watkinson, 1966).

Primary manifestations of human vitamin E deficiency include spinocerebellar ataxia, skeletal myopathy, and pigmented retinopathy. Similarly, rats and monkeys develop ataxia and neuroaxonal degeneration in the brain stem, spinal cord, and peripheral nerves and retinal dystrophy.

II. Vitamin E Deficient Experiment

Materials and Methods

Male and female Wistar Kyoto rats were fed a vitamin E deficient diet starting 20 days after birth: 38% corn starch, 25% vitamin free casein, 10% α-wheat starch, 8% purified fibrin, 6% purified lard oil, 6% mineral mixture, 5% sugar, and 2% vitamin mixture containing 1,000 I.U. of vitamin A and less than 0.5mg of d-α-tocopherol per 100g of final diet. Some rats were killed late in the afternoon by luxation of the neck after 6, 8.5, 12, 14, 16, 18 or 24 months. Fourteen-month-vitamin E-deficient rats were given 100mg of vitamin E once a week four times and killed one week after the last administration. Control rats were maintained on a solid rat chow diet containing 5mg vitamin E/100g of diet and all other nutrients obtained from Oriental Yeast, Tokyo, Japan.

Clinical Features of the Vitamin E Deficient Animal

In general, the diets produced excellent growth in both groups of rats throughout the experimental period, although slight weight loss occurred in the terminal stages in the rats fed the vitamin E-deficient diet. However, there was no statistically significant difference in body weights between the two groups. Weight loss in the rats fed the vitamin E-deficient diet was associated with decreased food intake, which occurred only when plasma tocopherol concentrations fell below 1.5-2.0μl/ml. Rats fed the vitamin E-deficient diet for more than 8 months developed severe myoparesis, limb ataxia and vaginal splinter bleeding (in female rats). Slight corneal opacity was recognized with formation of corneal ulcers and lens opacity after 12 months on the vitamin E-deficient diet. No fundus abnormalities were detected by indirect ophthalmoscopy. Fourteen months after the start of the experiments, the systolic blood pressure was in the normal range (115±8.4mnHg; mean±SD) in all control and vitamin E-deficient rats.

The serum level of vitamin E in rats fed the vitamin E-deficient diet for 12 months was 1.0±0.49μg/ml, while that of rats fed the normal diet was 13.7±1.0μg/ml. The difference is statistically significant at $p<0.0001$.

III. The Conjunctiva and Cornea

Results

The Conjunctiva

The Transmission Electron Microscopic (TEM) Findings

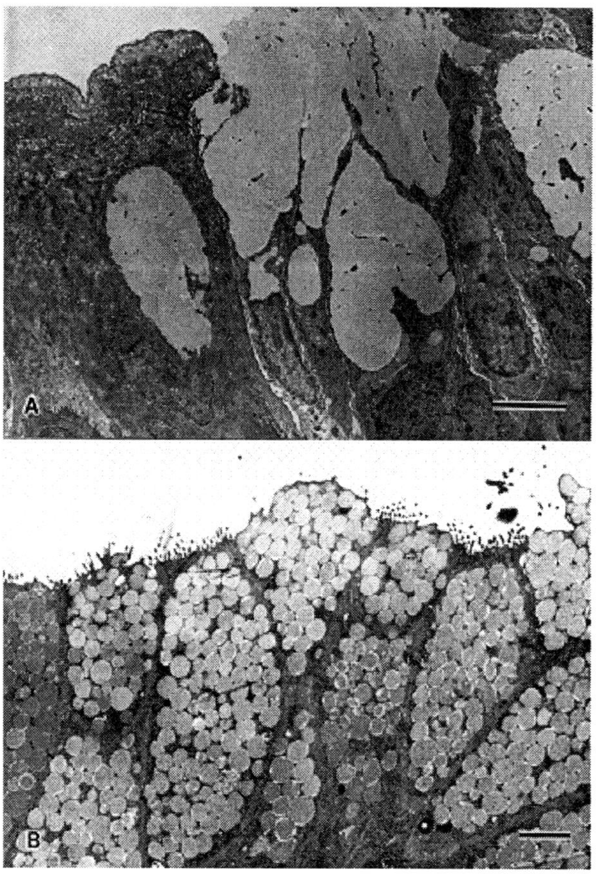

Figure 9.3.1. TEM micrograph of the conjunctiva of a 16-month-vitamin E-deficient rat. Goblet cells show no secretory granules and look atrophic. The epithelium has scarce microvilli and microplicae (A). In control rat, many goblet cells are filled with secretory granules and the most superficial epithelial layer has many microvilli (B). Bar: 5μm (A), 2μm (B).

In the conjunctiva of rats fed a vitamin E deficient diet for 16 months, the most superficial epithelium had scarce microvilli and microplicae, and goblet cells had no secretory granules (Fig. 9.3.1A). On the other hand, control rats had many goblet cells filled with secretory granules and many microvilli and microplicae in the epithelium (Fig. 9. 3. 1B).

The Cornea

Scanning Electron Microscopic (SEM) Findings

In the cornea of rats fed a vitamin E deficient diet for 16 months, the majority of the most superficial epithelial cells were dark cells with scarce microvilli and microplicae (Fig. 9.3.2).

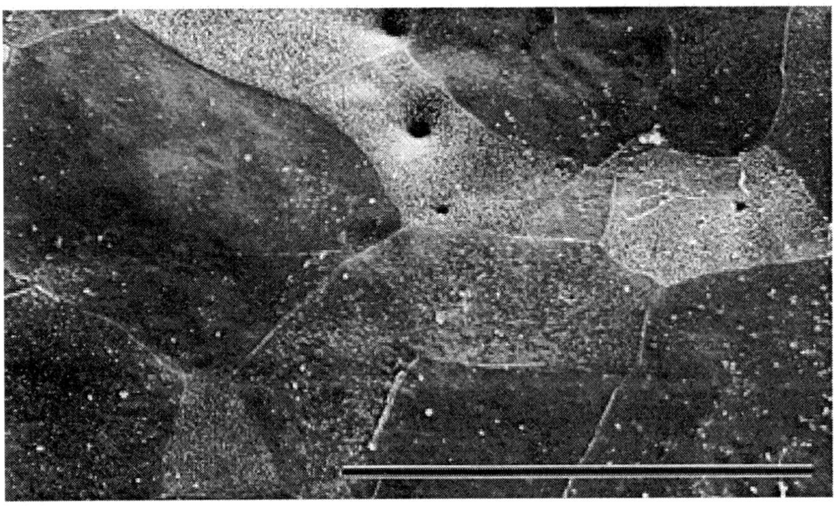

Figure 9.3.2. SEM micrograph of the surface of the corneal epithelium of a 16-month-vitamin E-deficient rat. Most of the superficial epithelial cells are dark cells and have scarce microvilli and microplicae. Bar: 50μm.

TEM Findings

In rats fed a vitamin E deficient diet for 16 months, the cornea showed scarce microvilli in the most superficial epithelium and decreased fibrils in the cytoplasm, and intercellular junctions were ambiguous (Fig. 9.3.3). Nuclei of the epithelial cells were prominently invaginated and some looked pyknotic (Fig. 9.3.3,4). The basal cells were releasing dense materials from the basal portion and dense materials were deposited under the basement membrane (Fig. 9. 3. 5). The corneal stroma had many depositions, but no abnormalities in collagen fibers and keratocytes (Fig. 9. 3. 5, 6). The Descemet's membrane and endothelium showed no abnormalities (Fig 9. 3. 7).

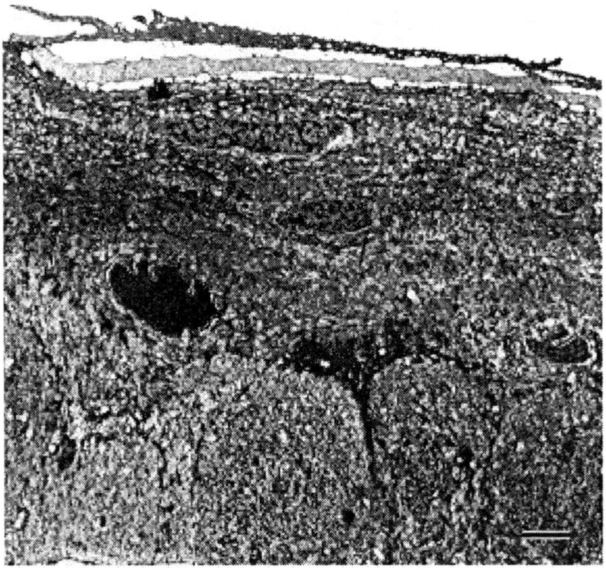

Figure 9.3.3. TEM micrograph of the corneal epithelium of a 16-month-vitamin E-deficient rat. Most superficial epithelial cells are dark and have scarce microvilli. One of them is about to desquamate. Nuclei are irregular in contour and some are pyknotic. The cytoplasm contains scarce fibrils. Bar: 2μm.

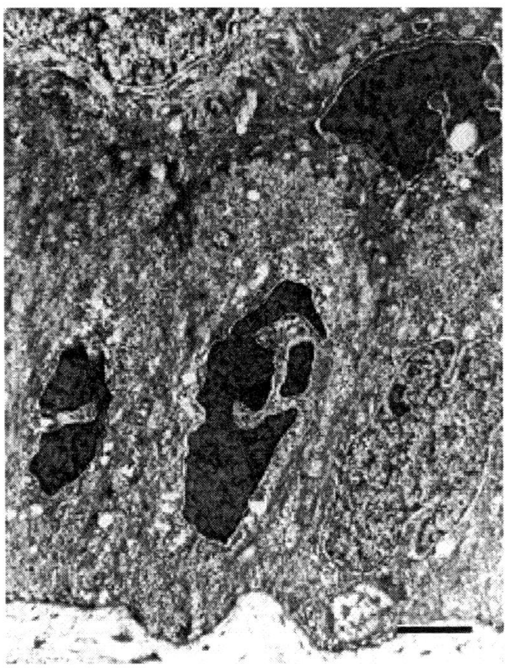

Figure 9.3.4. Basal cells in the corneal epithelium of a 16-month-vitamin E-deficient rat. Nuclei are deeply invaginated and some are pyknotic. Basement membrane and hemidesmosomes look intact. Bar: 2μm.

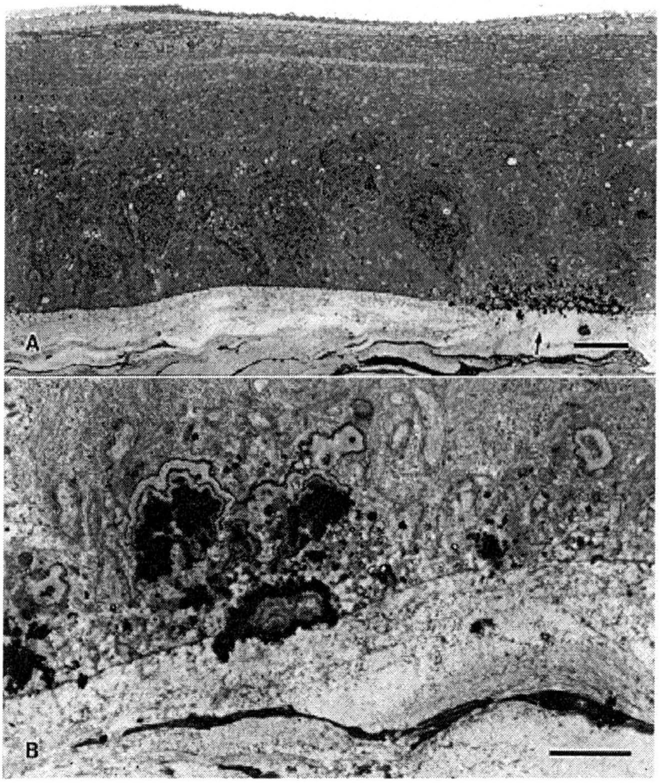

Figure 9.3.5. TEM micrograph of the cornea of 16-month-vitamin E-deficient rats. The epithelial cells are dark and basal cells have many dense materials (arrows) at the basal portion (A). These dense materials are releasing from the basal portion of the basal cell to the subepithelium (B). Bar: 5μm (A), 1μm (B).

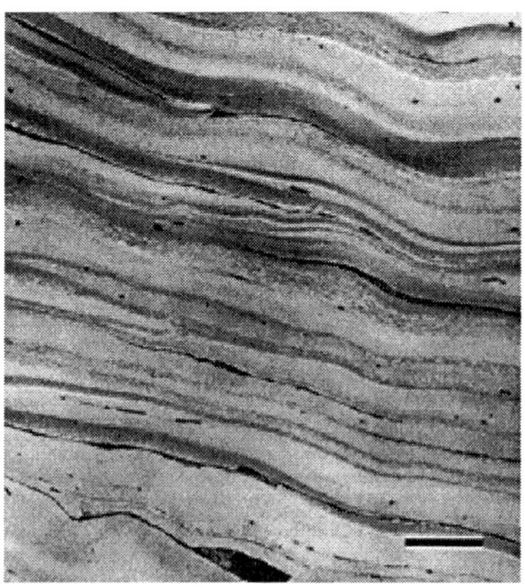

Figure 9.3.6. The corneal stroma of a 16-month-vitamin E-deficient rat has many dot-like dense materials, but collagen fibers and keratocytes show no abnormalitics. Bar: 5μm.

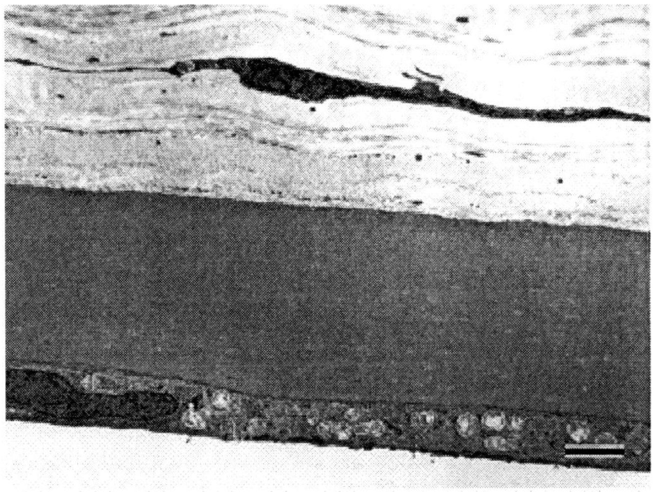

Figure 9.3.7. Descemet's membrane and endothelium of a 16-month-vitamin E-deficient rat show no abnormalities. Bar: 5μm.

IV. The Retina

Light Mitcroscopic Findings

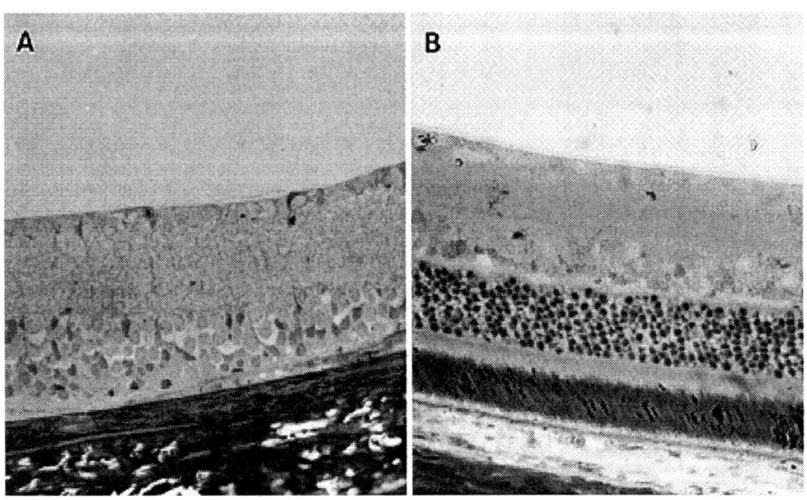

Figure 9.4.1. (A) Light micrograph of a 14-month-old vitamin E-deficient rat showing degenerated retina half as thick as normal retina. A very few photoreceptor cell nuclei are seen. (B) Light micrograph of a 14-month-old control rat showing full-thickness retina with all layers well defined. Toluidine blue, × 200.

In 14-month-old vitamin E-deficient rats light microscopy showed thin degenerated retinas half as thick as the control retinas. The outer plexiform layer was very thin; photoreceptor cell nuclei in the outer nuclear layer decreased to one layer, and the outer and inner segments completely disappeared (Fig. 9.4.1A). As a result, the retinal pigment epithelial (RPE) cells were almost in contact with the inner nuclear layer nuclei. In contrast, light microscopy of control rat retinas showed full-thickness and well-defined layers that could be identified easily (Fig. 9.4.1B).

TEM Findings

In rats fed the vitamin E-deficient diet for 6 months starting 20 days after birth, the discs in the distal regions of photoreceptor outer segments were vesiculated (Fig. 9.4.2) and RPE contained many secondary lysosomes and elongated mitochondria. In rats given 100mg of vitamin E once a week four times after vitamin E deficiency for 6 months, the photoreceptor outer segments showed normal discs (Fig. 9.4.3). However, the RPE still contained many secondary lysosomes including lipofuscin granules (Fig. 9.4.3). The mitochondria looked normal.

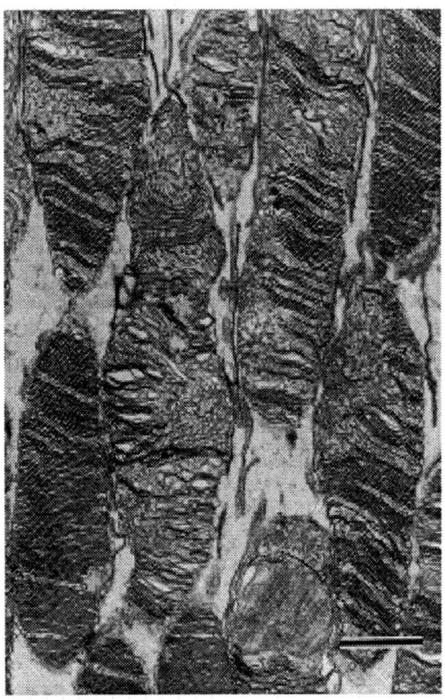

Figure 9.4.2. SEM micrograph of the photoreceptor outer segments of a rat fed a vitamin E-deficient diet for 6 months. The discs of the photoreceptor outer segments are vesiculated. Bar: 100 nm.

In rats fed a vitamin E-deficient diet for 8.5 months, the retina was thin, especially the outer nuclear layer (Fig 9.4.4). The photoreceptor outer segment was greatly decreased and the RPE was filled and swollen with numerous lysosomes containing phagocytized discs. In rats fed the vitamin E-deficient diet for more than 14 months, the retina had almost lost the outer nuclear layer. The photoreceptor outer and inner segments had disappeared, and the microvilli of the RPE had direct contact with inner nuclear layer nuclei (Fig. 9.4.5). The retinal capillary was in almost direct contact with the RPE cells (Fig. 9.4.6) or invaded between the RPE cells (Fig. 9.5.4). More severely ill rats lost the retinal components from the photoreceptor outer segment to the inner nuclear layer nuclei (Fig. 9.4.6, 7). In rats given 100 mg of vitamin E once a week four times after vitamin E deficiency for 8.5, 12, 14 or 18 months, the retina had the same appearance as before vitamin E administration (Fig. 9.4.8).

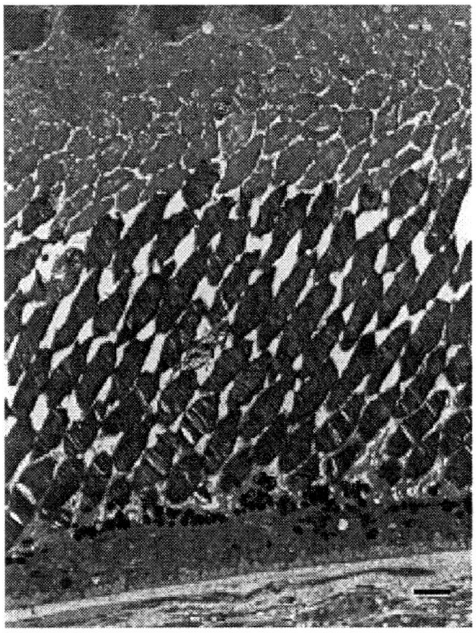

Figure 9.4.3. Photoreceptor outer segment (OS) and RPE of a rat given 100mg of vitamin E once a week four times after being fed a vitamin E-deficient diet for 6 months. Many lipofusin granules still remain and are situated mainly in the apical portion of the RPE. The mitochondria are almost round. The OS discs look normal. Bar: 1μm.

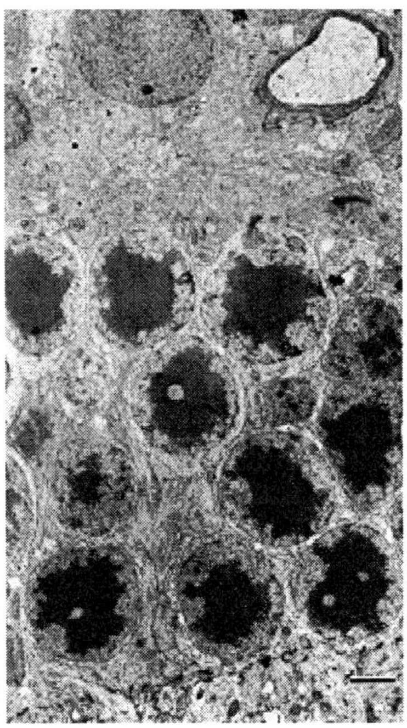

Figure 9.4.4. The outer nuclear layer of a rat fed a vitamin E-deficient diet for 8.5 months is prominently decreased to three lines. Bar: 1μm.

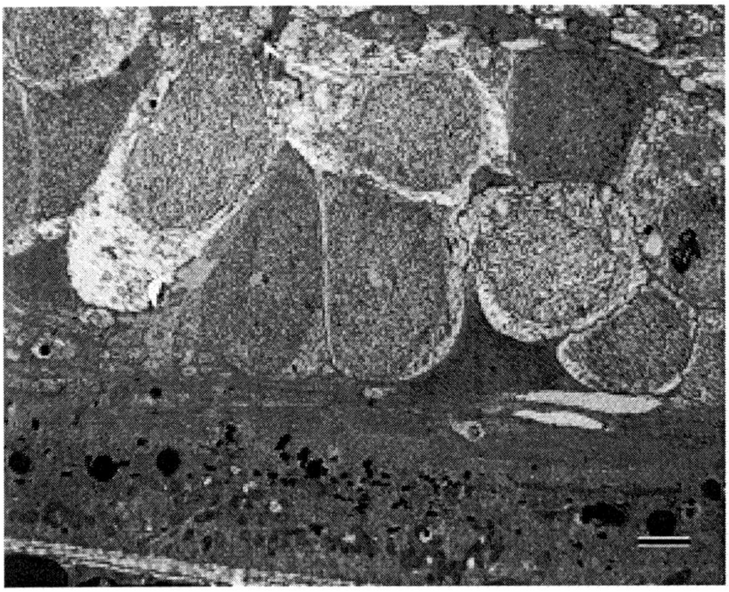

Figure 9.4.5. In the retina of a rat fed a vitamin E-deficient diet for 18 months, extended microvilli of the RPE have direct contact with two lines of inner nuclear layer nuclei. The RPE contains many lipofuscin granules. No photoreceptor outer or inner segments are seen. Bar: 2μm.

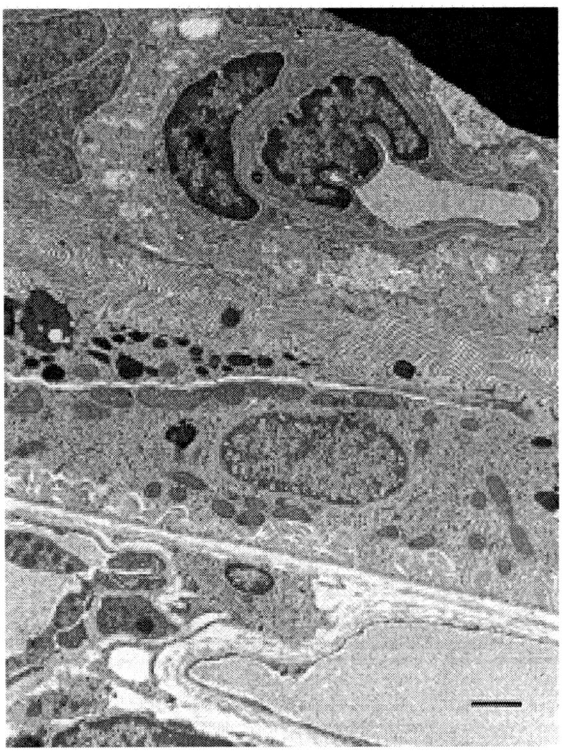

Figure 9.4.6. The retina of a rat fed a vitamin E-deficient diet for 18 months loses photoreceptor outer and inner segments and nuclei and is in contact with a capillary. The inner nuclear layer nuclei are very near the RPE. Bar: 1 μm.

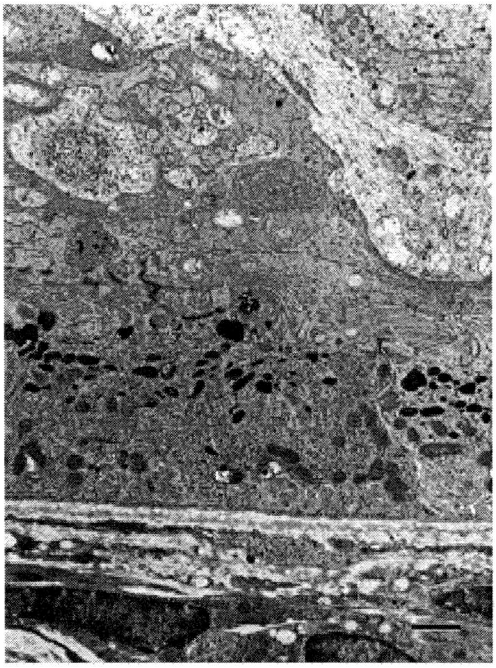

Figure 9.4.7. The retina of a rat fed a vitamin E-deficient diet for 18 months shows the RPE cells in contact with Müller cell, dendrites and neurons in the inner plexiform layer. Bar: 1μm.

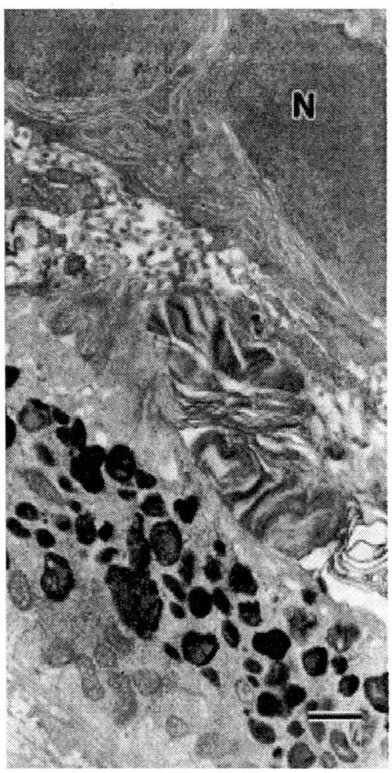

Figure 9.4.8. In a rat given 100mg of vitamin E once a week four times after being fed a vitamin E-deficient diet for 12 months, lost retinal photoreceptor cells are not recovered. Bar: 100nm.

Retinal Vascular Architecture

TEM Findings

In rats fed a vitamin E deficient diet for more than 12 months, retinal capillaries had narrow lumen with irregularly thickened endothelial basement membranes (Fig. 9.4.9) (Table 9.4.1). The endothelial cells were thickened and had scarce cytoplasmic components. The capillary pericytes remained vacuoles.

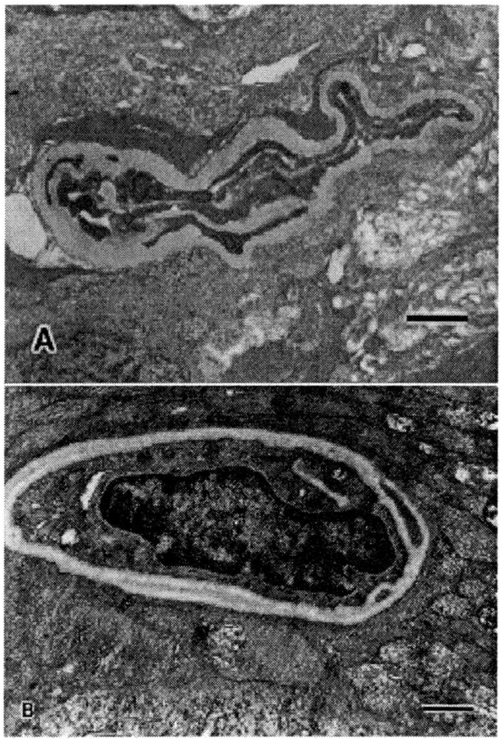

Figure 9.4.9. TEM of a capillary in the retina of a rat fed a vitamin E-deficient diet for 18 months shows irregularly thickened basement membranes and narrow lumen near the RPE (A) and near the nerve fiber layer (B). Bar: 100nm (A), 500nm (B).

SEM and TEM Findings

SEM of vascular casts of the retinas of 14-month-old vitamin E-deficient rats revealed no remarkable micrographic abnormalities in the large retinal vessels other than arterial caliber changes. The mean caliber of the arteries and veins is shown in Table 9.4.2. The difference in arterial caliber between the vitamin E-deficient and the control Wistar Kyoto rats is statistically significant ($p<0.022$). Some of the arterioles in the pericapillary region showed slight tortuosity. However, retinal capillary changes were more evident. The retinal capillaries of the entire retina were decreased in number and scattered. Capillaries showed localized narrowing, caliber irregularity and frequent loop formation (Fig. 9.4.10). In the posterior pole of the retina, some capillaries showed clusters of small tortuous knots (Fig. 9.4.11) and few endothelial cell nuclear impressions (Fig. 9.4.12). SEM micrograph of a 15-month-old control rat retina shows complicated capillary networks with numerous capillaries

(Fig. 9.4.13). The mean caliber of the retinal capillaries is shown in Table 9.4.2. The difference in capillary diameter between the rats fed the vitamin E-deficient diet and the control rats is statistically significant ($p<0.0001$). There were fewer capillary branches (9.3±4.6, n=20 fields examined) in 14-month-old vitamin E-deficient rats than in 14-month-old control rats (21.6±11.2, n=20 fields examined) in a 200μm square ($p<0.0001$). Superficial (innermost) capillaries ran parallel to the large retinal vessels. The capillaries were decreased in number but apparently maintained their two layers (Fig. 9.4.11). The endothelial nuclear impressions on capillary surfaces were more scarce in vitamin E-deficient rats than in control rats (Fig. 9.4.12, 13). No arteriovenous shunts, crossing defects or microaneurysms were seen. In contrast, none of the control rats showed any abnormalities (Fig. 9. 4. 13).

Table 9.4.1 Width of basement membrane of retinal capillary endothelial cells.

Experimental group	n	Width
		Mean±SD (nm)
Control	740	12.7±0.46*
(18months old)		
Vitamin E-deficient	620	22.9±0.32*,**
(18 months old)		
Selenium deficient	540	17.1±0.99**
(18 months old)		

n, number of fields examined. *,** P<0.0000006

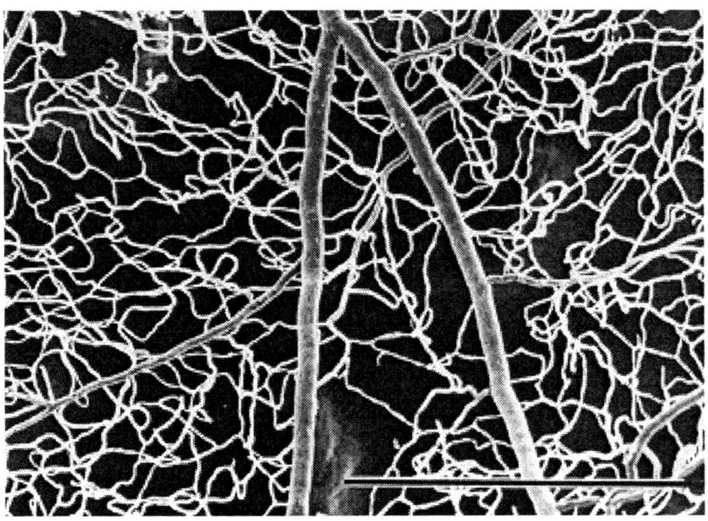

Figure 9.4.10. SEM of retinal vessels and capillary networks of a 14-month-vitamin E-deficient rat showing a sparse capillary network, frequent loop formations (arrows) and local narrowing of capillaries (arrowheads). Bar: 500μm.

Table 9. 4. 2 Mean caliber of retinal vessels and capillaries.

Rat	Artery	Vein	Capillary
Vitamin E-deficient	36.73±1.04μm	47.07±1.47μm	3.98±0.15μm
(14 months old)	n=46	n=46	n=60
Control	38.56±4.24μm	48.75±6.21μm	8.52±0.21μm
(14 months old)	n=46	n=46	n=60
	P<0.022	P=0.147	P<0.0001

n, number of fields examined.

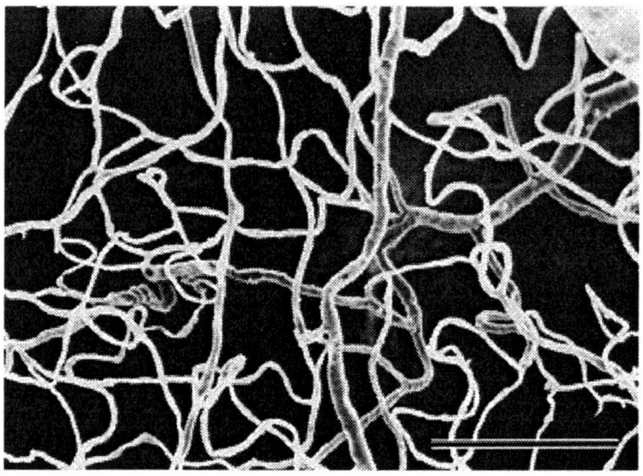

Figure 9.4.11. SEM micrograph of a 14-month-vitamin E-deficient rat showing sparse thin capillaries. Some of the capillaries are clustered into small tortuous knots (arrows), loop formations and irregular calibers. Bar: 100μm.

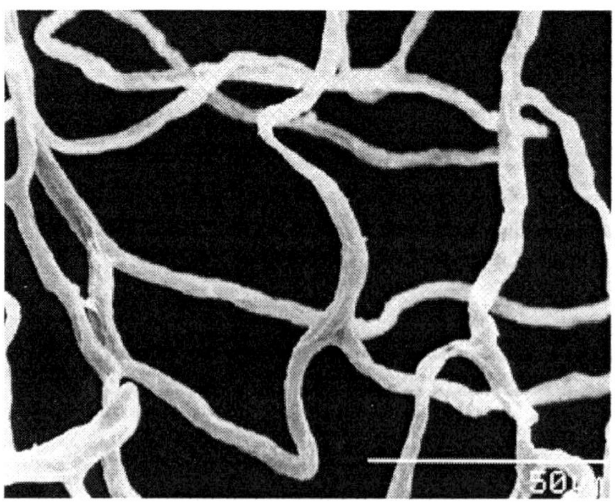

Figure 9.4.12. A magnified view of retinal capillaries of a 14-month-vitamin E-deficient rat showing few endothelial cell nuclear impressions. Bar: 50μm.

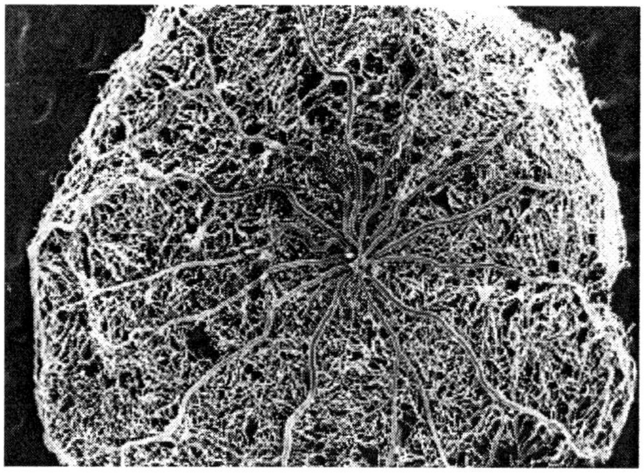

Figure 9.4.13. SEM micrograph of a 15-month-old control rat retina shows complicated retinal capillary networks. Bar: 2mm.

Discussion

In the vitamin E-deficient retina, the photoreceptor outer segment shows disc degeneration, while the RPE contains many secondary lysosomes (Amemiya, 1978; Hayes, 1974; Robison, Kuwabara and Bieri, 1979). Vitamin E may play a role in membrane stabilization by the prevention of lipid peroxidation (Lucy, 1978; McCay, Fong, Lai et al, 1978), although much evidence against the antioxidant theory has been presented (Schwarz, 1972). The fact that the discs of the photoreceptor outer segment contain much polyunsaturated lipids and vitamin E suggests that the photoreceptor outer segment disc degeneration may be due to peroxidation of the disc containing polyunsaturated lipids induced by vitamin E deficiency (Farnsworth and Dratz, 1976). The author's previous paper (Amemiya, 1981) showing spread of acid phosphatase to the disc membrane and increase of secondary lysosomes in the RPE suggested that the release of lysosomal enzymes due to rupture of the lysosome membrane in vitamin E deficiency results in disc degeneration and enhanced phagocytosis in the RPE.

There have been few studies of recovery from vitamin E deficiency. The cytoplasmic membranes of the jejunal epithelial cells of two patients with low serum vitamin E levels showed less stainability with osmium tetroxide, perhaps because of a decrease in the lipid content of the membranes. This alteration was reported to disappear upon vitamin E administration (Molenaar, Hommes, Braams et al, 1968). It has not been confirmed that retinal changes due to vitamin E deficiency can be repaired by vitamin E administration. Our study revealed that mild vitamin E deficiency can be cured morphologically, but severe alterations in long-term deficiency cannot be repaired (Amemiya, 1981). The photoreceptor cells in the central nervous system could not regenerate when the nucleus was damaged, but partly damaged photoreceptor cells could be repaired. There is, however, quite a difference in the RPE between vitamin A and E deficiencies. In vitamin A deficiency, secondary lysosomes are absent in the RPE with a phagocytotic function (Amemiya, 1968; Dowling and Gibbons, 1961). In severe vitamin E deficiency, on the other hand, the RPE contains many lipofuscin granules although no photoreceptor outer segment remains. This suggests that damage to lysosomes caused by long-term vitamin E deficiency results in the accumulation of lipofuscin granules following the loss of the digestive function for engulfed materials. Thus, severe vitamin E deficiency may give rise to irreversible dysfunction of the phagocytotic cells, probably because of damage to the lysosomes. The accumulation of lipofuscin in the RPE of the rat recovered from moderate vitamin E deficiency may mean one of the aging signs accelerated by vitamin E deficiency (Hochshild, 1971). Cells in the central nervous system, such as photoreceptor cells, can be repaired after slight damage, but they cannot be regenerated after severe changes with nuclear damage (Kuwabara, 1970).

The retinas of rats fed a vitamin E-deficient diet for 14 months were very thin because of the disappearance of the photoreceptor cells and outer plexiform layer. Normally the retinal vessels are present from the outer plexiform layer to the nerve fiber layer. The photoreceptor cells, i.e. the retina from the outer nuclear layer to the outer segments, have no vasculature and are supplied with oxygen and nutrients from the vessels in the outer plexiform and choriocapillaries through the RPE. It is very interesting to consider what happens to the blood vessel architecture in the retina when blood vessels lose their target of blood supply in retinal degeneration such as that seen in vitamin E-deficient rat retinas. The current study showed that the two layer capillary network was maintained: the deep retinal capillary bed was brought into close proximity with the RPE as a consequence of degeneration of the outer neuroretinal layers. The sparsity of capillaries is understandable because capillaries themselves degenerate in vitamin E deficiency and because retinal thinning and degeneration and loss of retinal structures result in a reduced need for oxygen and nutrient supplies. The vascular changes in the vitamin E-deficient rat retina were similar to those previously reported in rats with spontaneous diabetes (WBN/kob) with hereditary retinal degeneration (Bhutto, Miyamura and Amemiya, 1999): a two-layer capillary network is maintained in the thin degenerated retina. Although the cause of retinal degeneration may be different in each animal model, gradual disappearance of a retinal capillary network is considered to be one of the common pathologies in the degenerated retina.

Since vessel distribution may be determined by the blood requirements of degenerated tissue, it is mysterious that the deep capillaries persist. These findings are surprising because retinal thickness and vascularity are normally positively correlated. Davson (1979) and Bellhorn (1980) believe that vessel morphology is determined by the requirements of the tissue it subserves. Thus, if a vessel is placed in an unusual environment, the morphology of that vessel may change. The superficial capillary network in the rat retina comes essentially from arterioles, while deep layer capillaries of the network are more regularly and densely arranged and are connected mainly with venules (Bhutto and Amemiya 1995). This anatomical structure may explain why the deep capillaries of the network may not act as feeders; even if they have a role in feeding the RPE, it would be a small role because the RPE is nourished by choriocapillaries. Since the superficial capillaries are distributed to the whole retina, the deep capillaries are necessary for the retina pathway. This might be why the two-layer network is maintained.

On the other hand, retinal vessels themselves were affected by vitamin E deficiency: decrease of capillaries, capillary membrane thickening, capillary lumen narrowing due to thickened endothelium, pericyte damage, irregular caliber of capillaries and tortuous large vessels. Most of these findings have also been reported (Amemiya, 1989). Since vascular cells are damaged by free radicals and lipid peroxides generated by oxidation, vitamin E may act on the vascular wall to prevent cellular damage and maintain function (Tappel, 1972).

In spite of degeneration throughout the retina, a decrease in number of retinal capillaries and irregularity of retinal caliber in vitamin E deficiency, the two-layer pattern of the capillary network was maintained. This means that the basic pattern of retinal vascular architecture may be maintained in retinal degeneration despite local changes such as the decrease in the number of capillaries and changes in the entire retina with thickening or thinning of layers (Butto and Amemiya, 2001).

V. The Choroids

Results

SEM Findings

In rats fed a 14-month-vitamin E-deficient diet, choroidal vessels were sparse. Arterioles and collecting venules decreased in number. Thus, the choriocapillaris is clearly visible under the sparse vessels (Fig. 9.5.1). The choriocapillaris was elongated, engorged, and packed from the center to the periphery and had lost its normal orientation (Fig. 9.5.2). The choriocapillaris showed irregular caliber and dilatation. Intercapillary spaces were wider (Fig. 9.5.3).

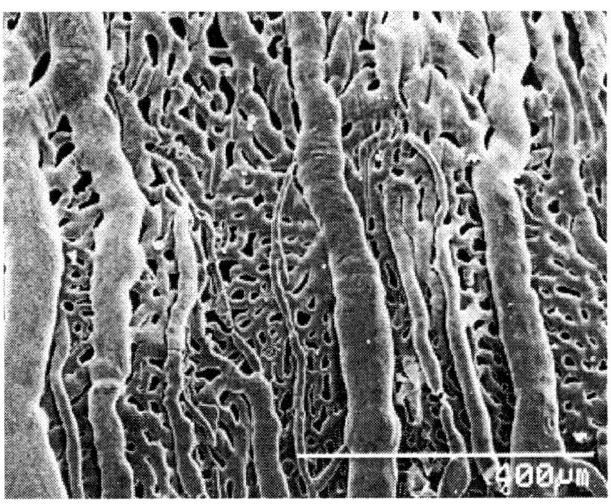

Figure 9.5.1. SEM micrograph of choroidal vasculature at the posterior pole of a rat fed a vitamin E-deficient diet for 14 months. Arterial branches and collecting venules are scarce between the arteries and veins. Thus, choriocapillaris are clearly seen.

TEM Findings

In 14-month-vitamin E-deficient rats, the choriocapillaris was flat and large, and had normal endothelial fenestration (Fig. 9.5.4). Arterioles were very near the choriocapillaries.

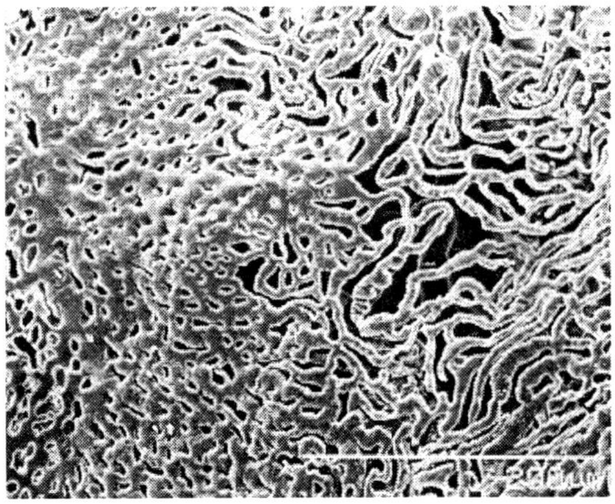

Figure 9.5.2. SEM image of choriocapillaris of a 14-month-vitamin E-deficient rat. Capillary networks are decreased and irregular, and intercapillary spaces are wide.

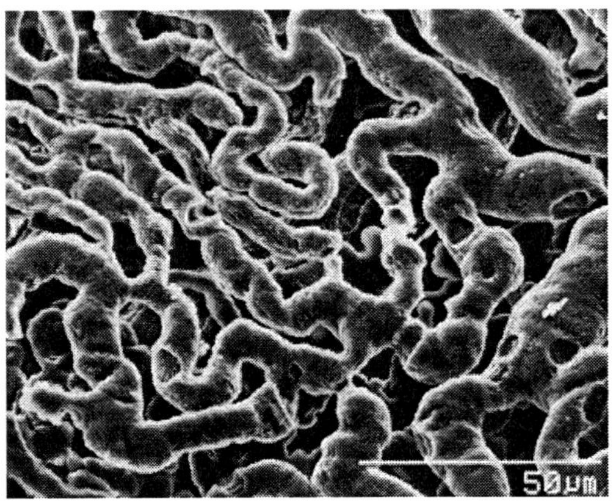

Figure 9.5.3. Choriocapillary network image of a 14-month-vitamin E-defficient rat. Intercapillary spaces are wide.

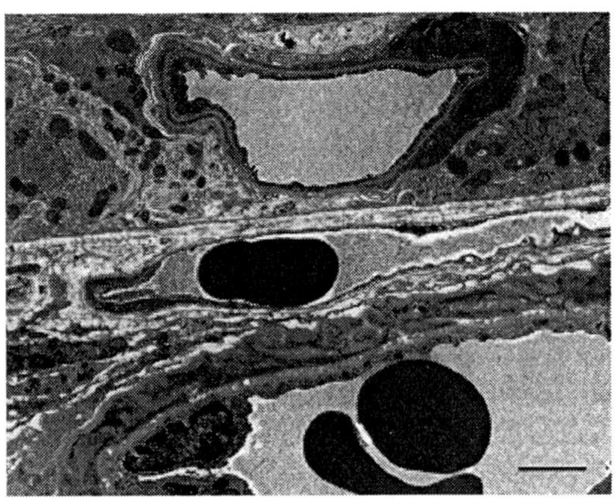

Figure 9.5.4. TEM micrograph of the RPE and choroid of a 14-month-vitamin E-deficient rat. A choriocapillary is flat and endothelial fenestrations are kept. An arteriole is seen near a choriocapillary and looks intact. A retinal capillary invades between the retinal epithelial cells. Bar: 1µm.

VI. THE OPTIC NERVE

Results

TEM Findings

In the postlaminar part of the optic nerve of rats on the vitamin E-deficient diet for 16 months, destruction of the myelin sheath and proliferation of glial cells were diffuse (Fig 9.6.1). Myelinated axons were decreased (Fig. 9.6.1). Glial cells were mainly astrocytes. The mylein was thin and its lamellae were detached and clumped (Fig. 9.6.2). The axonal cytoplasm contained vacuoles and few neurofilaments (Fig. 9.6.2).

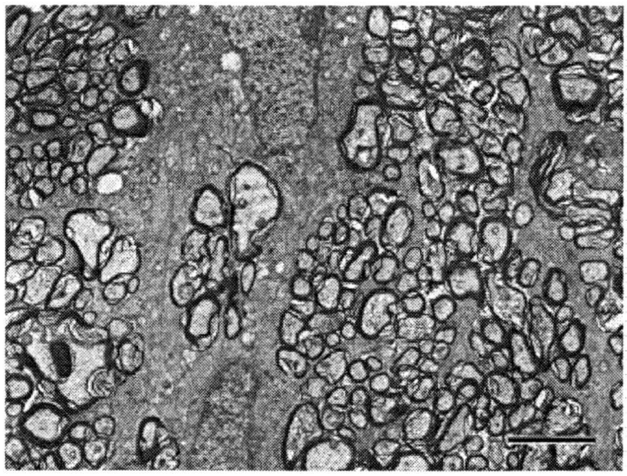

Figure 9.6.1. TEM micrograph of the optic nerve in a 16-month-vitamin E-deficient rat. Myelinated optic nerve fibers are decreased in number and myelin sheath is irregular and thin and clumped glial cells proliferate. Bar: 1μm.

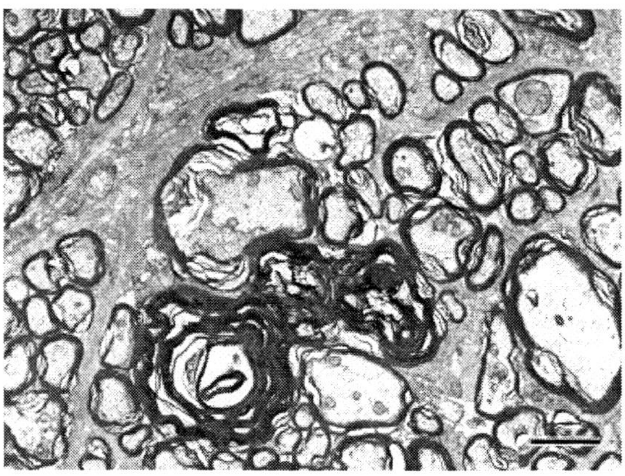

Figure 9.6.2. TEM micrograph of the optic nerve in a 16-month-vitamin E-deficient rat. Lamellae of myelin are degenerated and irregular in arrangement, and detached from the axoplasmic membrane. Some myelin sheaths are clumped. Neurotubulus and mitochondria are destructed in the axon. Bar: 1μm.

Discussion

In vitamin E-deficient rats, the myelin sheath was severely destroyed. The myelin sheath is composed of lipids. Vitamin E is well-known to be a strong antioxidant as a proxyl radical scavenger which prevents lipid membrane peroxidation, especially polyunsaturated fatty acids of the biomembrane. In rats of vitamin B_2 and B_{12} deficiencies, myelinated optic nerve fibers are severely degenerated and/or disappear. These degenerations may be caused by disturbed myelin formation because vitamins B_2 and B_{12} are related to myelin synthesis as coenzymes (Weir and Scott, 1999; van der Westhuyzen, 1983). However, the damage of the myelin sheath in vitamin E deficiency may be caused by peroxidation of the lipid sheath.

VII. The Recti Muscle

Results

Electron Microscopic Findings

In rats fed a vitamin E deficient diet for 6 months, the capillary endothelium in the rectus muscle contained many vacuoles and fewer mitochondria than did that of controls.

In rats fed a vitamin E-deficient diet for 12 months, pigment granules began to appear in the sarcoplasm, and A-Z bands and muscles fibers showed a slightly irregular arrangement.

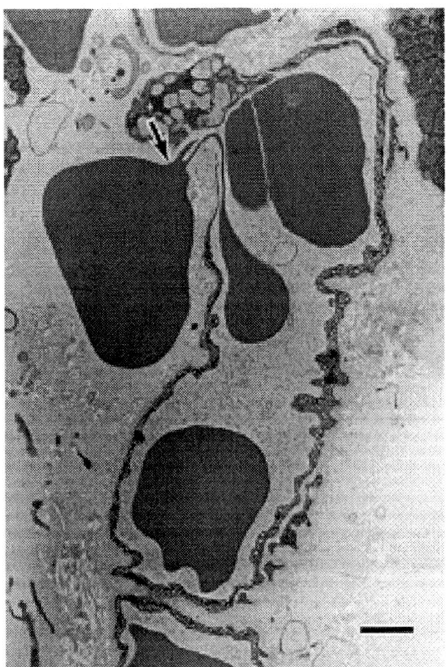

Figure 9.7.1. TEM micrograph of a capillary in a rectus muscle of a rat on a vitamin E-deficient diet for 18 months. The endothelial cells show thinning of the basement membrane and disruption, with escaping of blood cells. Bar: 1μm.

Rats fed a vitamin E-deficient diet for 18 or 24 months showed thinning of the basement membrane in the capillary endothelium and distruption of the endothelium (Fig 9.7.1) (Table 9.7.1). The endothelium contained electron dense materials and vacuoles and scarce cytoplasmic organelles such as mitochondria and ribosomes (Fig. 9.7.2). Muscle cells contained electron dense materials, degenerated mitochondria and irregular arrangements of A-Z bands and muscle fibers (Fig. 9.7.3). The nuclei looked normal.

Table 9.7.1. Width of basement membrane of capillary endothelial cells in rectus muscles.

Experimental group	n	Width
		M±SD (nm)
Controls	200	86.8±21.64*
(18 months old)		
Vitamin E-deficient	250	35.3±13.64*,**
(18 months old)		
Selenium deficient	200	72.8±21.9**
(18 months old)		

n, number of fields examined. *,** P<0.0000006.

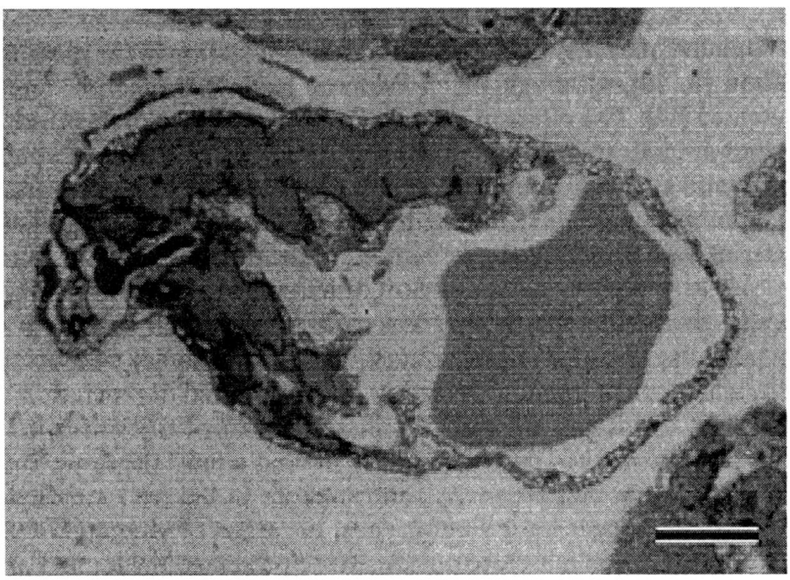

Figure 9.7.2. TEM micrograph of the capillary in the rectus muscle of a rat fed a vitamin E-deficient diet for 18 months. The endothelium contains many vacuoles and electron dense materials. Cytoplasmic materials are scarcely seen. Nuclei show irregular contour. Bar: 1μm.

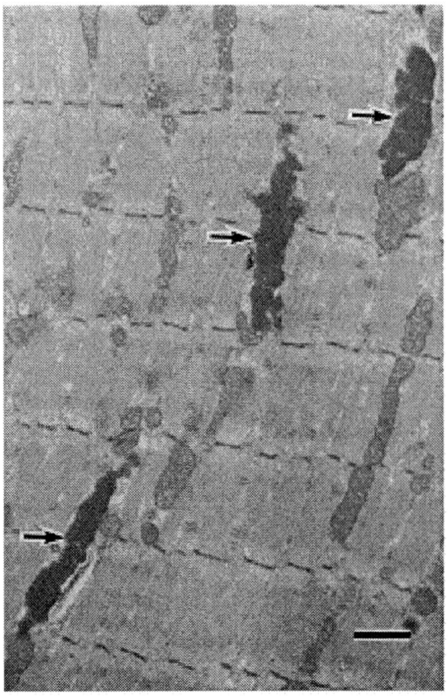

Figure 9.7.3. TEM micrograph of the rectus muscle of a rat fed a vitamin E-deficient diet for 24 months. Muscle fibers show irregular arrangements and are decreased in number. Electron dense materials and degenerated mitochondria are seen. A-Z bands are irregular. Bar: 1μm.

Discussion

The effect of vitamin E deficiency on muscle cells has been studied in various animals such as rats, rabbits, guinea pigs, cows, sheep, chickens, pigs, horses, dogs, ducks, goats and guppy fish (West and Mason, 1958). The skeletal muscle changes seen in these animals are characterized by hyaline or Zenker's degeneration of contractile material, sarcolemmal tube formation, dystrophic carcification, and macrophagic invasion with phagocytosis and lysis of degenerated sarcoplasm (Van Vleet, Ruth and Ferrans, 1976; West and Mason, 1958). Electron microscopic findings in the skeletal and cardiac muscles in vitamin E deficiency are endothelial degeneration, basement membrane thickening and extracellular appearance of macrophages, and pigment granule formation, mitochondrial degeneration, irregular arrangement of A-Z bands and muscular fibrils and increased ribosomes in the sarcoplasm (Howes, Price and Blumberg, 1964; Van Vleet, Ruth and Ferrans, 1976). The current study on recti muscles showed almost the same findings as in cardiac and skeletal muscles. However, abnormalities in the recti muscles seemed to be less severe and appear more slowly. Thus, the effect of vitamin E deficiency on muscle cells may vary from muscle to muscle. Muscle damage in vitamin E deficiency has been considered to be due to insufficient antioxidant action.

References

Alvarez F, Landrieu P, Laget P, Lemonnier F, Odievre M, Alagille D. Nervous and ocular disorders in children with cholestasis and vitamin A and E deficiencies. *Hepatology.* 1983;3:410-414.

Amemiya T. Cytochemical and electron microscopic examination of the retina of rats with hypovitaminosis A. *Acta Soc Ophthalmol Jpn.* 1968;72:1074-1099.

Amemiya T. Effect of vitamin E deficiency on photoreceptor outer segment and pigment epithelium of the rat retina. *Acta Soc Ophthalmol Jpn.* 1978;82:822-826.

Amemiya T. Retinal recovery from vitamin E deficiency. *Acta Soc Ophthalmol Jpn.* 1981a;85:410-414.

Amemiya T. Effect of vitamin E administration on photoreceptor outer segment and retinal pigment epithelium of vitamin E deficient rats. *Int J Vit Nutr Res.* 1981b;51:114-118.

Amemiya T. Photoreceptor outer segment and retinal pigment epithelium in vitamin E deficient rats. An electron microscopic and electron histochemical study. *Graefes Arch Clin Exp Ophthalmol.* 198c1;216:103-109.

Amemiya T. Effect of vitamin E and selenium deficiencies on rat capillaries. *Int J Vit Nutr Res.* 1989;59:122-126.

Bellhorn RW. Control of blood vessel development. *Trans Ophthalmol Soc UK.* 1980;100:328-331.

Bhutto IA, Amemiya T. Corrosion cast demonstration of retinal vasculature of normal Wistar Kyoto rats. *Acta Anat.* 1995;153:290-300.

Bhutto IA, Miyamura N, Amemiya T. Vascular architecture of degenerated retina in WBN/kob rats: corrosion cast and scanning electron microscopic study. *Ophthalmic Res.* 1999;31:367-377.

Bhutto IA, Amemiya T. Retinal vasculature is maintained in retinal degeneration: corrosion cast and electron microscopic study. *Eye.* 2001;15:531-538.

Burton GW, Joyce A, Ingold KU. Is vitamin E the only lipid-soluble, chain-breaking antioxidant in human blood plasma and erythrocyte membranes? *Arch Biochem Biophys.* 1983;221:281-290.

Davson H. The Bowman lecture. The little brain. *Trans Ophthalmol Soc UK.* 1979;99:21-37.

Dowling JE, Gibbons IR. The effect of vitamin A deficiency on the fine structure of the retina. In : Smelser GK, ed. *The Structure of the Eye.* New York:Academic Press Inc;1961:85-99.

Farnsworth CC, Dratz EA. Oxidative damage of retinal rod outer segment membranes and the role of vitamin E. *Biochim Biophys Acta.* 1976;433:556-570.

Friedrichson T. Kalbach HLV, Buck P, van Kuijk FJGM. Vitamin E in macular and peripheral tissues of the human eye. *Curr Eye Res.* 1995;14:693-701.

Fryer MJ. Evidence for the photoprotective effects of vitamin E. *Photochem Photobiol.* 1993;58:304-312.

Grant CA. Morphological and etiological studies of diabetic microangiopathy in pigs ('mulberry heart'). *Acta Vet Scand.* 1961;2(Suppl 3):1-107.

Hayes KC. Retinal degeneration in monkeys induced by deficiencies of vitamin E or A. *Invest Ophthalmol Vis Sci.* 1974;13:499-510.

Hawes EL, Price HM, Blumberg JM. The effects of a diet producing lipochrome pigment (ceroid) on the ultrastructure of skeletal muscle in the rat. *Am J Pathol.* 1964;45:599-631.

Hochschild R. Lysosomes, membranes and aging. *Exp Gerontol.* 1971;6:153-166.

Howard L, Ovesen L, Satya-Murti S, Chu R. Reversible neurological symptoms caused by vitamin E deficiency in a patient with short bowel syndrome. *Am J Clin Nutr.* 1982;36:1243-1249.

Ingold KU, Webb AC, Witter D, Burton GW, Metcalfe TA, Müller DP. Vitamin E remains the major lipid-soluble, chain-breaking antioxidant in human plasma even in individuals suffering severe vitamin E deficiency. *Arch Biochem Biophys.* 1987;259:224-225.

Kuwabara T. Retinal recovery from exposure to light. *Am J Ophthalmol.* 1970;70:187-198.

Lucy JA. Structural interactions between vitamin E and polyunsaturated phospho-lipids. In de Duve C, Hayaishi O, ed. Tocopherol, *Oxygen and Biomembranes.* Amsterdam:Elsevier/North-Holland Biomedical Press;1978:109-120.

Mahan DC, Jones JE, Cline JH, Cross RF, Teague HS, Grifo AP Jr. Efficacy of selenium and vitamin E injections in the prevention of white muscle disease in young swine. *J Am Sc.* 1973; 36:1104-1108.

Mares-Perlman JA, Bredy WE, Klein R, Klein BEK, Bowen P, Stacewicz-Sapuntzakis M, Petta M. Serum antioxidants and age-related macular degeneration in a population-based case-control study. *Arch Ophthalmol.* 1995;113:743-748.

McCay PB, Fong K-L, Lai EK, King MM. Possible role of vitamin E as a free radical scavenger and singlet oxygen quencher in biological systems which initiate radical-mediated reactions. In de Duve C, Hayaishi O, ed. *Tocopherol, Oxygen and Biomembranes.* Amsterdam:Elsevier/North-Holland Biomedical Press;1978:41-57.

Mojon D, Boscoboinic D, Haas A, Bohnke M, Azgi A. Vitamin E inhibits retinal pigment epithelium cell proliferation in vitro. *Ophthalmic Res.* 1994;26:304-309.

Molenaar I, Hommes FA, Braams WG, Polman HA. Effect of vitamin E on membranes of the intestinal cell. *Proc Natl Acad Sci USA.* 1968;61:982-988.

Müller DP, Lloyd JK, Bird AC. Long-term management of abetalipoproteinaemia. Possible role for vitamin E. *Arch Dis Child.* 1977;52:209-214.

Obel AL. Studies on the morphology and etiology of so-called toxic liver dystrophy (hepatosis dietelica) in swine. *Acta Pathol Microbiol Scand.* 1953;94(Suppl):1-119.

Owens WC, Owens EU. Retrolental fibroplasias in premature infants. ii. Studies on the prophylaxis of the disease. The use of alpha tocopheryl acetate. *Am J Ophthalmol.* 1949;32:1631-1637.

Robison WG, Kuwabara T, Bieri JG. Vitamin E deficiency and the retina: Photoreceptor and pigment epithelial changes. *Invest Ophthalmol Vis Sci.* 1979; 18:683-690.

Schwarz K, Foltz CM. Selenium as initial part of α-factor 3 against dietary necrotic liver degeneration. *J Am Chem Soc.* 1957;79:3292-3293.

Schwarz K. The cellular mechanisms of vitamin E action: Direct and indirect effects of α-tocopherol on mitochondrial respiration. *Ann NY Acad Sci.* 1972;203:45-52.

Tappel AL. Vitamin E as the biological lipid antioxidant. *Vitam Horm.* 1962;20:493-510.

Tappel AL. Vitamin E and free radical peroxidation of lipids. *Ann NY Acad Sci.* 1972;203:12-28.

Tauber MG, Packer L. Vitamin E: beyond antioxidant function. *Am J Clin Nutr.* 1995;62(Suppl):1501S-1509S.

Van der Westhuyzen J. Effect of vitamin B_{12} deficient on lipid and fatty acid composition of spinal cord myelin in the fruit bat. *J Nutr.* 1983;113:531-537.

Van Vleet JF, Carlton W, Olander HJ. Hepatosis dietetica and mulberry heart disease associated with selenium deficiency in Indian swine. *J Am Vet Med Associ.* 1970;157:1208-1219.

Van Vleet JF, Ruth G, Ferrans VJ. Ultrastructural alterations in skeletal muscles of pigs with selenium–vitamin E deficiency. *Am J Vet Res.* 1976;37:911-922.

Watkinson JH. Fluometric determination of selenium in biological material with 2,3-diaminonaphthalene. *Anal Chem.* 1966;38:92-97.

Wefers H, Sies H. The protection by ascorbate and glutathione against microsomal lipid peroxidation is dependent on vitamin E. *Eur J Biochem.* 1988;174:353-357.

Weir DG, Scott JM. Vitamin B_{12} "cobalamin". In: Maurice E, Shils ME, Olson JA, Shike M, Ross AC, ed. *Modern Nutrition in Health and disease.* 9th ed. Philadelphia:Lippincott Williams & Wilkins;1999:447-458.

West WT, Mason KE. Histopathology of muscular dystrophy in the vitamin E-deficient hamster. *Am J Anat.* 1958;102:323-363.

West S, Vitale S, Hallfrisch J, Munoz B, Muller D, Bressler S, Bressler NM. Are antioxidants or supplements protective for age-related macular degeneration? *Arch Ophthalmol.* 1994;112:222-227.

Chapter 10

VITAMIN B_2 (RIBOFLAVIN)

I. SIGNIFICANCE

Riboflavin (vitamin B_2) is chemically specified as 7, 8-dimethyl-10-(1-D-ribilyl) isoalloxazine. In bound coenzyme form, riboflavin participates in oxidation-reduction reactions in numerous metabolic pathways and in energy production via the respiratory chain. A variety of chemical reactions are catalyzed by flavoproteins. Riboflavin is contained in many enzymes called flavoproteins and several coenzymes which take on hydrogen and pass it on to other substances in the long chain of oxidation-reductions by which hydrogen is finally combined with oxgen to form water (Goodman and Gilman, 1985). In this way, riboflavin-containing enzymes contribute to the metabolism of carbohydrates, amino acids and fats (Bogert, Briggs and Calloway, 1973).

In rats, a prolonged lack of riboflavin induces eye symptoms varying in severity from an inflamed condition of the cornea to its complete opacity (Day, Langston and O'Brien, 1931; Miller, Johnson, Hoeffer et al, 1954; Bietti, 1977; Lee and Hart, 1944). Usually it takes several months for signs of riboflavin deficiency to appear.

Riboflavin deficiency is rare in humans, but is occasionally reported to be induced by dietary deficiency or drugs (Goodman and Gilman, 1985). Many people live for long periods on low intake and minor signs of deficiency are consequently common in many parts of the world (Bates, 1987). However, the deficiency encountered seems to occur in combination with deficiency of other water-soluble vitamins (McCormick, 1989). For instance, "Shibigachaki disease", an endemic disease in Tsugaru district, Japan several decades ago (Masuda and Aoyama, 1951) seems to be caused by a vitamin B complex deficiency, not by an independent riboflavin deficiency. The clinical syndrome is characterized by sore throat, hyperemia and edema of the pharyngeal and oral mucous membranes, cheilosis, angular stomatitis, glossitis (magenta tongue), seborrheic dermatitis, and normochromic, normocytic anemia associated with pure red cell cytoplasia of the bone marrow (Wilson, 1982). In humans, on the other hand, riboflavin deficiency gives rise to ocular signs and symptoms such as tearing, foreign body sensation, photophobia and blepharitis (Goodman and Gilman, 1985; Bietti, 1977).

In adult rabbits fed a high-riboflavin diet, the cornea has the highest riboflavin content (Batey and Eckhert, 1991). Flavins are light sensitive and are rapidly degraded when exposed to light in near ultraviolet and visible wavelengths. Some of the byproducts of flavin photodegradation are toxic, but this toxicity could be used to treat corneal ulcers (Schnitzler, Sporl and Seiler, 2000). The effect of riboflavin deficiency on the cornea was studied about 70 years ago. Although knowledge of riboflavin biochemistry has advanced considerably, studies of ocular tissue in riboflavin deficiency have not increased since 1966. For instance, Medline shows only one paper on the cornea in riboflavin deficiency. It seems that the symptoms and findings in ocular tissues have been defined and established in the cornea and the lens: as corneal opacity with neovascularization (Bessey and Wolbach, 1939; Fromer and Klintworth, 1975) and cataract in experimental animals (Day, Langston and Cosgrove, 1934). But the pathologic findings were based on light microscopy and were never studied by electron microscopy; and the conjunctiva of riboflavin-deficient animals have not been described.

Human Riboflavin Deficiency

Riboflavin deficiency is rare in humans, but is occasionally reported to be induced by diet or drugs (Goodman and Gilman, 1985). However, it seems to be caused by a vitamin B complex deficiency not by an independent riboflavin deficiency. Generally speaking, ariboflavinosis seldom occurs in the United States (Goodman and Gilman, 1985) or in Japan as a discrete deficiency, but may accompany other nutritional disorders like "Shibigatchaki disease" an endemic disease in Japan, several decade ago (Masuda and Aoyama, 1951). In human riboflavin deficiency gives rise to ocular signs and symptoms such as tearing, foreign body sensation, photophobia and blepharitis (Goodman and Gilman, 1985). These clinical signs and symptoms make us suppose damage of the ocular surface. To our surprise, the study on the riboflavin deficiency to the conjunctiva is scarcely found.

II. Riboflavin-Deficient Experiment

Material and Methods

Twenty-one-day-old male Wistar Kyoto rats were divided into a riboflavin-deficient and a control group. All animals were fed a riboflavin-deficient powdered diet made by ourselves. The riboflavin-deficient diet is the AIN-93G formula-based diet containing sucrose instead of riboflavin. It contains no riboflavin and is complete in all other nutrients, and distilled and deionized water. The riboflavin concentrations of the riboflavin-deficient and control diets were measured by high performance liquid chromatography. The riboflavin content was less than 0.05mg/100g in the riboflavin-deficient diet and 0.37mg/100g in the control diet. All the rats were killed after 3 months on the deficient diet.

In the recovery experiment rats fed a riboflavin-deficient diet for 3 months were continued on the same diet but given distilled and deionized water supplemented with 1mg riboflavin /300ml for 2 months.

Clinical Features of the Riboflavin-Deficient Animals

In rats, riboflavin deficiency induces slight coarsening of fur and abnormal eye secretion in the 3rd month of the experiment.

Body weight: In the 3rd month of the experiment the weight of the riboflavin-deficient rats was lower than that of the controls ($p<0.0001$); 3-month-old controls 498±36.3g, n=5 and deficient rats 328±45.9g, n=5; and 5-month-old control rats 488±31.1g, n=5 and recovery rats 481±37.5g, n=3. The difference between the 5-month-old control rats and the recovery rats was not significant ($p=0.8039$).

Serum riboflavin: In the 3rd month of the experiment the serum riboflavin level was 12.8±1.70µg/dl, n=5 in the 3-month-old control rats and 8.6±0.96µg/dl, n=5 in the deficient rats ($p=0.0147$). In the recovered rats it was 6.4±1.41µg/dl, n=3 and 9.4±0.64µg/dl, n=5 in the 5-month-old control rats. The difference between the control and recovered rats was not significant ($p=0.8039$).

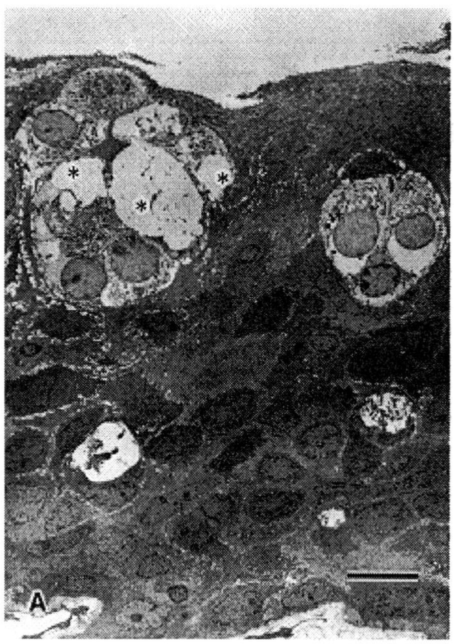

Figure 10.3.1A. TEM micrograph of conjunctiva of a control rat. Goblet cells are filled with secretory granules (arrows). Bar: 5µm.

III. The Conjunctiva and Cornea

Results

Electron Microscopic Findings

The surface of the conjunctiva of the control rats showed numerous microvilli and microplicae and many goblet cells filled with secretory granules (Fig. 10.3.1A- C, Table 10.3.1), while the surface of the cornea showed numerous microvilli and microplicae and many light cells (Fig. 10.3.2A,B ; Table 10.3.2). TEM micrographs of the control rat cornea showed normal features: many microvilli in the superficial epithelial cells, regularly arranged epithelial cells, hemidesmosomes and basement membrane in the basal epithelium and no evidence of apoptosis or subepithelial deposits (Fig. 10.3.2C).

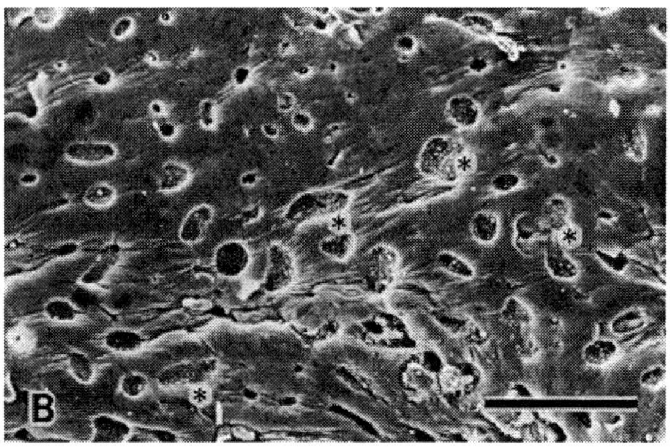

Figure 10.3.1B. SEM micrograph of conjunctional surface of a control rat. Many goblet cells (asterisks) are seen to contain secretory granules. Bar: 100nm.

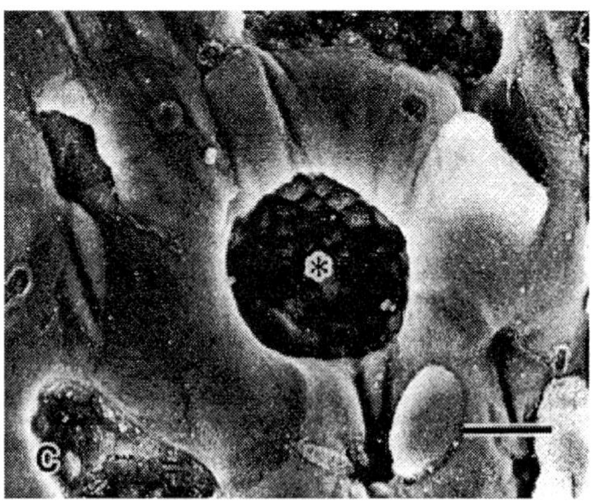

Figure 10.3.1C. Higher magnification of conjunctival surface of a control rat. Surface epithelial cells have numerous microvilli and microplicae. A goblet cell contains secretory granules (asterisk). Bar: 10μm.

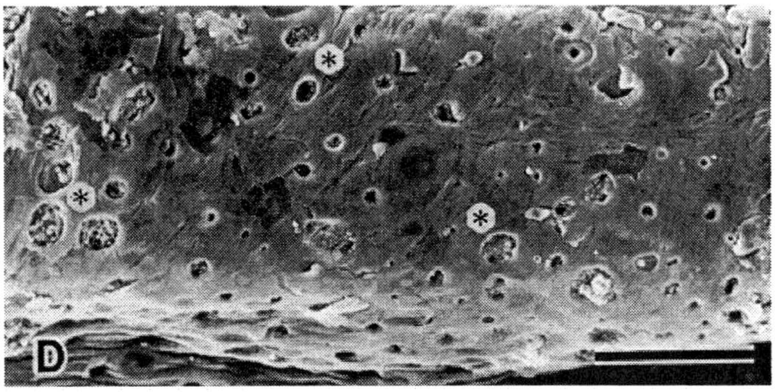

Figure 10.3.1D. SEM micrograph of conjunctival surface of a 3-month-old riboflavin-deficient rat. Goblet cells (asterisks) are fewer compared to those in the control rats, and they have fewer secretory granules. Bar: 100nm.

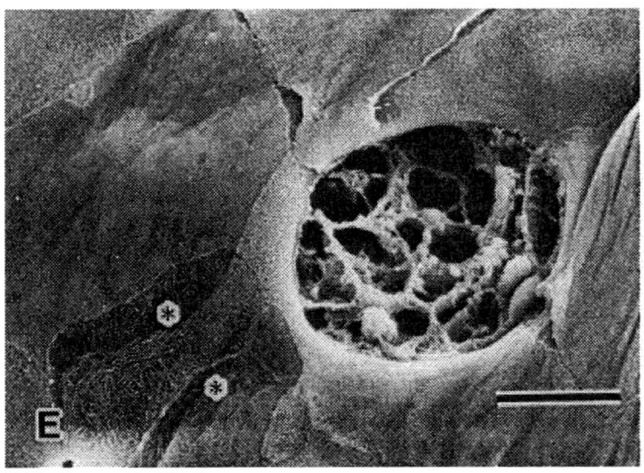

Figure 10.3.1E. Higher magnification of the conjunctival surface of a 3-month-old riboflavin-deficient rat. Microvilli are decreased and only microplicae remain in some cells (asterisks). A goblet cell contains scarce secretory granules. Bar: 10μm.

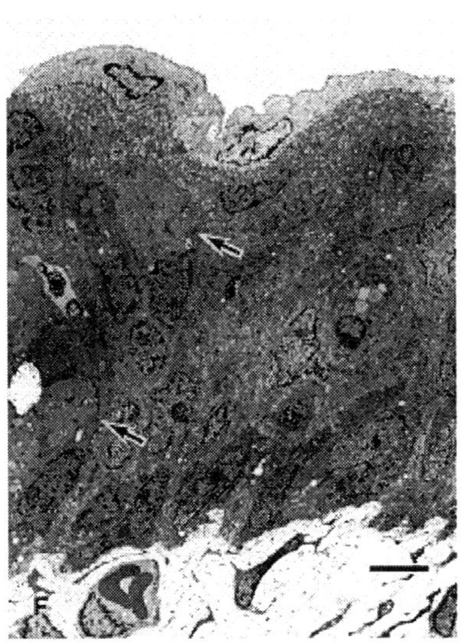

Figure 10.3.1F. TEM micrograph of conjunctiva of a 3-month-old riboflavin-deficient rat. Goblet cells have poorly developed secretory granules (asterisks). Bar: 10μm.

Table 10.3.1. Number of goblet cells per 40,000μm² standard field (mean±SD).

Groups	Number of field examined	Number of goblet cells (40,000μm²)
Control	10	19.6±3.2 *, **
Deficient	10	13.8±2.3 *
Recovery	10	14.2±2.8 **

* p=0.0002, ** p=0.0008.

In the riboflavin-deficient rat, the conjunctiva had a decreased number of goblet cells of various sizes (Fig. 10.3.1D, Table 10.3.1) and a prominent decrease in microvilli and microplicae in the most superficial epithelial cells (Fig. 10.3.1E). The orifices of the goblet cells looked empty (Fig. 10.3.1E). TEM of the riboflavin-deficient rat conjunctiva confirmed the SEM findings: secretory granules in the goblet cells were poorly developed (Fig. 10.3.1E, F).

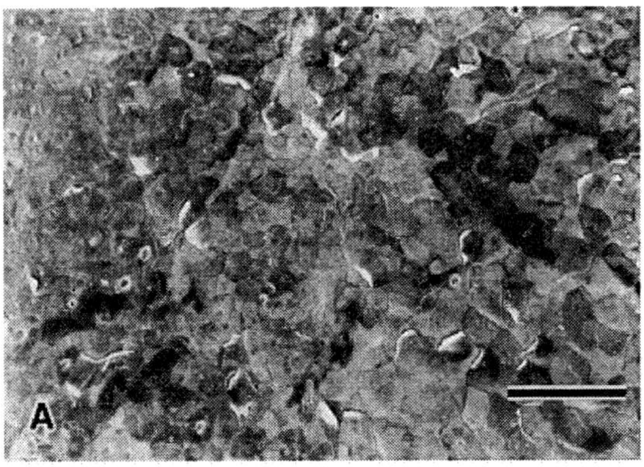

Figure 10.3.2A. SEM micrograph of corneal surface of a control rat. Light cells are in the majority. Bar: 100μm.

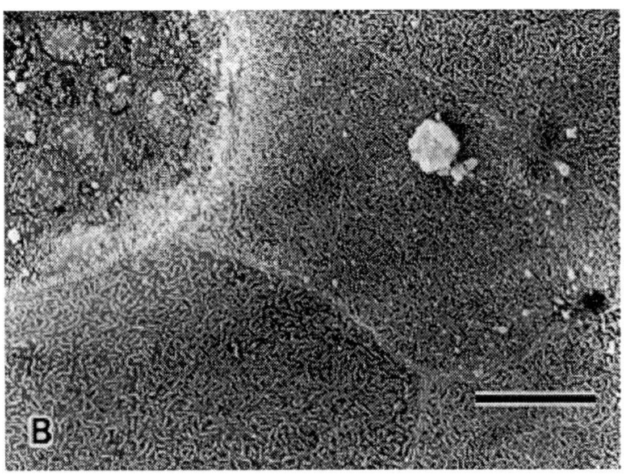

Figure 10.3.2B. Higher magnification of light cells of a control rat cornea. Light cells have numerous microvilli. Bar: 5μm.

Table 10.3.2. Ratio of light cell/light cells plus dark cells in the cornea (mean±SD).

Groups	Number of field examined	ratio of light cell/light cells plus dark cells
Control	10	0.55 ±0.03 *, **
Deficient	10	0.369±0.04 *, ***
Recovery	10	0.627±0.07 **, ***

*, *** $p<0.0001$, ** $p=0.0048$.

On the other hand, the cornea of the riboflavin-deficient rats showed an increase of dark cells with scarce microvilli and microplicae by SEM (Fig. 10.3.2D, E, Table 10.3.2), although the central and limbal cornea had no neovascularization. TEM showed undeveloped microvilli and microplicae and dark wing cells (Fig. 10.3.2F, G). In the subepithelial layer, there was much cellular debris with high density cytoplasmic debris (Fig. 10.3.2G) and high density granular and round structures with cores (Fig. 10.3.2H). Basal cells lost their basement membranes and hemidesmosomes (Fig. 10.3.2G). Stroma cells were degenerative, and dense deposits were scattered through the stroma (Fig. 10.3.2I).

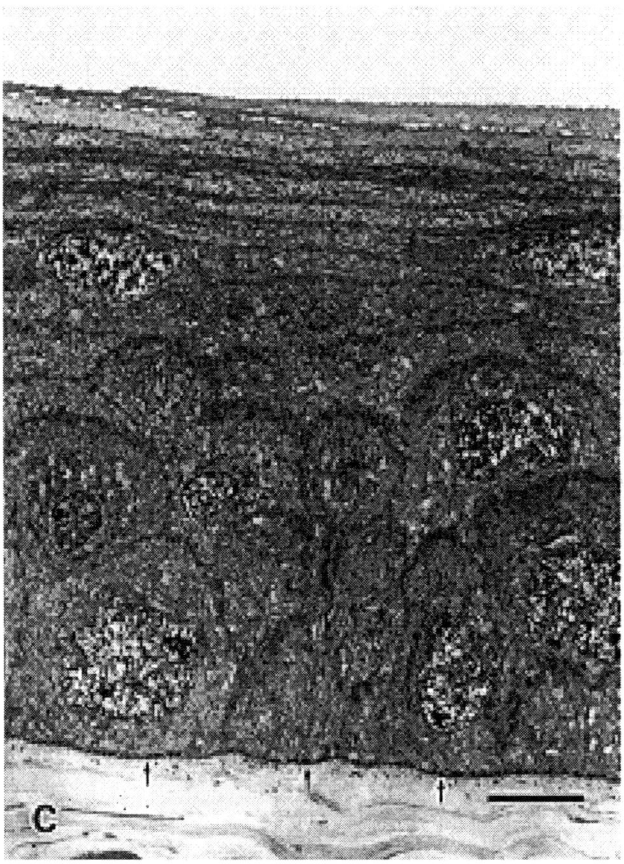

Figure 10.3.2C. TEM micrograph of the subepithelial stroma and the basal cell of a control rat. The basal cells have hemidesmosomes (arrows) and basement membrane. No deposits are seen in the subepithelial stroma. Bar: 5μm.

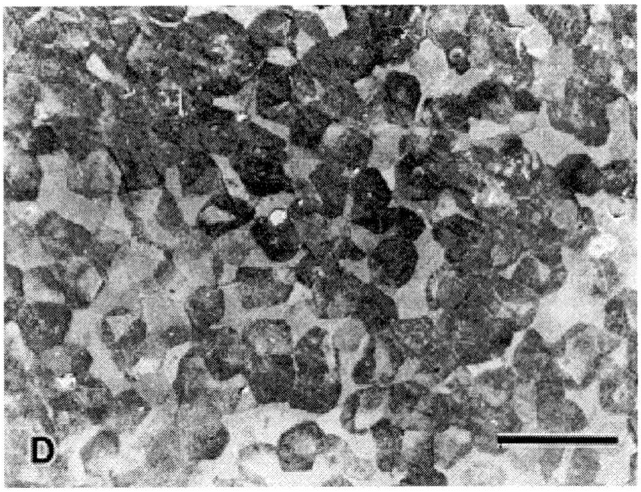

Figure 10.3.2D. SEM micrograph of corneal surface of a 3-month-old riboflavin-deficient rat. Many dark cells are present. Bar: 1μm.

When rats fed a riboflavin-deficient diet for 3 months were continued on the same diet but given distilled and deionized water supplemented with 1mg riboflavin/300ml for 2 months, the conjunctiva and cornea showed almost the same features as in the controls; many light cells (Table 10.3.2, 3) and regularly arranged microvilli in the conjunctiva (Figs 10.3.3A, B) and cornea (Figs 10.3.4A, B): an apparently slight increase in the number of goblet cells with well-developed secretory granules in the conjunctiva but no actually statistically significant difference between the control and recovery rats and recovery and deficient rats (Fig 10.3.3C, Table 10.3.1); normal basement membranes and hemidesmosomes and normal stroma in the cornea (Fig. 10.3.4C).

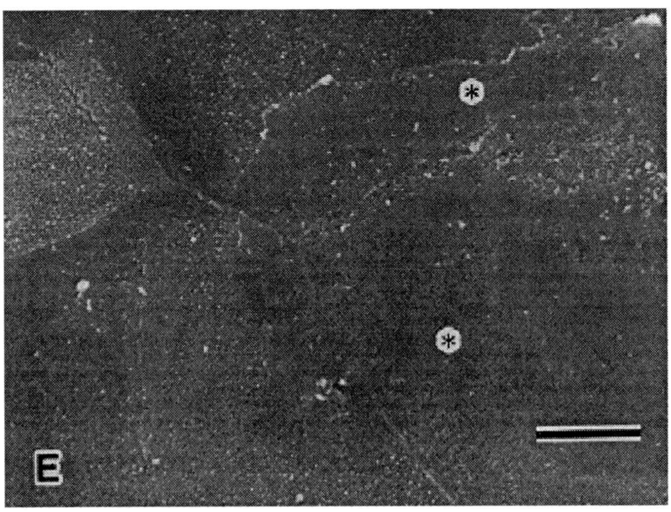

Figure 10.3.2E. Higher magnification of corneal surface of a riboflavin-deficient rat. Dark cells (asterisks) have fewer microvilli. Bar: 5μm.

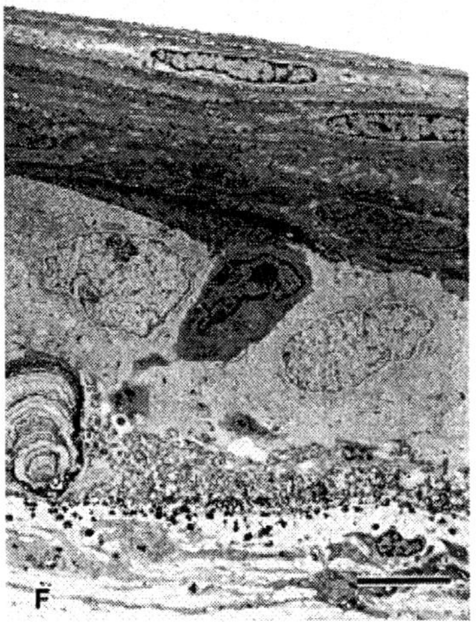

Figure 10.3.2F. TEM micrograph of corneal epithelium and subepithelial stroma of a 3-month-old riboflavin-deficient rat. The most superficial epithelial cells have decreased microvilli. Some basal cells and wing cells are dark and their cytoplasmic organelles and nuclei are condensed. In the subepithelial stroma, there are numerous dense bodies and some cellular debris. Bar: 5μm.

Table 10.3.3. Ratio of light cell/light cells plus dark cells in the conjunctiva (mean±SD).

Groups	Number of field examined	Ratio of light cell/light cells plus dark cells
Control	15	0.86 ±0.08 *, ***
Deficient	15	0.49±0.08 *, **
Recovery	15	0.80±0.17 **, ***

*, ** $p<0.0001$, *** $p=0.202$.

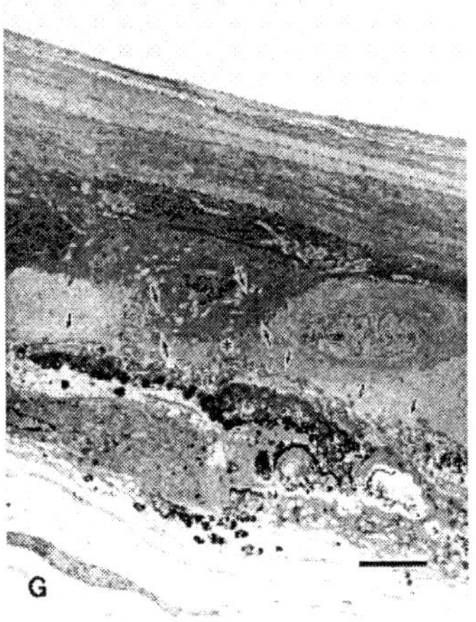

Figure 10.3.2G. TEM micrograph of the corneal epithelium and subepithelial stroma of a 3-month-old-riboflavin-deficient rat. Microvilli are scarce in the most superficial epithelial cells. Wing cells are dark and its cytoplasmic organelles are condensed. Some of the cells (thick arrows) are migrating toward the subepithelium. Some cellular debris being released from the basal cell layer to the subepithelial stroma (asterisks). Basal cells lose the basement membrane and hemidesmosomes (arrows). Bar: 5μm.

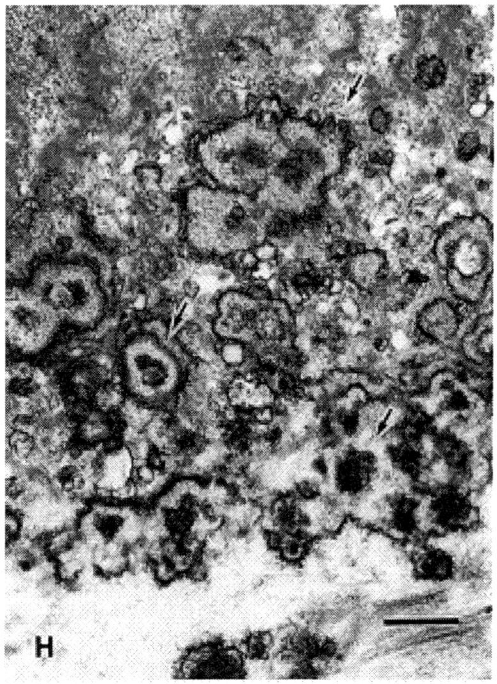

Figure 10.3.2H. Higher magnification of dense bodies in subepithelial stroma. Granular and round structures (arrows) are seen. Bar: 500nm.

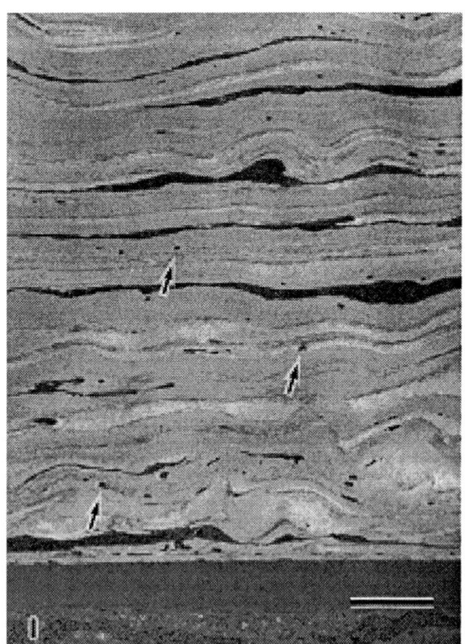

Figure 10.3.2I. TEM micrograph of Descemet membrane and endothelium of a 3-month-old riboflavin-deficient rat. The stroma shows dense deposits (arrows) and many stroma cells. The endothelial cells look intact. Bar: 5μm.

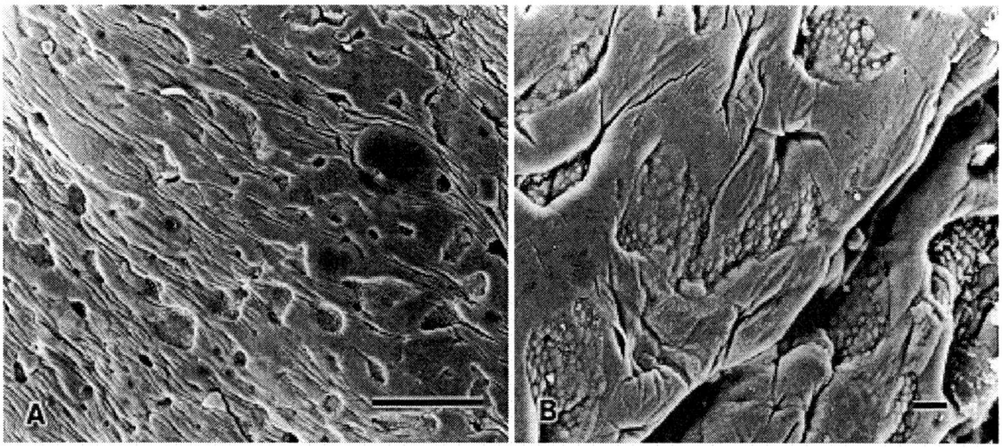

Figure 10.3.3. SEM micrographs of conjunctival surface of a recovery rat. There are many light cells and goblet cells (3A). Light cells have numerous microvilli and microplicae, and goblet cells have secretory granules (3B). Bar: 100µm (A), 10µm (B).

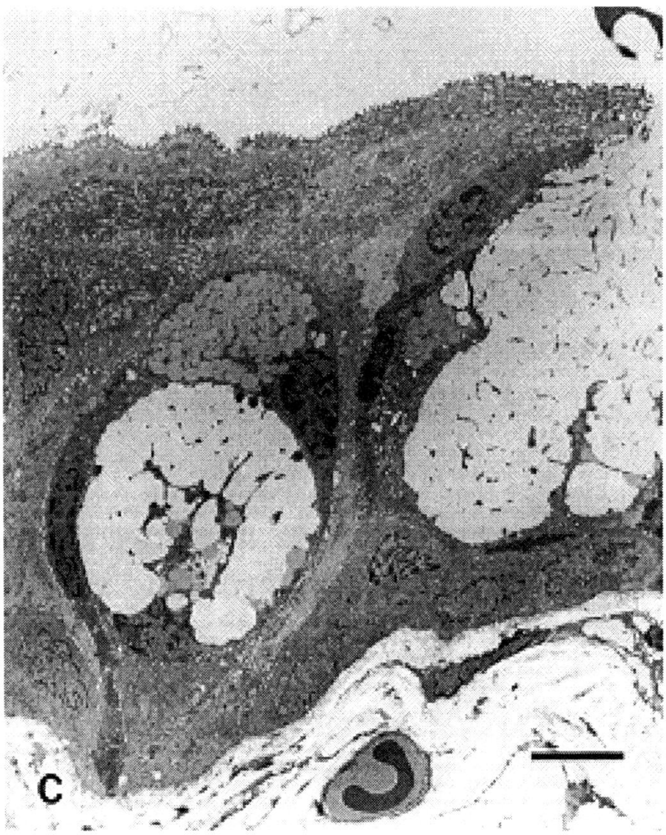

Figure 10.3.3C. TEM micrograph of conjunctiva of a recovery rat. Three to 4 layers of epithelial cells are seen, and the cytoplasm has many fibrils and normal nuclei. Goblet cells are seen, and they contain many secretory granules. Bar: 5µm.

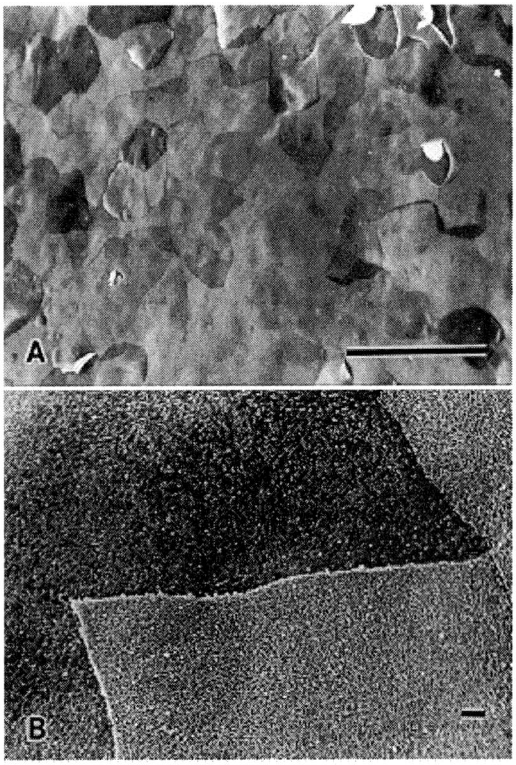

Figure 10.3.4. SEM micrographs of corneal surface of a recovery rat. Many light cells occupy the corneal surface (4A) and have numerous microvilli and microplicae (4B). Bar: 100μm (A), 1μm (B).

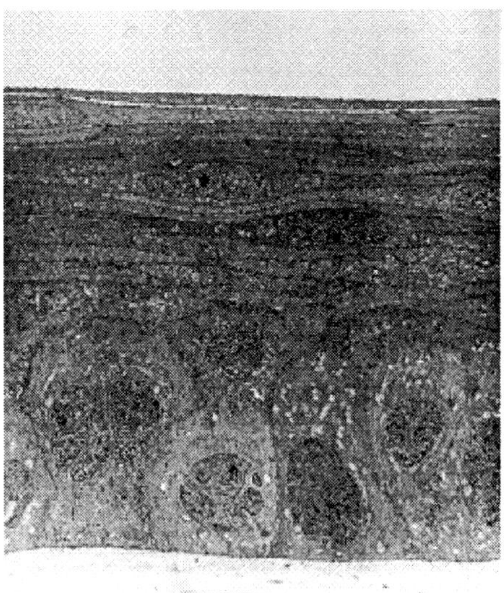

Figure 10.3.4C. TEM micrographs of corneal surface of a recovery rat. There are many microvilli in the most superficial layer of the epithelium and no degeneration in the corneal epithelium. The basement membrane and hemidesmosomes are seen. Bar: 5μm.

Discussion

Although the old literature on the cornea of experimentally induced riboflavin-deficient animals reported neovascularization at the corneal limbus (Day, Langston and O'Brien, 1931), it was not seen in the present study using an electron microscope. This discrepancy might be due to differences in the duration or content of the diets because the diet in this study is a better scientifically qualified AIN-93G formula-based diet (Reeves, Nielsen and Fahey, 1993). Another possibility is that the riboflavin-deficient diets used in older studies lack some micronutrients as well as riboflavin. Current results may reflect relatively early riboflavin deficiency, and neovascularization in the corneal limbus may be a severe later result.

The main conjunctival and corneal changes are degenerative changes of the wing and basal epithelial cells, decrease or disappearance of microvilli and microplicae in the most superficial epithelial cells and increased dark cells in the most superficial epithelial cells. Generally speaking, the dark cell-light cell phenomenon is seen in both normal and pathologic tissues, and it is occasionally seen in poorly fixed tissues, immature cells such as embryonic and developing cells, technical artifacts, dead or dying cells, dehydrated cells and degenerating cells. Thus, the dark cell-light cell phenomenon may vary from species to species, from experiment to experiment, from procedure to procedure, and from researcher to researcher. The surfaces of conjunctival and corneal epithelial cells with scarce and incomplete microvilli and microplicae may appear dark by SEM and TEM. Dark wing cells may be degenerated and transferred to the basal cell layer. The marked decrease of goblet cells may induce poor development of the glycocarix layer on the conjunctival surface and dry-eye syndrome in addition to the corneal changes. Abnormal secretion in riboflavin deficiency may be one of these ocular surface disturbances.

The changes in the cornea are specific for riboflavin deficiency and are not seen in other micronutrient deficiencies such as those of Zn (Mizoguchi and Amemiya, 1992; Gong, Takami, Amemiya et al, 2004), Mn (Gong and Amemiya, 1999), Mg (Gong, Takami, Kitaoka et al, 2003), Cr and vitamin A (Kanazawa, Kitaoka, Ueda et al, 2002) and C. The reduction of microvilli and microplicae in the corneal surface is common in those micronutrient deficiencies, but only riboflavin deficiency induces degenerative changes of the wing cells, onion-shaped dense deposits in the subepithelial area, and degenerative stroma cells. The significance of dense deposits in the subepithelial stroma is unclear, but the author assumes that degenerative wing cells are released to the subepithelial stroma through basal cells and dense deposits represent cellular debris, because epithelial cells generally release waste products from the basal portion like the dense deposits in Bruch's membrane (Hogan and Alvarado, 1967; Farkas, Sylnester and Arher, 1971). On the other hand, it has been assumed that degenerated superficial epithelial cells are desquamated. The epithelial keratinization induced by vitamin A deficiency is never seen in riboflavin deficiency. These different changes suggest riboflavin specific activity in the conjunctiva and cornea.

A series of studies on Zn (Mizoguchi and Amemiya, 1992; Gong, Takami, Amemiya et al, 2004), Mg (Gong, Takami, Kitaoka et al, 2003), Mn (Gong and Amemiya, 1999), vitamin A (Kanazawa, Kitaoka, Ueda et al, 2002), vitamin E (Fujikawa, Gong and Amemiya, 2003) and vitamin C deficiencies have shown some corneal changes similar to those seen in riboflavin deficiency. The deficiency of these essential trace elements and vitamins may lead to cell degeneration as well as lowered activity of the superoxide dismutases (SOD) Zn·Cu-SOD and Mn-SOD (Keen and Zindenberg-Cherr, 1994). Riboflavin also has antioxidant action as a flavoenzyme. The antioxidant action of riboflavin is performed through the reduced activity of flavoenzyme and glutathione reductase (Batey and Eckhert, 1991). An adequate amount of dietary riboflavin is required for optimal activity of GSSG (oxidized glutathione reductase) (Schnizler, Sporl and Seiler, 2000).

Patients with accidentally induced riboflavin deficiency have photophobia, foreign body sensation and tearing (Bietti, 1977; Lee and Hart, 1944). The present experiment indicates that these symptoms may be induced by the decrease and dysfunction of the goblet cells and incomplete formation of the tear film due to loss of microvilli and microplicae in the ocular surface. Riboflavin is known to be effective in making the skin smooth, and moist and the fur glossy. This vitamin might aid in epithelial development as do vitamins A and Zn, and probably helps to maintain healthy ocular development and functioning.

IV. THE RETINA

Results

Electron Microscopic Findings

In the control rats, the retinal pigment epithelial (RPE) cells had no lamellar structures 7h after exposure to light (Fig.10.4.1B). The photoreceptor outer segment, inner segment and nucleus showed no abnormalities. The outer nuclear layer nuclei were compactly arranged (Fig. 10.4.2B).

In the riboflavin-deficient rats, the RPE cells still contained lamellar structures 7h after exposure to light (Fig. 10.4.1A). Although the tip of the outer segments appeared to be destructed (Fig. 10.4.1A), the photoreceptor inner segment and nucleus showed no changes. However, Müller's fibers in the outer nuclear layer of the deficient rats were edematous and vacuolated (Fig. 10.4.2A). Vacuolated parts contained amorphous materials. Nuclei in the inner nuclear layer was arranged in 3-4 lines (Fig. 10.4.3).

In the recovered rats, no lamellar structures were found in the RPE cells 7h after exposure to light (Fig. 10.4.1C) and Müller's fibers were filled between photoreceptor cell nuclei (Fig. 10.4.2B).

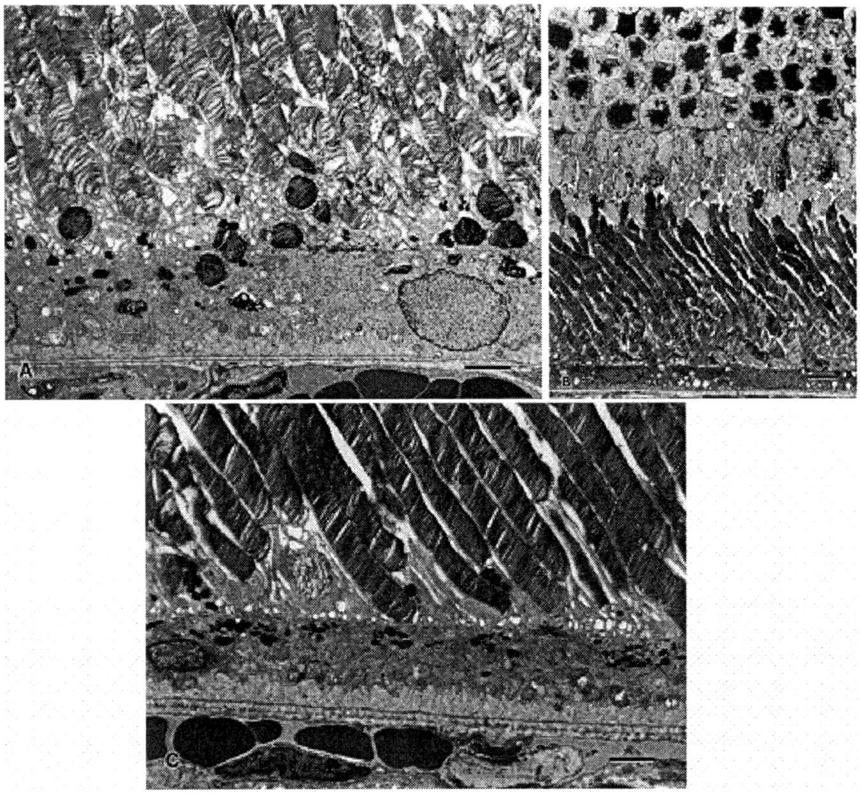

Figure 10.4.1. TEM micrographs of rat retinas 7h after exposure to light. In a rat fed a riboflavin-deficient diet for 3 months, photoreceptor outer segment discs are degenerated at the tip and separated. The RPE still contains phagocytized lamellar structures (A). B shows the control rat retina (B). Neither separated discs nor phagocytized lamellar structures are seen. Photoreceptor cell nuclei are regularly arranged and Müller cell processes extend well. C shows the retina of a rat recovered from riboflavin deficiency, which is almost the same as that of B. Bar: 2μm (A, C), 10μm (B).

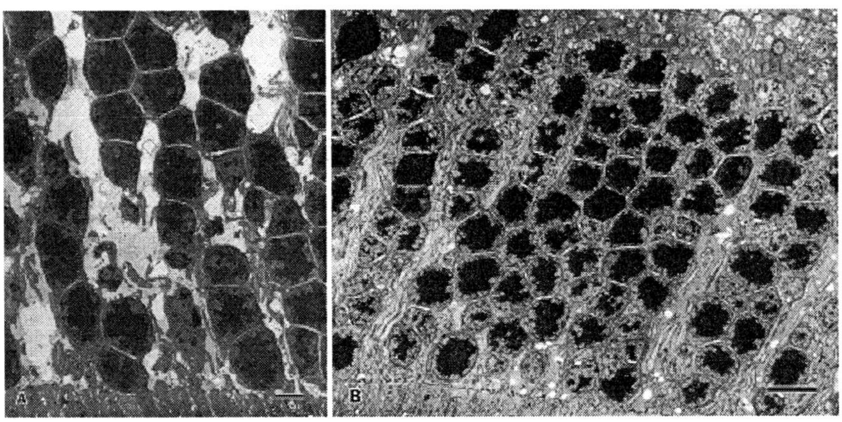

Figure 10.4.2. TEM micrographs of outer nuclear layers of rats. In a rat fed a riboflavin-deficient diet for 3 months, Müller cells are edematous and destroyed, but the number of lines of nuclei is kept. The space of Müller cells after damage contains cellular debrises and amorphous substances (A). B shows the outer nuclear layer of a rat recovered from riboflavin deficiency. Nuclei and Müller cells are compactly arranged. Bar: 2μm (A), 5μm (B).

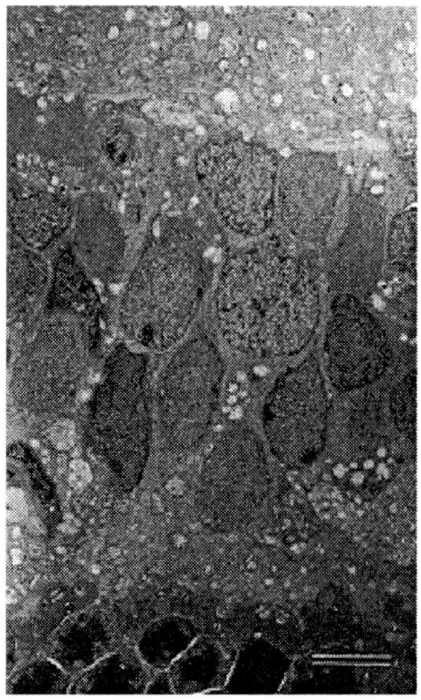

Figure 10.4.3. TEM micrograph of inner nuclear layer of a rat fed a riboflavin-deficient diet for 3 months. The number of nuclei is 3-4 lines. Bar: 5μm.

Discussion

The riboflavin deficiency seemed to affect the retina very slightly: edematous swelling of Müller cells in the outer nuclear layer and; increased phagocytosis of photoreceptor cell outer segment discs even 7h after light exposure. It has been established that rod shedding in the rat and mouse occurs at the beginning of the light cycle and cone shedding at the beginning of the dark cycle. These sheddings follow a circadian rhythm (La Vail, 1976). Phagocytosis of the rat RPE begins at the start of light exposure: the peak of phagocytosis is 2 to 3 hours later and almost no phagocytosis occurs after 6h. The normal circadian rhythm is disturbed by some vitamins and trace elements. Vitamin B_{12} deficiency induces the maximal phagocytosis in the RPE 3h after the start of light exposure (Imamura and Amemiya, 1995). However, the circardian rhythm with one-hour-behind maximum of phagocytosis in vitamin B_{12}-deficient rats recovers by administration with vitamin B_{12}. Thus vitamin B_{12} might be related to circadian rhythm regulation. In addition, vitamin B_{12} deficiency affects no morphological photoreceptor cell changes, despite the decrease of ganglion cells and disappearance of myelinated nerve fibers. Another type of disturbed circadian rhythm is continuous phagocytosis with the maximum at 3h after the start of light exposure under Cr deficiency. In Cr deficiency morphological alterations suggest increased phagocytosis of the outer segment discs and very slight degeneration of the photoreceptor cell under the abnormal phagocytosis of the RPE at the initial stage. But in the late stage the whole retina is led to degeneration (Ueda, Kanazawa, Gong et al, 2002). In riboflavin deficiency, slight degeneration of the outer segment discs may induce enhanced phagocytosis due to increased disc degradation. It remains unclear whether enhanced phagocytosis in the RPE in riboflavin deficiency is a sign of the beginning of degeneration of the photoreceptor cell because of no existing data on long-term riboflavin deficiency.

Riboflavin has antioxidant action through the activity of flavoenzyme and glutathione reductase (Batey and Eckhert, 1991). According to author's research, main antioxidative actions to polyunsaturated fatty acids in the outer segment discs may be related to vitamins A and E and trace elements such as Zn and Mn. Riboflavin might play less of a role for the prevention of peroxidation of disc membranes.

V. THE OPTIC NERVE

Results

Electron Microscopic Findings

In the 3rd month of the experiment the control rat optic nerve had numerous myelinated nerve fibers (Fig. 10.5.1A), and myelin sheaths and myelinated axons showed no abnormality. Riboflavin-deficient rats also had numerous myelinated nerve fibers as much as the controls (Table 10.5.1). Myelin lamellae showed almost the same amount and thickness as those of the controls, but were slightly irregularly arranged. The myelin axon contained neurotubules and fibrils, and a few vacuoles (Fig.10.5.B, C). The recovered rats had more damages and deformed myelin lamellae (Fig. 10.5.1D,E).

Table 10.5.1. Number of myelinated nerve fibers in the optic nerve per 600μm²

Groups	Number of fields examined	Number of myelinated nerve fibers
Control rat	20	233.7±22.6
3-month-riboflavin-deficient rat	20	247.1±34.0
2-month-recovery rat	20	227.0±27.1

No significant difference

Discussion

A series of the studies on vitamins and trace elements revealed that deficiencies of vitamins A, B_{12} (Amemiya, Kawata and Maekawa, 1987), C (Tsuda, 2002) and E and trace elements such as Zn (Gong and Amemiya, 2001), Mn (Gong and Amemiya, 1999), Mg (Gong, Takami and Amemiya, 2003), and Cu (Dake and Amemiya, 1991; Mishima, Dake and Amemiya, 1996) destruct the myelin sheath and axons. However, riboflavin deficiency induced very slight changes in the optic nerve. Riboflavin might have the least action to maintain the retinal and optic nerve architectures, although riboflavin-containing enzymes are related to the metabolism of carbohydrates, amino acids and fat (Bogert, Briggs and Calloway, 1973).

Since vitamin B_2 deficiency caused only slight damage to the retina and the duration of deficiency in the current experiment seemed to be too short, it might be difficult to induce retrograde loss of axons initiated by the loss of retinal fibers.

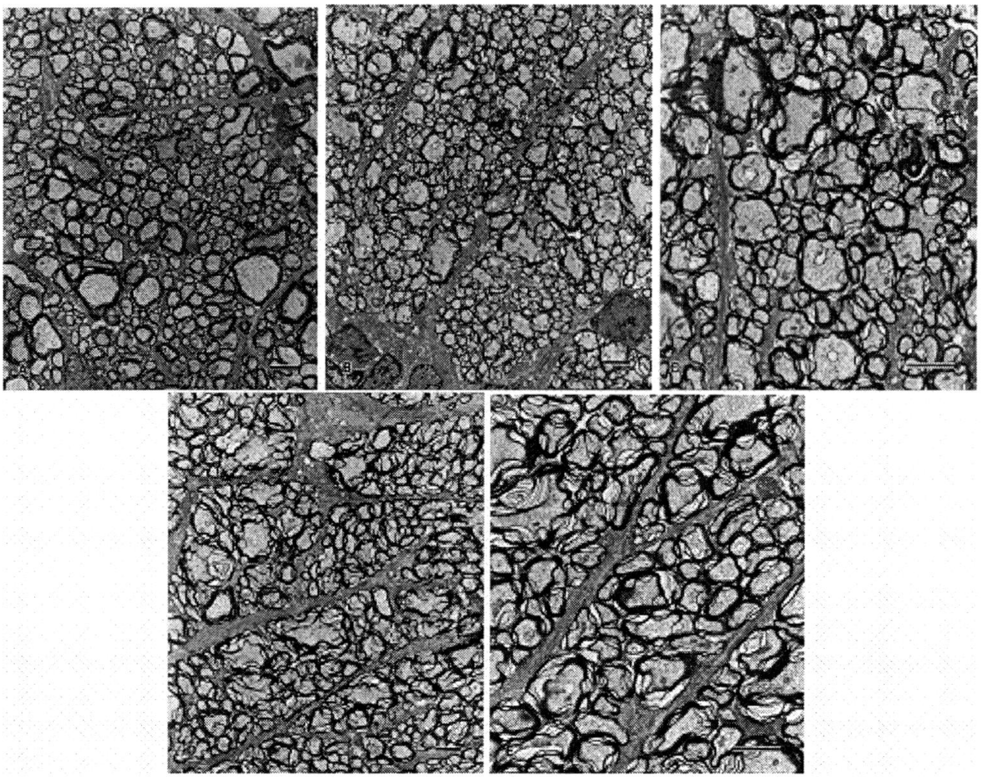

Figure 10.5.1. TEM micrographs of optic nerves of the riboflavin-deficient, recovery and control rats. (A) A control rat optic nerve shows no abnormal findings. In rats fed a riboflavin-deficient diet for 3 months, the optic nerve looks no decrease of myelinated nerve fibers, but myelin lamellae are slightly irregular in arrangement and axoplasmal components are degenerated (B). Myelinated axons of a deficient rat show a few vacuoles, slightly destructed neurotubules and mitochondria and irregular arrangement of myelin sheath (C). In rats recovered from riboflavin deficiency, myelinated nerve fibers look normal in number (D). Myelin lamellae are still irregular in arrangement,and axoplasmic components seem to have more damages (E). Bar: 2μm (A-E).

References

Amemiya T, Kawata T, Maekawa A. Ocular pathology of vitamin B_{12}-deficient rats. In Takaku F, Uchino H, ed. *Kyoto Symposium on Methyl B_{12}*. Tokyo: Kyodo Tsushin; 1987: 80-85.

Bates CJ. Human riboflavin requirements, and metabolic consequences of deficiency in man and animals. *World Rev Nutr Diet*. 1987;50:215-265.

Batey DW, Eckert CD. Analysis of flavins in ocular tissues of the rabbit. *Invest Ophthalmol Vis Sci*. 1991;32:1981-1985.

Bessey OA, Wolbach SH. Vascularization of the cornea of the rat in riboflavin deficiency with a note on corneal vascularization in vitamin A deficiency. *J Exp Med*. 1939;69:1-12.

Bietti G. Ocular manifestation of vitamin deficiencies and disordered vitamin metabolism. *Metabol Ophthalmol*. 1977;1:81-89.

Bogert LJ, Briggs GM, Calloway DH. *Nutrition and Physical Fitness*, 9th. ed. Philadelphia. Saunders Comp; 1973:127-133.

Dake Y, Amemiya T. Electron microscopic study of the optic nerve in copper deficient rats. *Exp Eye Res*. 1991;52:277-281.

Day PL, Langston WC, O'Brien LS. Cataract and other ocular changes in vitamin G deficiency. *Am J Ohthalmol*. 1931;14:1005-1009.

Day PL, Langston WC, Cosgrove KW. Further experiments with cataract in albino rats resulting from withdrawal of vitamin G. *J Nutr*. 1934;7:97-104.

Farkas TG, Sylnester V, Arher D. The ultrastructure of drusen. *Am J Ophthalmol*. 1971;71;1196-1205.

Fromer CH, Klintworth GK. An evaluation of the role of leucocytes in the pathogenesis of experimentally induced corneal vascularization. *Am J Pathol*. 1975;79: 537-550.

Fujikawa A, Gong H, Amemiya T. Vitamin E prevents changes in the cornea and conjunctiva due to vitamin A deficiency. *Graefes Arch Clin Exp Ophthalmol*. 2003;241:287-297.

Gong H, Amemiya T. Corneal changes in manganese-deficient rats. *Cornea*. 1999;18:472-482.

Gong H, Amemiya T. Optic nerve changes in zinc-deficient rats. *Exp Eye Res*. 2001;72:361-369.

Gong H, Takami Y, Kitaoka T, Amemiya T. Corneal changes in magnesium-deficient rats. *Cornea*. 2003;22:448-456.

Gong H, Takami Y, Amemiya T, Tozu M, Ohashi Y. Ocular surface in Zn-deficient rats. *Ophthalmic Res*. 2004;36:129-138.

Goodman LS, Gilman AG. Water-soluble vitamins. In Gilman AG, Goodman LS, Rall TW, Mural F, ed. *Goodman and Gilman's the Pharmacological Basis of Therapeutics*, 7th ed. New York:Macmillan Publishing Comp;1985:1552-1557.

Hogan MJ, Alvarado J. Studies on the human macula. IV. Aging changes in Bruch's membrane. *Arch Ophthalmol*. 1967;77:410-420.

Imamura N, Dake Y, Amemiya T. Circadian rhythm in the retinal pigment epithelium related to vitamin B_{12}. *Life Sci*. 1995;57:1317-1323.

Kanazawa S, Kitaoka T, Ueda Y, Gong H, Amemiya T. Interaction of zinc and vitamin A on the ocular surface. *Graefes Arch Clin Exp Ophthalmol*. 2002;240:1011-1021.

Keen CL, Zindenberg-Cherr S. Trace element and vitamin interactions in free radical defence. In Wahlqvist ML, Truswell AS, Smith R, Nestel PJ, ed. Nutrition in a Sustainable Environment. *Proceedings of the XV International Congress of Nutrition*. Adelaide, London:Smith-Gordon and Company Limited;1994:799-803.

LaVail MM. Rod outer segment disk shedding in rat retina: relationship to cyclic lighting. *Science*. 1976;194:1071-1074.

Lee OS, Hart WM. The metabolism of the cornea. *Am J Ophthalmol*. 1944;27:488-500.

Masuda K, Aoyama J. Endemic occurrence of ariboflavinosis and pellagra. Clinical observations of so-called "Sibi" or "Gatchaki" in Tsugaru district. *Tohoku J Exp Med*. 1951;55:1-5.

McComic DB. Two interconnected B vitamins: Riboflavin and pyridoxine. *Physiol Rev*. 1989;69:1170-1198.

Miller PJ, Johnson RL, Hoeffer JA, Luecre RW. The riboflavin requirement of the bay pig. *J Nutr*. 1954;52:405-413.

Mishima K, Dake Y, Amemiya T. Electron microscopic study of optic nerves of macular mice. *Exp Eye Res*. 1996;63:85-90.

Mizoguchi T, Amemiya T. Ultrastructure of the corneal epithelium of zinc deficient rats —deficiency and recovery. *Trace Element Med*. 1992;9:84-89.

Reeves PG, Nielsen FH, Fahey GC. AIN-93G purified diets for laboratory rodents: final report of the American Institute of Nutrition Ad Hoc writing committee on the reformulation of the AIN-76A rodent diet. *J Nutr*. 1993;123:1939-1951.

Schnitzler E, Sporl E, Seiler T. Bestrahlung der Hornhaut mit UV-Licht und Ribo-flavingabe als neuer Behandlungsversuch bei einschmerzenden Hornhautprozessen, erste Ergebnisse bei vier Patienten. *Klin Monatsbl Augenheilkd*. 2000;217:190-193.

Tsuda Y. Optic nerve changes in ascorbic acid-deficient rats. *Acta Med Nagasaki*. 2002;47:161-166.

Ueda Y, Kanazawa S, Gong H, Miyamura N, Kitaoka T, Amemiya T. The retinal pigment epithelium of Cr-deficient rats. *Life Sci*. 2002;71:1569-1577.

Wilson JA. In Petersdorf RG, ed. Harrison's *Principles of Internal Medicine*. 10th ed. 1982:461-470.

Chapter 11

VITAMIN B_{12} (COBALAMIN)

I. SIGNIFICANCE

Vitamin B_{12} was isolated in 1948 and subsequently it was determined that adenosylcobalamin and methylcobalamin are the two active cofactor forms of vitamin B_{12} in a carbon-cobalt bond. Vitamin B_{12} deficiency induces megaloblastic anemia and a specific neuropathy; vitamin B_{12}-associated neuropathy or subacute combined degeneration of the cord.

Vitamin B_{12} is synthesized by bacteria, which is its only source. It is present in virtually all forms of animal tissues, which acquire the vitamin indirectly from bacteria. Thus, vitamin B_{12} is not present in plants (Weir and Scott, 1999).

Methylmalonyl-CoA mutase and methionine synthase need vitamin B_{12} as a coenzyme in mammalian cells (Weir and Scott, 1999). Methylmalonyl-CoA mutase is involved in the conversion of propionic to succinic acid, which is necessary for fatty acid metabolism. Methionine synthase plays important roles for nucleic acid synthesis and the methylation reactions of the body.

The effect of vitamin B_{12} on the eye is scarcely reported (Amemiya, Kawata and Maekawa, 1987). Agamanolis et al (1976) showed demyelination and proliferation of astrocytes in the optic nerve of a monkey with dietary vitamin B_{12}-deficiency. Rob et al (1984) reported retinal degeneration in a patient with methylmalonic aciduria and sulfur amino acid abnormalities. Sandyk (1984) presented paralysis of upward gaze as a presenting symptom of vitamin B_{12} deficiency.

II. Vitamin B_{12}-Deficient Experiment

Materials and Methods

Male Wistar Kyoto rats were fed a vitamin B_{12}-deficient diet for 3 months starting 20 days after birth. After having been on a vitamin B_{12}-deficient diet for 3 months, some of the vitamin B_{12}-deficient rats were injected intraperitoneally with vitamin B_{12} (1μg per g body weight) 1 day, 2 and 3 weeks after deficiency and fed the normal diet for these 3 weeks as a recovery experiment. Controls were 3- to 4-month-old male normal Wistar Kyoto rats.

Clinical Features of the Vitamin B_{12}-Deficient Animals

The rats fed a vitamin B_{12}-deficient diet for 3 months had lower serum levels of vitamin B_{12} than did the control group (Table 11.2.1). There was no statistically significant difference in the serum level of vitamin B_{12} between the recovered and control groups. However, the injected group is one-half the levels found in the normal group, although the standard deviation for the normal control group covers a large range. Controls were 3- to 4-month old male normal Wistar Kyoto rats.

Table 11. 2. 1. Serum vitamin B_{12} levels in B_{12}-deficient, B_{12} injected and normal control rats.

	Mean±SD	Number of rats examined
Control group	1164.3±435.7	13
B_{12}-deficient group	55.6±35.6	11
B_{12} injected group	588.9±82.4	9

There is a significant difference ($p<0.05$) between the control group and the B_{12}-deficient group, and also there is a significant difference ($p<0.05$) between the B_{12} injected group and the B_{12}-deficient group.

III. The Retina

Experiment

For the experiment of the circadian rhythm, the eyes were enucleated under Nembutal anesthesia immediately before and 1, 2 or 3, 4, 6, 10, 11 or 12h after the start of light exposure and 1, 2 or 3h after dark.

Results

Light Microscopic Findings

There were 4-5 layers of inner nuclear layer nuclei and 8-9 layers of outer nuclear layer nuclei in rats fed a vitamin B_{12}-deficient diet for 3 months. The retina looked normal, but a separation was present between the nerve fiber and ganglion cell layers (Fig. 11.3.1).

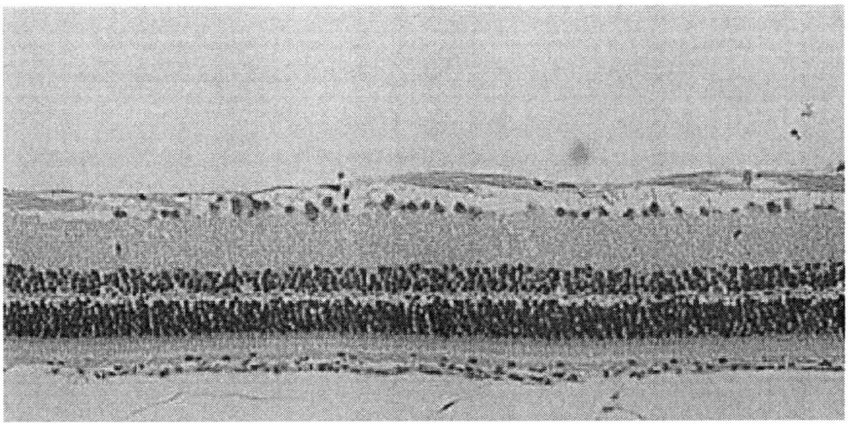

Figure. 11.3.1. Light micrograph of the retina of a vitamin B_{12}-deficient rat. A separation between the nerve fiber and ganglion cell layers is seen. HE stain, × 200.

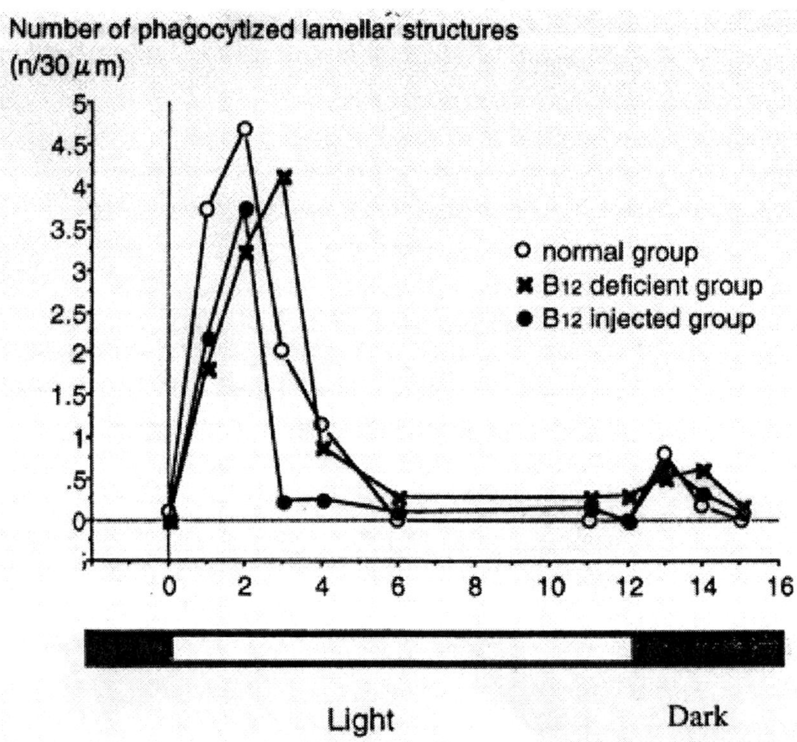

Figure 11.3.2. Number of phagocytized lamellar structures after the start of light exposure and darkness.

Electron Microscopic Findings

There were many lamellar structures, probably phagocytized by the retinal pigment epithelium (RPE), in the RPE. Fig. 11.3.2 shows the changes in the number of lamellar structures phagocytized by the RPE. The number of phagocytized lamellar structures reached a peak 2h after the start of light exposure in the control and vitamin B_{12}-injected groups. After the start of darkness another peak of lamellar structures appeared at 1h in the control and B_{12} injected groups. However, the vitamin B_{12}-deficient group showed a peak of phagocytized lamellar structures in the RPE at 3h after the start of light exposure (Fig. 11.3. 3-5) and a small peak 2h after the start of darkness. The peak of the number of phagocytized lamellar structures showed a statistically significant difference ($P<0.01$) at 2 and 3h after the start of light exposure between the control and vitamin B_{12}-deficient groups, but no significant difference at 1 and 2h after the start of darkness. There were no morphological findings in the 3 groups and no significant electron microscopic differences in the RPE between the normal control and vitamin B_{12}-deficient groups.

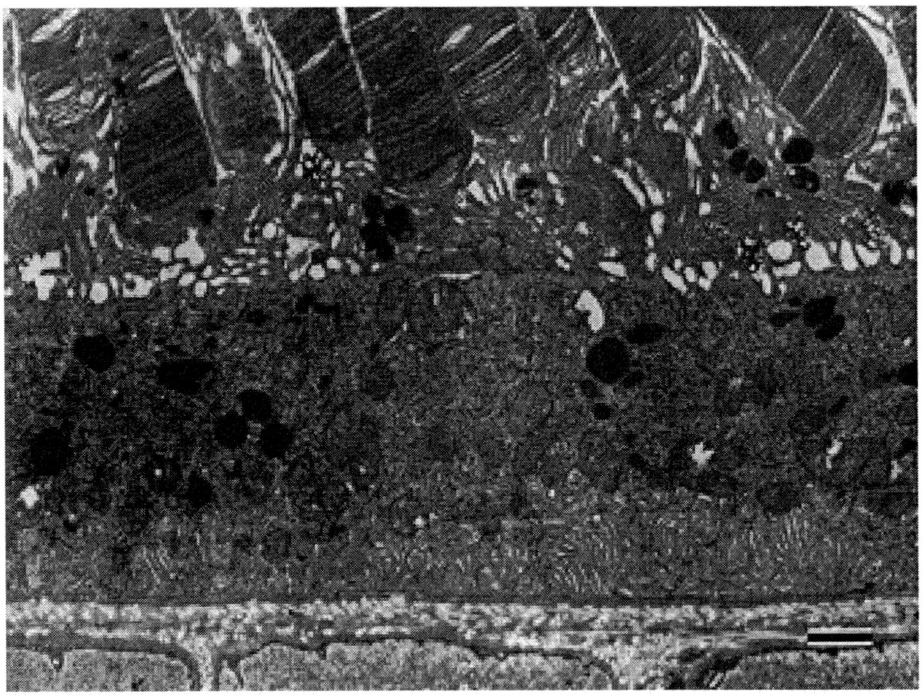

Figure 11.3.3. Electron micrograph of lamellar structures in the retinal pigment epithelium of a normal control rat 3h after start of light exposure. Bar: 1μm.

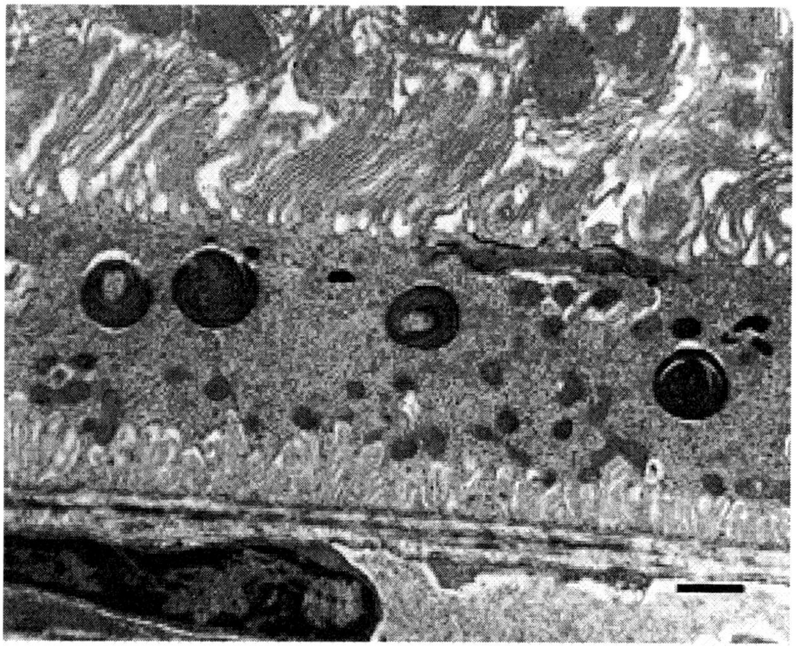

Figure 11.3.4. Electron micrograph of lamellar structures in the retinal pigment epithelium of a vitamin B_{12}-deficient rat 3h after start of light exposure. Bar: 1μm.

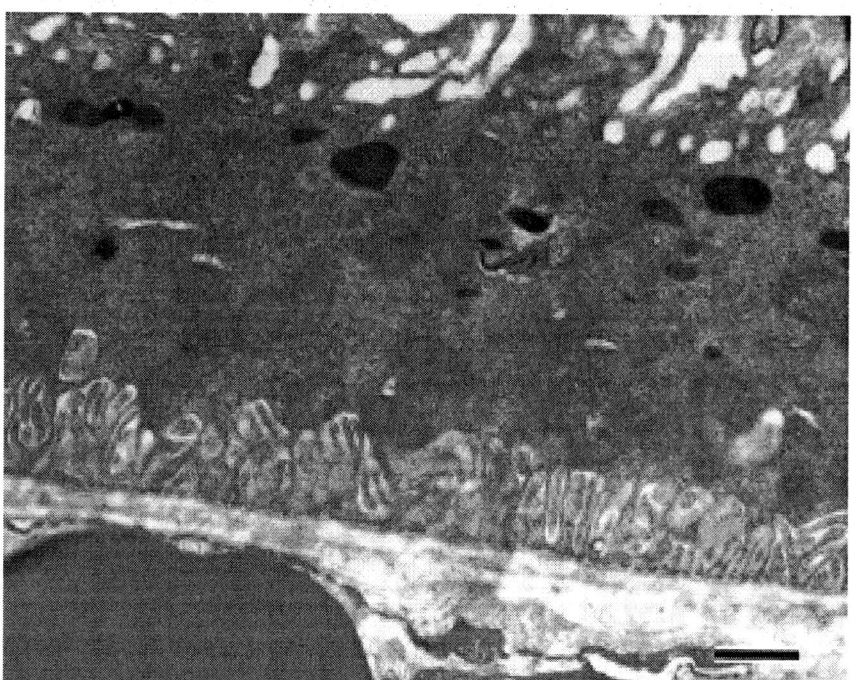

Figure 11.3.5. Electron micrograph of lamellar structures in the retinal pigment epithelium of a vitamin B_{12}-injected rat 3h after start of light exposure. Bar: 1μm.

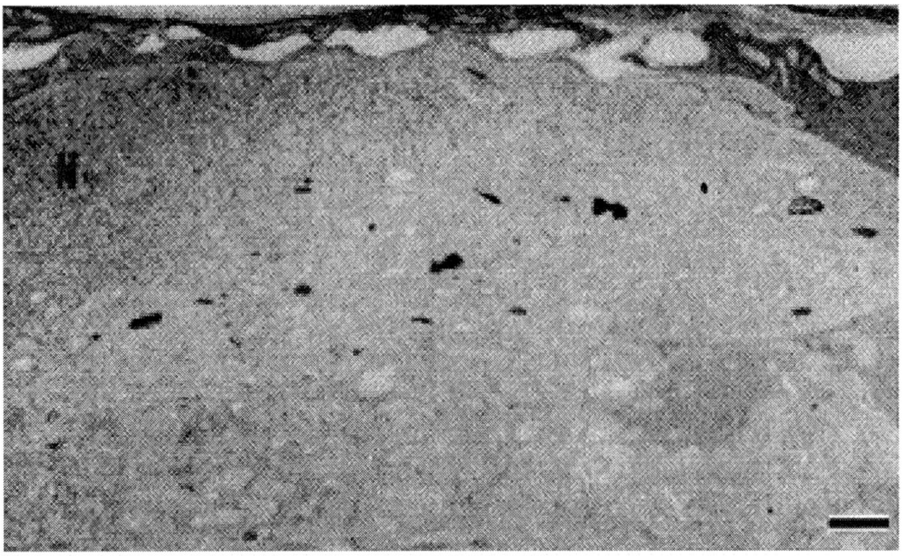

Figure 11.3.6. Electron micrograph of the retina of a vitamin B_{12}-deficient rat. Separations are seen between the nerve fiber and ganglion cell layers, but Müller cell dendrites extend to ganglion cells. Bar: 1μm.

The electron microscopy showed no morphological abnormalities in the photoreceptor cell, outer and inner plexiform layers, inner nuclear layer; 8 or 9 layers in the outer nuclear layer and 4 or 5 layers in the inner nuclear layer. However, there were empty spaces between the nerve fiber layer and ganglion cell layer, but Müller cell dendrites extended to ganglion cells and prevented a separation between the two layers (Fig.11.3.6). Ganglion cells and nerve fibers were decreased in number (Fig. 11.3.7).

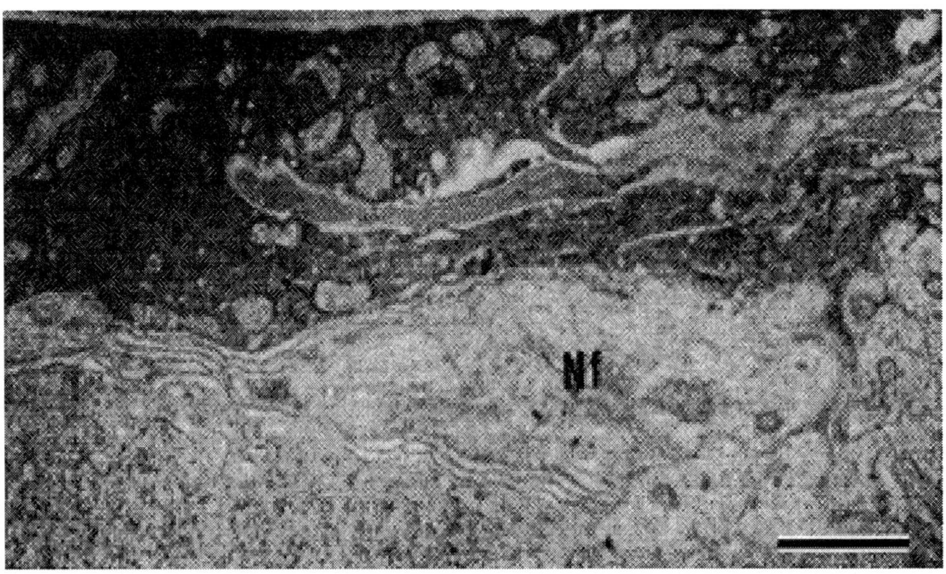

Figure 11.3.7. Electron micrograph of the ganglion cell and nerve fiber layers of the retina of a vitamin B_{12}-deficient rat. Nerve fibers are scarce and no ganglion cells are seen. Bar: 1μm.

Discussion

It is well known that some organs and systems of all animals have circadian rhythm. For example, the wake-sleep rhythm is a typical circadian rhythm. Animals have their own wake-sleep rhythms. The rhythm is controlled by its own center. The pineal body of the chicken, which is famous as a biological clock, shows a circadian rhythm in vitro (Okawa, Mishima, Nanami et al, 1978). Some circadian rhythms have their own control center. The structural changes in the retina may not have any effect on the retinal circadian rhythm since electron microscopic examination failed to show morphological differences between the control and vitamin B_{12}-deficient groups.

There are two kinds of photoreceptor cells, cones for light adaptation and rods for dark adaptation. The tips of cone and rod outer segments are shedding in the RPE. It has been established that rod shedding in the rat and mouse occurs at the beginning of the light cycle and cone shedding at the beginning of the dark cycle. This shedding follows a circadian rhythm. LaVail (1976) reported that the rat RPE begins to phagocytize the outer segment disc immediately after the start of light exposure, and the peak of phagocytization is 2 to 3h later. Our normal group showed the same peak, but the peak of phagocytosis in the vitamin B_{12}-deficient group was delayed about 1h. On the other hand, the recovered group showed the same pattern of retinal circadian rhythm of photoreceptor disc shedding in the retina. While the peak of the rod shedding showed a statistically significant difference 2 and 3h after the start of light between the control and vitamin B_{12}-deficient groups, the peak of cone shedding was lower than that of rod shedding and looked different in the vitamin B_{12}-deficient group. But, there was no statistically significant difference in the number of phagocytized lamellar structures at 1 and 2h after the start of darkness. Since the rat and mouse are nocturnal and exhibit a rod-rich retina with few cones, the peak after dark may be low. Thus, in the rat, cones are too scarce for a difference in shedded cones to be clear. Phagocytization of outer segments in the RPE may be controlled by the center of circadian rhythm and the endophthalmic center. Korenbrot and Fernald (1989) reported that in toad and fish retinas the level of mRNA for opsin, the most abundant protein in rod discs, fluctuates with a daily rhythm and is regulated by both light and a circadian oscillator. It is also said that the center of circadian rhythm may be situated in the pineal body, suprachiasmatic nucleus and/or other circadian centers. As yet, investigators have been unable to find a link between circadian centers and the rhythm of disc shedding (Stetson and Watson-Whitmyre, 1976), since neither pinealectomy, superior cervical ganglionectomy and hypophysectomy nor thyroidectomy and parathyroidectomy alter disc shedding (Tamai, Teirstein, Goldman et al, 1978). Teirstein et al (1980) reported that the patched eye, shielded from the direct effect of 24h continuous light, continues cyclical shedding of the photoreceptor disc. This means that the inhibitory effect of 24 hours of continuous light can influence one eye without affecting the other eye. It is said that there are some enzymes and hormones related to light (LaVail and Ward, 1978; Mathews and Basinger, 1980; Cardinal and Rosner, 1971; Schaffer, Brownstein and Axelrod, 1977; Iuvone, Galli, Garrison-Gund et al, 1978). There is no evidence, however, of a relationship between vitamin B_{12} and circadian rhythm.

Kamgar-Parsi et al (1983) first prescribed vitamin B_{12} for a patient who had a non-24-h-sleep-wake rhythm. Since this patient incidentally had mild hypothyroidism, he was given vitamin B_{12}, which had a very favorable effect on the sleep-wake disturbance. Since then, there have been many reports of similar favorable effects of vitamin B_{12} on wake-sleep disturbance (Okawa, Mishima, Nanami et al, 1990). The mechanism by which vitamin B_{12} produces beneficial effects on circadian rhythm disturbances is unclear. Some possible mechanisms are as follows (Imamura and Amemiya, 1995); vitamin B_{12} may change the timing of the circadian rhythm; vitamin B_{12} may increase sensitivity to light; vitamin B_{12} may increase sensitivity to synchronization factors other than light. The auther assumes that the circadian rhythm in the RPE was changed by the decrease of synchronizing factors following vitamin B_{12} deficiency. When vitamin B_{12}-deficient rats received vitamin B_{12}, they regained the normal rhythm of phagocytosis of outer segments. Since many phenomena such as blood pressure, ocular tension and sleep-wake rhythm follow circadian rhythm, vitamin B_{12} may be useful to regulate or relieve pathologic conditions such as hypertension, glaucoma and sleep-wake disturbance.

IV. The Optic Nerve

Results

Light Microscopic Findings

In rats fed a vitamin B_{12}-defecient diet for 3 months, Klüver-Barrera staining method, which stains myelin, failed to demonstrate myelin in the optic nerve posterior to the lamina cribrosa (Fig. 11.4.1).

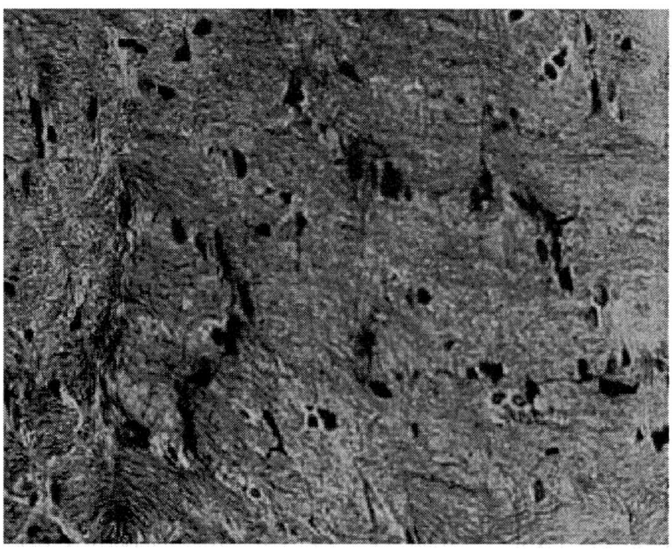

Figure 11.4.1. Light micrograph of the optic nerve of a vitamin B_{12}-deficient rat. Myelin is not stained with Klüver-Barrera stain for myelin. × 400.

Electron Microscopic Findings

In the control rat optic nerve, clusters of numerous myelinated nerve fibers were surrounded by astrocytes. On the other hand, the optic nerves of vitamin B_{12}-deficient and vitamin B_{12}-injected rats showed unmyelinated nerve fibers and proliferated astrocytes were seen (Fig. 11.4.2), but myelinated nerve fibers were not.

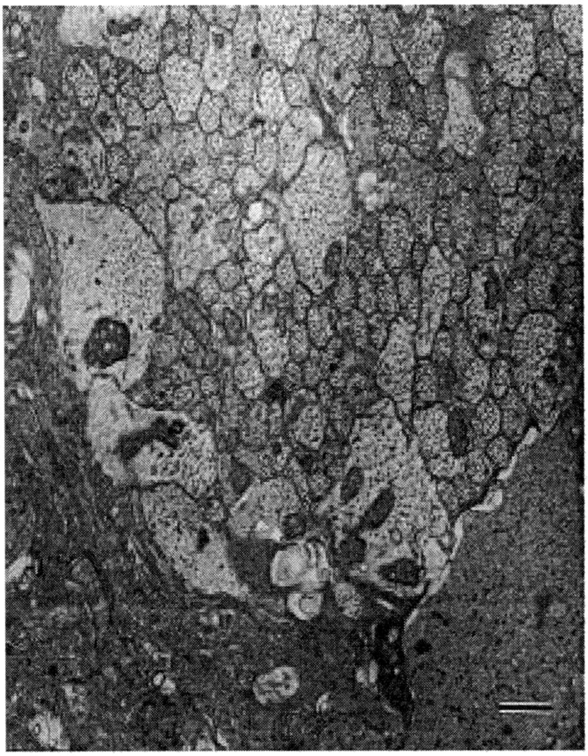

Figure 11.4.2. Electron micrograph of the optic nerve of a vitamin B_{12}-deficient rat. No myelinated nerve fibers are seen, but most are unmyelinated nerve fibers. Bar: 1μm.

Discussion

Ishikawa (1967) reported light microscopic findings in the optic nerve of vitamin B_{12}-deficient rats: edematous swelling and hemorrhage localized in the nerve fiber, ganglion cell and inner plexiform layers, irregular swelling, fragmentation and vacuoles in axons, and incomplete destruction of the myelin sheath. Agamanolis et al (1976) reported that the monkey takes five years to suffer from dietary vitamin B_{12} deficiency and showed demyelination and astrocyte proliferation in the optic nerve by light microscopy. In spite of the difficulty of inducing dietary vitamin B_{12} deficiency in humans and animals, the current experiment shows that the rat can relatively easily be induced to vitamin B_{12} deficiency and is available for this kind of experiment. The vitamin B_{12}-deficient rat showed the same light microscopic finding in the optic nerve as did Agamanolis et al (1976) by light microscopy. Electron microscopy confirmed the disappearance of myelin structures and proliferation of astrocytes.

The enzymes for which vitamin B_{12} is a coenzyme in mammalian cells are methylmalonyl-CoA mutase and methionine synthase. When methionine synthase is inhibited due to vitamin B_{12} deficiency, homocysteine and S-D adenosyl homocysteine accumulate, and methionine and S-adenosylmethionine synthesis is impaired, causing the methylation ratio to fall. The methylation reactions are inhibited, including a state of hypomethylation and impaired synthesis of myelin basic protein (Weir and Scott, 1999: van der Westhuyzen, 1983). Thus the myelin sheath in the optic nerve of vitamin B_{12}-deficient rats may be degenerated and disappear.

V. The Rectus Muscle

Results

Light Microscopic Findings

Light microscopy revealed no abnormalities in the rectus muscle of rats with vitamin B_{12}-deficiency.

Electron Microscopic Findings

In the rectus muscles of vitamin B_{12}-deficient rats, electron micrographs showed lipid droplet-like vacuoles near mitochondria in the cytoplasm of myocytes (Fig. 11.5.1), but neither irregular arrangement of myofilaments, A-Z bands nor abnormal mitochondria were present.

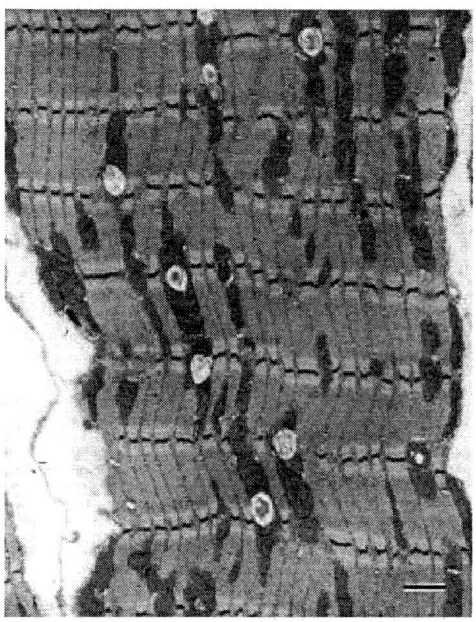

Figure 11.5.1. Electron micrograph of the rectus muscle of a vitamin B_{12}-deficient rat. Lipid-like droplets are present near mitochondria in the cytoplasm of a myocyte, but muscular bundles are regularly arranged. Bar: 1μm.

Discussion

Most of the ultrastructural lesions in humans and animals with vitamin B_{12} deficiency are concerned with changes in the number and presence of inclusions of mitochondria (Peterson and Vahouny, 1975; Frenkel, Mukherjee, Hackenbrock et al, 1976; Maltin, Duncan and Wilson, 1983). However, the current study showed no mitochondrial alterations in the rectus muscle. Further study is needed to confirm a difference in preponderance between rectus muscle and skeletal muscle. Paralysis of upward gaze was reported to be improved with the administration of cyanocobalamin (Sandyk, 1984). Defects of cellular methylcobalamin and adenosylcobalamin produce muscular hypotonia. Since decreased activities of methylmalonyl-CoA mutase and methionine synthase due to vitamin B_{12}-deficiency induce abnormal lipid and fatty acid metabolism, the appearance of lipid droplets may suggest fatty degeneration in the myocyte, while myopathy may be a specific neuropathy called vitamin B_{12}-associated neuropathy or subacute combined degeneration of the cord.

REFERENCES

Agamanolis DP, Chester EM, Victor M, Kark JA, Hines JD, Harris JW. Neuropathology of experimental vitamin B_{12} deficiency in monkeys. *Neurology.* 1976;26:905-914.

Amemiya T, Kawata T, Maekawa A. Ocular pathology of vitamin B_{12}-deficient rats. In Takaku F, Uchino H, ed. *Kyoto Symposium on Methyl B_{12}.* Tokyo: Kyodo Tsushin;1987:80-85.

Binkley SA, Riebman JB, Reilly KB. The pineal gland: a biological clock in vitro. *Science.* 1978;202:1198-1200.

Cardinaly DP, Rosner JM. Retinal localization of the hydroxyindol-O-methyl transferase (HIOMT) in the rat. *Endocrinology.* 1971;89:301-303.

Frenkel EP, Mukherjee A, Hackenbroch CR, Srere PA. Biochemical and ultrastructural hepatic changes during vitamin B_{12} deficiency in animals and man. *J Biol Chem.* 1976;251:2147-2154.

Imamura N, Dake Y, Amemiya T. Circadian rhythm in the retinal pigment epithelium related t vitamin B_{12}. *Life Sci.* 1995;57:1317-1323.

Ishikawa K. Histopathological studies on the experimental vitamin B_{12} neuropathy. *Acta Soc Ophthalmol Jpn.* 1967;71:1589-1606.

Iuvone PM, Galli CL, Garrison-Gund CK, Neff NH. Light stimulates tyrosine hydro-xylase activity and dopamine synthesis in retinal amacrine neurons. *Science.* 1978;202:901-902.

Kamgar-Parsi B, Wehr TA, Gillin JC. Successful treatment of human non-24-hour sleep-wake syndrome. *Sleep* 1983;6:257-264.

Korenbrot JI, Fernald RD. Circadian rthym and light regulate opsin mRNA in rod photoreceptors. *Nature.* 1989;337:454-457.

LaVail MM. Rod outer segment disk shedding in rat retina:relationship to cyclic lighting. *Science.* 1976;194:1071-1074.

LaVail MM, Ward PA. Studies on the hormonal control of circadian outer segment disc shedding in the rat retina. *Invest Ophthalmol Vis Sci.* 1978;17:1189-1183.

Maltin CA, Duncan L, Wilson AB. Mitochondrial abnormalities in muscle from vitamin B_{12}-deficient sheep. *J Comp Pathol.* 1983;93:429-435.

Matthews MT, Basinger SF. Myeloid body associations in the frog pigment epithelium. *Invest Ophthalmol Vis Sci.* 1980;19:298-302.

Okawa M, Mishima K, Nanami T, Iijima S, Hishikawa Y, Takahashi K. Vitamin B_{12} treatment for sleep-wake rhythm disorders. *Sleep.* 1990;13:15-23.

Peterson BJ, Vahouny GV. Cardiac structure and function in vitamin B_{12} deprived rats. *J Nutr.* 1975;105:1567-1577.

Robb RM, Dowton SB, Fulton AB, Levy HL. Retinal degeneration in vitamin B_{12} disorder associated with methylmalonic aciduria and sulfur amino acid abnormalities. *Am J Ophthalmol.* 1984;97:691-696.

Sandyk B. Paralysis of upward gaze as a presenting symptom of vitamin B_{12} deficiency. *Eur Neurol.* 1984;23:198-200.

Schaffer JM, Brownstein MJ, Axelrod J. Thyrothropin-releasing hormone-like material in the rat retina: changes due to environmental lighting. *Proc Natl Acad Sci USA.* 1977;74:3579-3581.

Stetson MH, Watson-Whitmyre M. Nucleus suprachiasmaticus: the biological clock in the hamster? *Science.* 1976;191:197-199.

Tamai M, Teirstein P, Goldman A, O'Brien P, Chader G. The pineal gland does not control rod outer segment shedding and phagocytosis in the rat retina and pigment epithelium. *Invest Ophthalmol Vis Sci.* 1978;17:558-562.

Teirstein PS, Goldman AI, O'Brien PJ. Evidence for both local and central regulation of rod outer segment disc shedding. *Invest Ophthalmol Vis Sci.* 1980;19:1268-1273.

van der Westhuyzen J. Effect of vitamin B_{12} deficient diet on lipid and fatty acid composition of spinal cord myelin in the fruit bat. *J Nutr.* 1983;113:531-537.

Weir DG, Scott JM. Vitamin B_{12} "cobalamin." In: Maurice E, Shils ME, Olson JA, Shike M, Ross AC, ed. *Modern Nutrition in Health and Disease.* 9th ed. Philadelphia: Lippincott Williams & Wilkins; 1999:447-458.

Chapter 12

ASCORBIC ACID (VITAMIN C)

I. SIGNIFICANCE

A deficiency of ascorbic acid (vitamin C) induces scurvy and hemorrhages in ocular tissues and the mucous membrane (Hoyt, 1979). Ascorbic acid provides reducing equivalents for various biological reactions, and plays as a cofactor for reactions requiring a reduced metal ion (Fe^{2+}, Cu^{1+}). Ascorbic acid serves as a protective antioxidant. Ascorbic acid is also essential for the formation of the mucopolysaccharide components of the ground substance of connective tissue, particularly hydroxyprolin. This may be related to corneal wound healing. Ascorbic acid is reported to be a coenzyme in collagen metabolism (Kurata, 1989). Ascorbic acid plays an important role for collagen formation as a reductive cofactor for posttranslational hydroxylation of peptide-bound proline and lysine residues. Ascorbic acid is a water-soluble dietary antioxidant and can readily donate electrons to quench various reactive free radical and oxidant species and is easily returned to its reduced state by such ubiquitous electron donors as glutathione and NADPH (May, Qu, Whitesell et al, 1996; Xu, Washburns, Sun et al, 1996). The antioxidant ascorbic acid is known to prevent cerebral tissue degeneration (Rice, Lee and Choy, 1995). In spite of these important roles of ascorbic acid, many physiological aspects of ascorbic acid remain obscure.

Most animals except humans, other primates and guinea pigs are capable of synthesizing ascorbic acid from carbohydrate precursors. Since most species of animals can produce ascorbic acid in the body, it is difficult to study the effect of ascorbic acid deficiency in the eyes of experimental animals.

II. ASCORBIC ACID DEFICIENCY

Material and Methods

A colony of mutant Wistar rats (OD rats) with a hereditary defect in ascorbic acid-synthesizing ability has been established (Mizushima, Harauchi, Yoshizaki et al, 1984; Horio, Ozaki, Yoshida et al, 1985). OD rats provided from Nippon Clea Incorporated, Tokyo were fed a usual diet containing no ascorbic acid and deionized distilled water starting 20 days after birth. These rats become ascorbic acid deficient since they cannot produce ascorbic acid. Ascorbic acid-deficient rats were killed 3 weeks after the start of the experiment because they rarely survive longer. Control rats were fed a usual diet and deionized water containing 2mg/ml of ascorbic acid. The rats were killed under Nembutal anesthesia. Blood was drawn from the heart or aorta for measurement of the serum levels of ascorbic acid, Cu, Zn and Mg by a standard atomic absorption spectrophotometer.

In the recovery experiment rats were fed the deficient diet for 3 weeks after weaning and then given deionized water containing 2mg/ml of ascorbic acid for 2 weeks.

In the pair-fed control group, infant rats were nursed by their normal mother rats for 3 weeks, then given the same amount of usual diet that ascorbic acid-deficient rats took on the previous day with free access to water containing 2mg/ml of ascorbic acid.

Clinical Features of Ascorbic Acid-Deficient Animals

Growth retardation was noted in the ascorbic acid-deficient rats by the end of the first week of the experiment. After 3 weeks on the diet, the ascorbic acid-deficient rats were much smaller than the controls (Fig. 12.2.1).

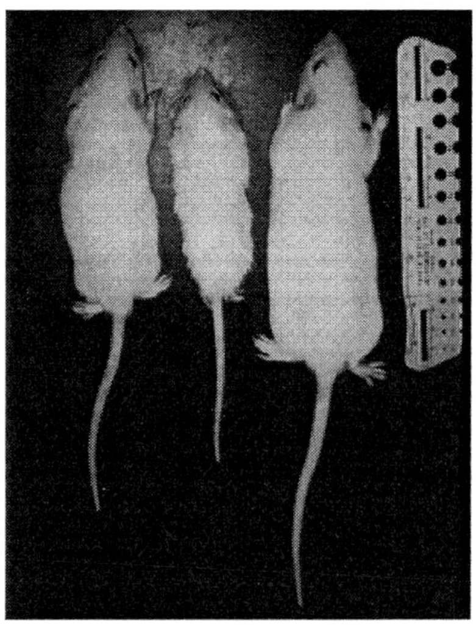

Figure 12.2.1. Gross appearance of the animals. There are obvious differences in a rat which has recovered from ascorbic-acid deficiency (left) (5 weeks after weaning), an ascorbic acid-deficient rat (center) (3 weeks after weaning) and a control rat (right) (3 weeks after weaning).

Most of the ascorbic acid-deficient rats showed hair loss and hemorrhages around the eyes and gait disturbance, and some had conjunctival secretions. By the end of 5th week of the experiment the ascorbic acid-deficient rats died. The pair-fed control rats were small, but looked healthy.

The body weight of the ascorbic acid-deficient rats was significantly lower than that of the controls ($p<0.0001$) (Table 12.2.1). The pair-fed control rats also weighed significantly lower than the controls ($p<0.0001$) (Table 12.2.1).

Table 12.2.1. Body weight.

Groups (n=12)	Weeks after start of experiment		
	1	3	5
Control	34.2±5.3	96.7±8.8 *, **, ***	161.1±13.2 *, **
Ascorbic acid-deficient	30.9±4.9	31.4±6.4 *	
Recovery	31.4±3.2	31.7±9.9 **	65.5±6.3 *
Pair-fed control	30.3±4.6	34.9±4.4 ***	68.3±7.7 **

*, **, *** $p<0.0001$.

Serum ascorbic acid and trace elements: At the end of the 3rd week the serum ascorbic acid level of the ascorbic acid-deficient rats was undetectable; in the control group it was 3.7μg/L. At the end of the 2 weeks of recovery, the serum ascorbic acid level was 2.3μg/L. The serum ascorbic acid level of the pair-fed control rats was 2.3 μg/L (Table 12.2.2). There was no significant difference in the serum ascorbic acid level between the recovery and control groups. There was no significant difference in the serum level of Zn, Cu and Mg in ascorbic acid-deficient, control and pair-fed control rats (Table 12.2.3).

Table 12.2.2. Serum ascorbic acid level.

Groups	n	Serum ascorbic acid (μg/ml)
Control	12	3.7±2.4
Ascorbic acid-deficient	12	undetectable
Recovery	12	2.3±0.6
Pair-fed control	12	2.3±1.0

Serum ascorbic acid level is not significantly different in control, recovery and pair-fed control groups ($p>0.1$).

Table 12.2.3. Serum Zn, Cu and Mg levels.

Groups	n	Serum Zn level	Serum Cu level	Serum Mg level
		(μg/ml)	(μg/ml)	(μg/ml)
Control	12	121±37	114±19	4.0±1.3
Ascorbic acid-deficient	7 *	119±17	108±9	4.1±1.2
Pair-fed control	12	131±9	119±16	3.2±0.6

* Enough blood was not taken in 5 rats.

Serum Zn, Cu and Mg levels are not significantly different in control, ascorbic acid-deficient and pair-fed control groups ($p>0.1$).

III. THE CONJUNCTIVA AND THE CORNEA

Results

1. The Conjunctiva

Scanning Electron Microscopic (SEM) Findings

In control and pair-fed control rats, the conjunctival surface showed many goblet cells with secretory granules, numerous microvilli and microplicae (Fig.12.3.1,2). On the other hand, ascorbic acid-deficient rats had empty goblet cells, and scarce microvilli and microplicae (Fig.12.3.3), but ascorbic acid-recovery rats exhibited goblet cells filled with secretory granules and many microvilli and microplicae (Fig.12.3.4).

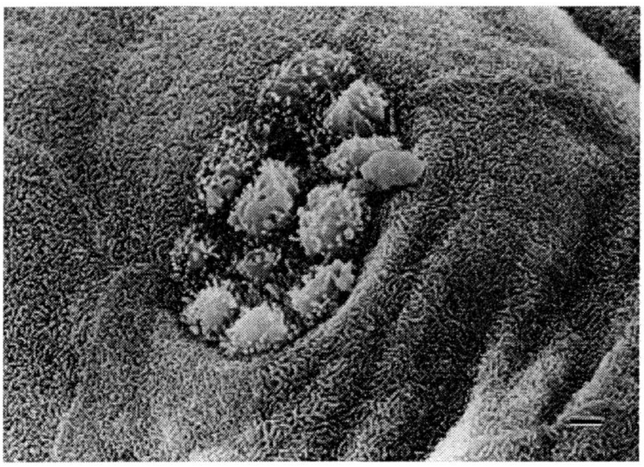

Figure 12.3.1. SEM micrograph of the conjunctival surface of a control rat. A goblet cell keeps many secretory granules at orifice and numerous microvilli and microplicae. Bar: 1μm.

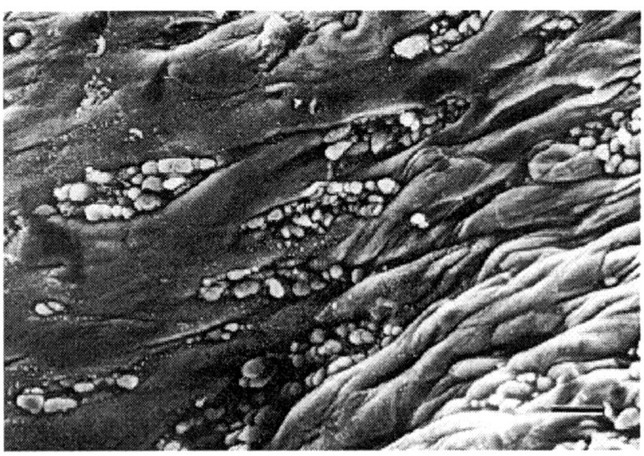

Figure 12.3.2. SEM micrograph of the conjunctival surface of a pair-fed control rat. There are many goblet cells with secretory granules and numerous microvilli and microplicae. Bar: 10μm.

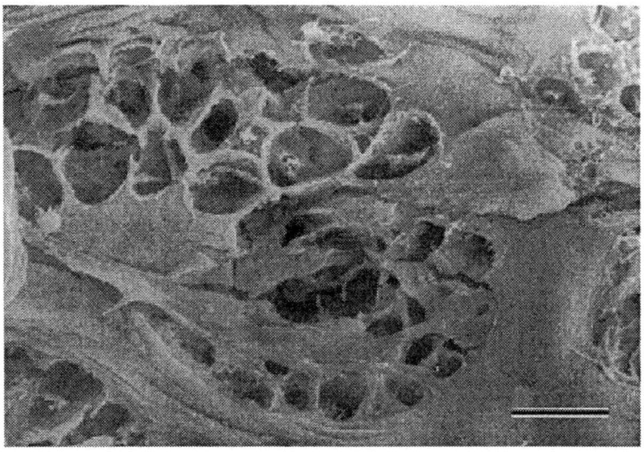

Figure 12.3.3. SEM micrograph of the conjunctival surface of an ascorbic acid-deficient rat. The orifices of goblet cells look empty. Bar: 10μm.

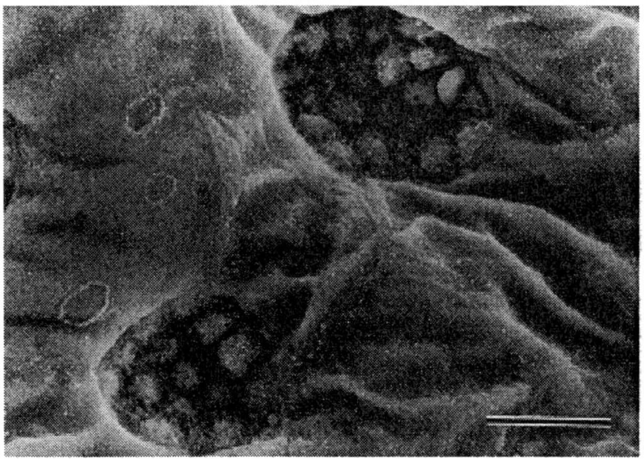

Figure 12.3.4. SEM micrograph of the conjunctival surface of an ascorbic acid recovery rat. Secretory granules are seen at the orifice of goblet cells. Numerous microvilli and microplicae are seen on the most superficial layer of epithelium. Bar: 10μm.

Transmission Electron Microscopic (TEM) Findings

In ascorbic acid-deficient rats, the most superficial epithelial layer had small goblet cells with less dense secretory granules and scarce microvilli (Fig 12.3.5).

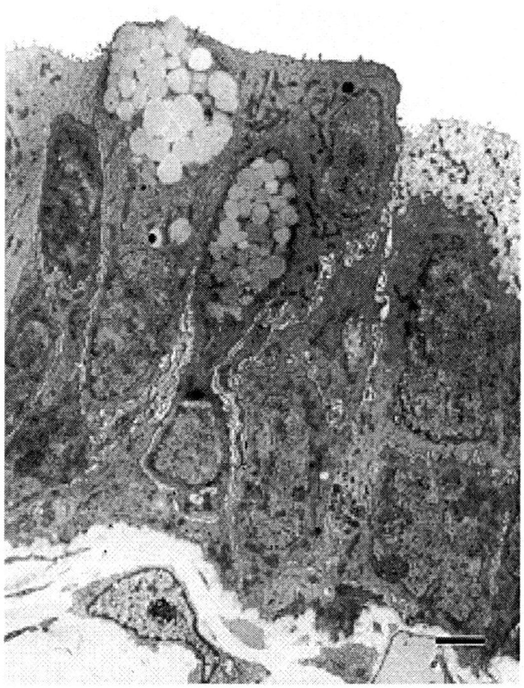

Figure 12.3.5. TEM micrograph of the conjunctiva of an ascorbic acid-deficient rat. The orifice of goblet cell is tiny and secretory granules are less dense. Microvilli are scarce in the most superficial layer of the epithelium. Bar: 2μm.

2. The Cornea

SEM Findings

In control and pair-fed control rats, SEM showed numerous microvilli and microplicae in the most superficial epithelial cells (Fig.12.3.6), while ascorbic acid-deficient rats had many dark cells with less microvilli and microplicae in the epithelium (Fig.12.3.7).

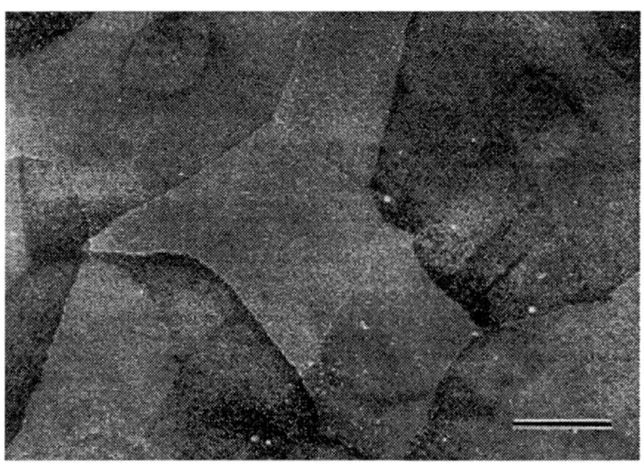

Figure 12.3.6. SEM micrograph of corneal surface of a pair-fed control rat. There are numerous microvilli and microplicae. Bar: 10μm.

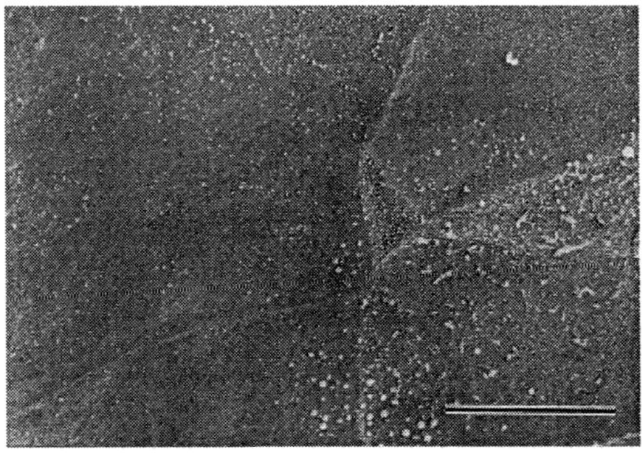

Figure 12.3.7. SEM micrograph of corneal surface of an ascorbic acid-deficient rat. Epithelial cells are dark and have less microvilli and microplicae. Bar: 10μm.

TEM Findings

In control and pair-fed control rats, the corneal epithelium had many ribosomes, fibrils, mitochondria and desmosome-like intercellular junctions and showed no abnormal findings in the subepithelium (Fig.12.3.8).

In ascorbic acid-deficient rats, on the other hand, TEM revealed scarce microvilli in the epithelium, but many intercellular junctions and well-developed cytoplasmic components (Fig.12.3.9).

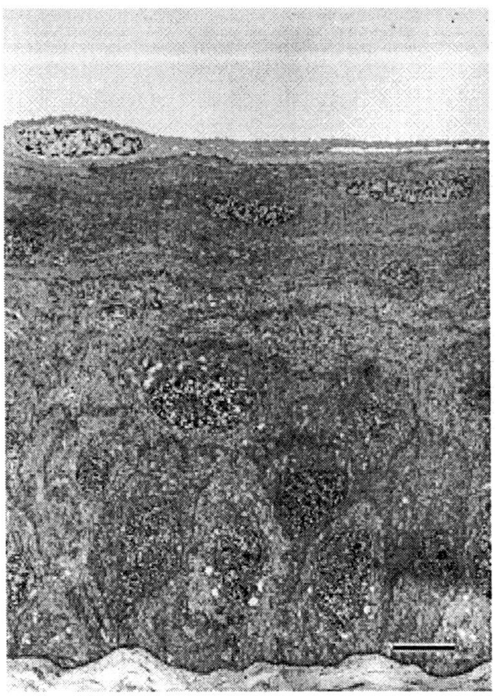

Figure 12.3.8. TEM micrograph of the corneal epithelium of a pair-fed control rat. Epithelial cells have many ribosomes, fibrils, mitochondria and desmosome-like intercellular junctions. The subepithelial layer shows no abnormalities. Bar: 5μm.

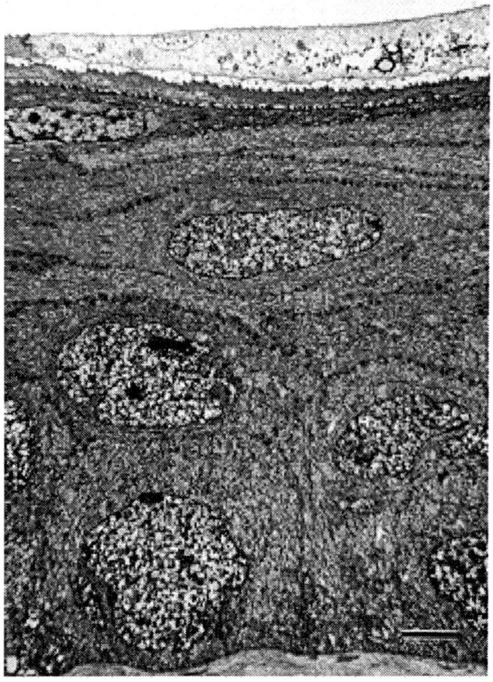

Figure 12.3.9. TEM micrograph of the corneal epithelium of an ascorbic acid-deficient rat. The epithelial cells have scarce microvilli, but intercellular junctions and cytoplasmic components are well-developed. Bar: 2μm.

Discussion

In ascorbic acid deficiency, the conjunctival changes were scarce microvilli and microplicae in the epithelium and small goblet cells with secretory granules in decreased density, while corneal changes were limited to decreased microvilli and microplicae. The changes are different from those in other vitamins and trace elements. For instance, vitamin A deficiency induces corneal keratinization (Carter-Dawson, Tanaka, Kuwabara et al, 1980; Van Horn, Schutten, Hyndiuk et al, 1980; Kanazawa, Kitaoka, Ueda et al, 2002; Fujikawa, Gong and Amemiya, 2003), vitamin B_2 (Riboflavin) deficiency (Bessey and Wolback, 1939; Takami, Gong and Amemiya, 2004) and vitamin E deficiency induce intercellular dehiscence of epithelial cells in the conjunctiva and cornea, and make cellular debris release to the subepithelial stroma from corneal basal cells; Mn (Gong and Amemiya, 1999), Mg (Gong, Takami, Kitaoka et al, 2003) and Zn (Gong, Takami, Amemiya et al, 2004) induce the decrease a microvilli and microplicae in the ocular surface and changes of the nucleus, fibrils and ribosomes in the corneal epithelium. The high levels of ascorbic acid have antioxidant protection against photolytically generated free radicals in ocular tissues such as the cornea, lens, retina and optic nerve.

Ascorbic acid can provide indirect antioxidant protection by supplying electrons to regenerate the active reduced form of other biologic antioxidants such as glutathione, tocopherol and flavonoids (Jacob, 1995).

Ascorbic acid plays roles in the formation of the mucous membrane (Hoyte, 1979) and collagen synthesis. Ascorbic acid plays a role in the production of the mucopolysaccharide components on the ground substance of connective tissue, particularly hydroxyprolin. This may be related to abnormal ocular surface structures and low-density secretory granules in the goblet cells due to ascorbic acid deficiency. The cornea contains much ascorbic acid, but its significance still remains unclear. However, considering slight or moderate changes in ocular tissue due to ascorbic acid deficiency, actions of this vitamin might be synergistic with other substances or vitamins. It is another possibility that ascorbic acid-deficient rats died before severe damages appeared in the ocular tissue.

IV. THE RETINA

Results

TEM Findings

In control and pair-fed control rats, photoreceptor outer segments extending from the inner segment to the apex of the retinal pigment epithelium (RPE) showed no vesiculation (Fig.12.4.1). However, ascorbic acid-deficient rats showed vesiculated discs and clumps of a few discs separated from the tip of the outer segments (Fig.12.4.2). In the RPE, lamellar structures and dense bodies appeared even at 6h after exposure to light (Fig.12.4.2). However, such findings disappeared in the photoreceptor outer segment and RPE in ascorbic acid-recovery rats (Fig.12.4.3). Although there were no apoptotic nuclei in the outer nuclear layer of the retina in control and pair-fed control rats (Fig.12.4.4), ascorbic acid-deficient rats had apoptotic nuclei in the outer nuclear layer (Fig.12.4.5). In ascorbic acid-recovery rats, the outer nuclear layer contained no apoptotic nuclei (Fig.12.4.6).

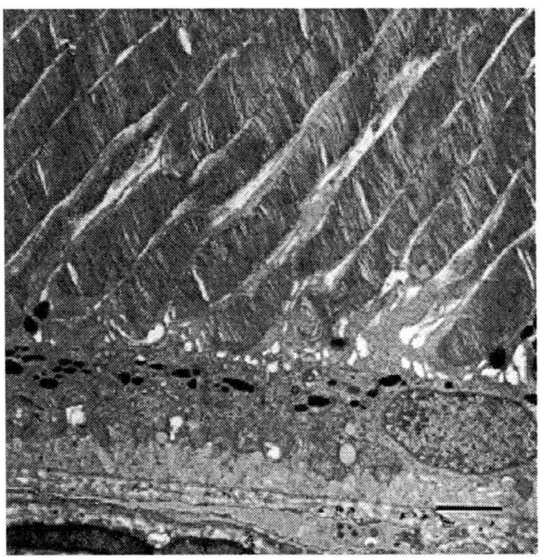

Figure 12.4.1. TEM micrograph of the photoreceptor outer segments and retinal pigment epithelium of a control rat. Outer segment discs show no vesiculation and well arrangement. No lamellar structures are seen in the pigment epithelium. Bar: 2μm.

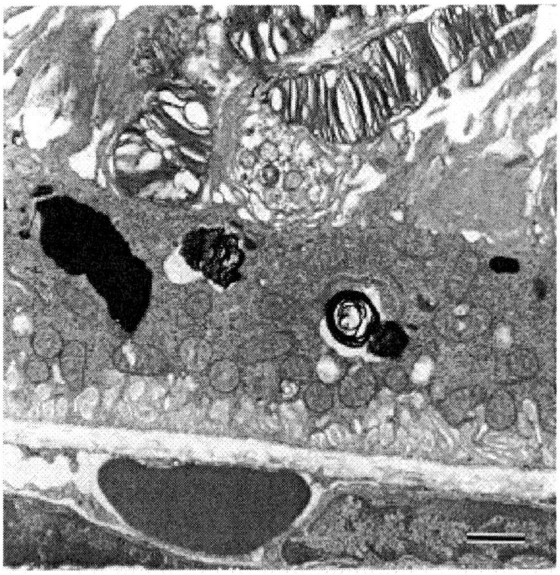

Figure 12.4.2. TEM micrograph of the photoreceptor outer segments and pigment epithelium of an ascorbic acid-deficient rat. Outer segment discs are vesiculated and separated. Lamellar structures and a clump of dense body are seen in the pigment epithelium. Bar: 1μm.

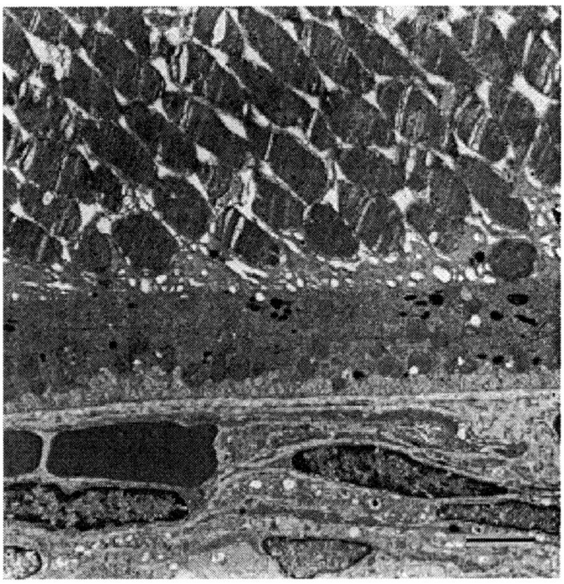

Figure 12.4.3. TEM micrograph of the photoreceptor outer segments and retinal pigment epithelium of an ascorbic acid-recovery rat. Outer segment discs are scarcely vesiculated and separated. No lamellar structures are seen in the pigment epithelium. Bar: 2μm.

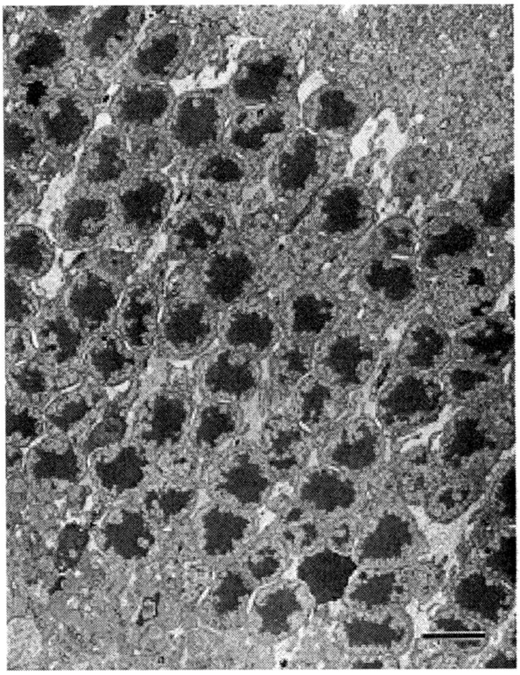

Figure 12.4.4. TEM micrograph of the outer nuclear layer of the retina of a pair-fed control rat. No apoptosis-like pyknotic nuclei are seen. Bar: 5μm.

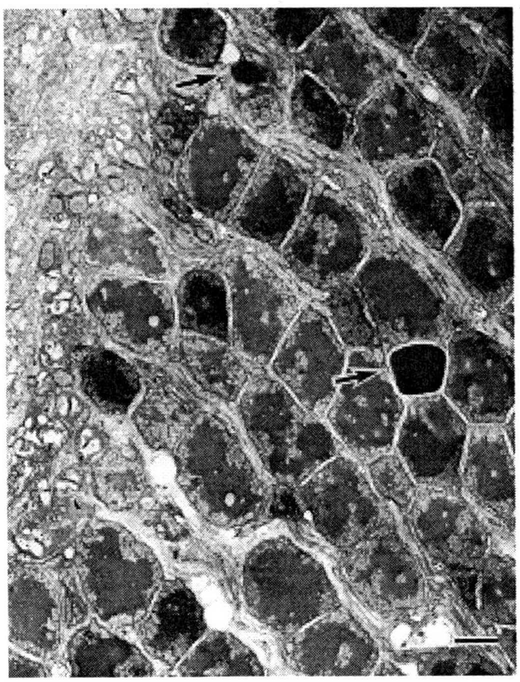

Figure 12.4.5. TEM micrograph of the outer nuclear layer of the retina of an ascorbic acid-deficient rat. Apoptosis-like pyknotic nuclei (arrows) appear. Bar: 2μm.

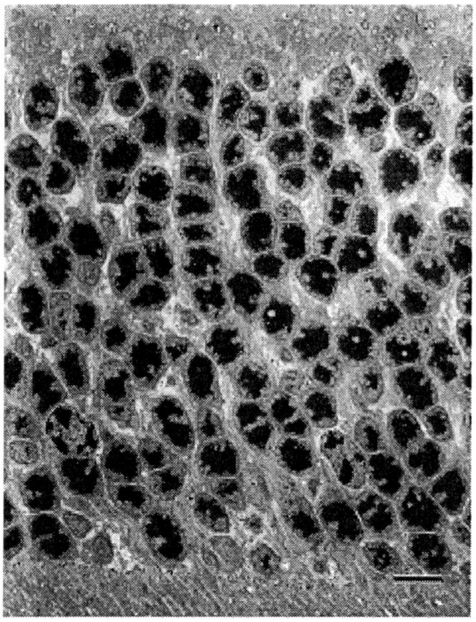

Figure 12.4.6. TEM micrograph of the outer nuclear layer of the retina of an ascorbic acid-recovery rat. No apoptosis-like pyknotic nuclei are seen. Bar: 5μm.

Discussion

Vesiculation of photoreceptor outer segment discs seen in ascorbic acid-deficient rats appears in vitamin A (Dowling and Gibbons, 1961; Amemiya, 1968) and E deficiencies (Amemiya, 1978; Robison, Kuwabara and Bieri; 1979) and masses of a few discs between the outer segment and RPE may be migrating to the RPE, which contains many lamellar structures phagocytized even at 6h after exposure to light. That is, enhanced phagocytosis of degenerated discs occurred in the RPE. Vitamin A deficiency induces the disc degeneration due to the decrease of vitamin A which consists of a disc membrane with fatty acids where vitamin A acts as an antioxidant. On the other hand, vitamin E is a strong antioxidant and vitamin E deficiency induces broken membrane stabilization to disc degeneration. Lysosomal dysfunction due to vitamin E deficiency leads to abundant accumulation of lipofuscin granules in the REP (Amemiya, 1978; Robison, Kuwabara and Bieri, 1979).

In deficiencies of Mn (Gong and Amemiya, 1996) and Zn, on the other hand, lowered activities of Mn superoxide dismutase and Cu·Zn superoxide dismutase containing Mn, Cu or Zn may induce peroxidation of the lipid-rich disc membrane. Ascorbic acid also has an antioxidant action. The tocopheroxyl radical reacts with ascorbic acid, thereby oxidizing the latter and returning the vitamin to its reduced state. Biologically important hydrogen donors, which have been demonstrated in vitro to regenerate tocopherom from the tocopheroxyl radical, include ascorbate and thiol (Webers and Sies, 1988), especially glutathione (Niki, 1987; Sies and Murphy, 1991; Sies, Stahl and Sundguist, 1992). Subsequently, the ascorbic acid and third radicals can be reduced via metabolic processes. Thus ascorbic acid has a synergistic function such as enhancing the antioxidant activity with its original antioxidant action. Therefore, ascorbic acid helps to offer protection. Compared to morphological damages due to deficiencies of vitamins A and E and of trace elements such as Mn and Zn, morphological damages due to ascorbic acid deficiency are lighter and its antioxidant action may be weaker than the action of other vitamins and trace elements.

V. The Optic Nerve

Results

Transmission Electron Microscopic (TEM) Findings

TEM revealed significantly fewer myelinated axons in the optic nerves of ascorbic acid-deficient (Fig. 12.5.2B, 2C) and ascorbic acid-recovery rats (Fig. 12.5.2D) than in those of control rats (Fig. 12.5.1A, 1B) (Table 12.5.1). In the controls (Fig. 12.5.1B) and pair-fed control rats (Fig. 12.5.2A), the axons of the myelinated optic nerve fibers contained mitochondria and neurotubulus, but ascorbic acid-deficient (Figs. 12.5.2B, 2C) and recovery rats (Fig. 12.5.2D) had vacuoles and destroyed mitochondria and tubules. The fiber density in the myelinated axons of ascorbic acid-deficient (Figs. 12.5.2B, 2C) and ascorbic acid-recovery rats (Fig. 12.5.2D) was obviously decreased. Unmyelinated axons in the optic nerve were more numerous in the ascorbic acid-deficient (Fig. 12.5.2B, 2C) and ascorbic acid-recovery rats (Fig. 12.5.2D) than in the control rats (Figs. 12.5.1A, 1B and 12.5.2A). In transverse sections of ascorbic acid-deficient (Fig. 12.5.1C) and ascorbic acid-recovery rats (Fig. 12.5.2D), the myelin sheaths of optic nerves were thin, and undeveloped axons were numerous.

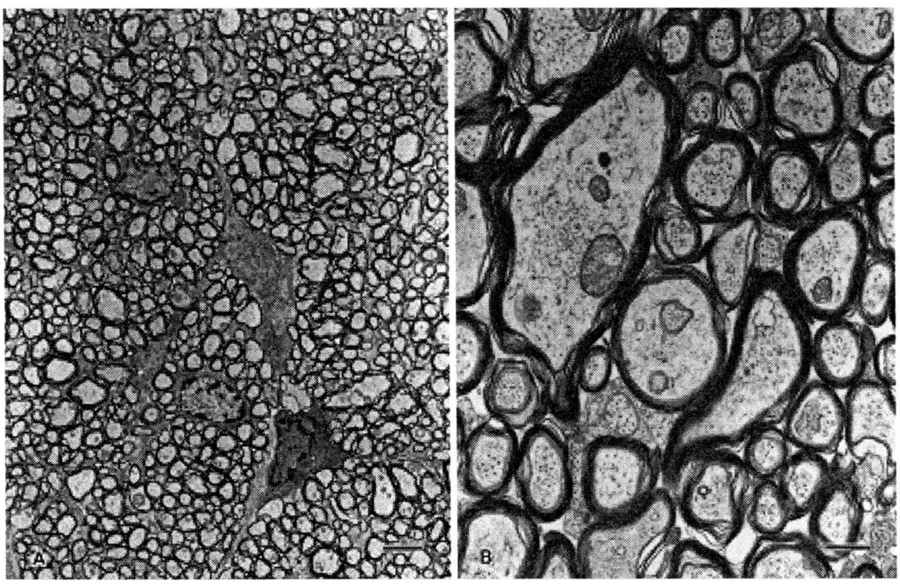

Figure 12.5.1. TEM micrographs of transverse sections of optic nerves of a control rat. (A) A low magnification view shows many myelinated nerve fibers and astrocytes. (B) A high magnification view shows mitochondria, neurotubules in axons and thick myelin lamellae. Bar: 2μm (A), 500nm (B).

The diameter of myelinated fibers was not significantly different between the ascorbic acid-deficient and recovery groups ($p>0.1$) (Table 12.5.2). Myelin sheath thickness and number of lamellae in ascorbic acid-deficient and ascorbic acid-recovery rats were significantly different from those of the control and pair-fed control rats ($p<0.01$) (Tables 12.5.3, 4). The myelin index (ratio of the axon diameter to the myelinated nerve fiber diameter) in ascorbic acid-deficient and ascorbic acid-recovery rats was significantly larger than that in the control and pair-fed control rats ($p<0.01$) (Table 12.5.5). The number of myelinated axons and of the lamellar layers of myelinated fibers and the thickness of the myelin sheath in the optic nerves were significantly reduced in the recovery and ascorbic acid-deficient rats, compared with those of the control and pair-fed control rats (Tables 12.5.1, 3, 4). The optic nerves of control and pair-fed control rats showed no abnormalities.

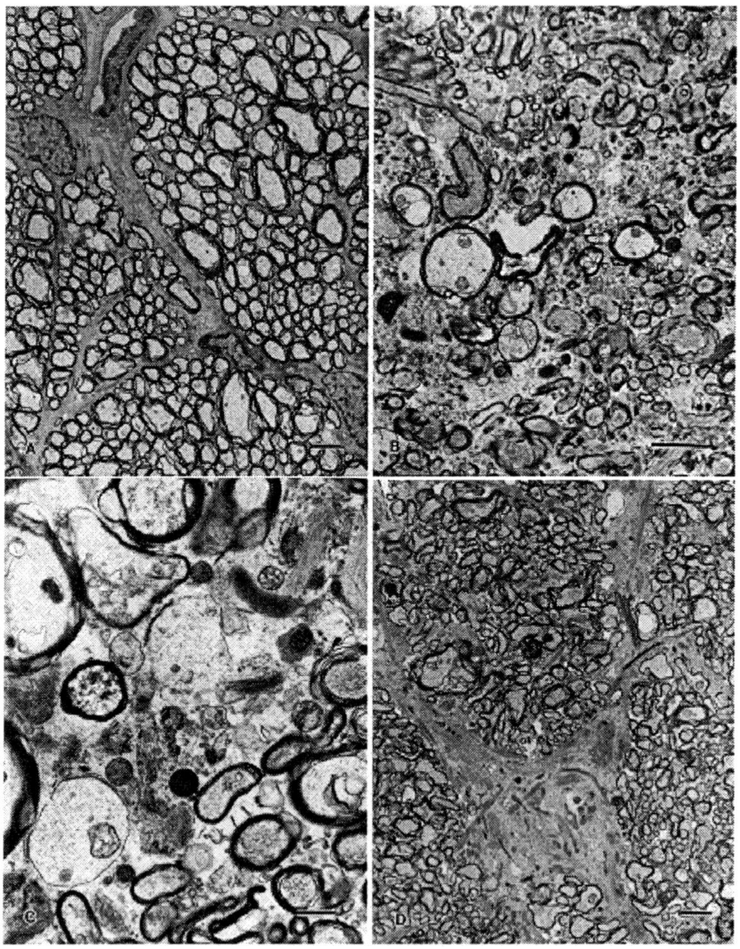

Figure 12.5.2. TEM micrographs of transverse sections of optic nerves. (A) A pair-fed control rat shows compactly packed myelinated nerve fibers demarcated by astrocyte processes. (B) An ascorbic acid-deficient rat shows that myelinated nerve fibers are prominently decreased and scattered in degenerative lesion. (C) A magnified view of degenerative lesion in an ascorbic acid-deficient rat shows thin myelin lamellae, degeneration of myelin lamellae and axonal components and extracellularly scattered cytoplasmic components. (D) An ascorbic acid-recovery rat shows degenerative myelin sheaths and axons and well-proliferated glial cells. Bar: 2μm (A, B, D), 500nm (C).

Table 12.5.1. Number of myelinated axons in optic nerve (600μm^2).

Groups	Number of fields examined	Number of myelinated axons
Control	121	147±20 *
Ascorbic acid-deficient	133	110±18 *, **, ***
Recovery	96	114±18 ***
Pair-fed control	78	148±35 **

- p<0.0001, ** p<0.0001, *** p=0.06.

Table 12.5.2. Diameter of myelinated nerve fibers in optic nerve (μm).

Groups	Number of myelinated fibers counted	Diameter
Control	154	0.81±0.25
Ascorbic acid-deficient	164	0.76±0.31
Recovery	146	0.78±0.28
Pair-fed control	123	0.84±0.32

The diameter of myelinated fibers in the 4 groups is not significantly different (p>0.1).

Table 12.5.3. Thickness of myelin sheath in optic nerve (nm).

Groups	Number of myelin sheath counted	Thickness
Control	123	142.1±33.9 *
Ascorbic acid-deficient	137	81.1±33.8 *, **, ***
Recovery	124	88.5±38.5 ***
Pair-fed control	115	143.7±39.5 **

* p<0.0001, ** p<0.0001, *** p=0.103.

Table 12.5.4. Thickness of lamellar layers of myelinated fibers in optic nerve (nm).

Groups	Number of myelin sheath counted	Number of layers
Control	148	10.9±2.8 *
Ascorbic acid-deficient	154	5.6±2.7 *, **, ***
Recovery	136	5.4±2.3 ***
Pair-fed control	115	11.8±3.2 **

* p<0.0001, ** p<0.0001, *** p=0.197.

Table 12.5.5. Myelin index (ratio of axon diameter to fiber to fiber diameter).

Groups	Number of myelinated nerve fibers counted	Myelin index
Control	154	0.71±0.12 *
Ascorbic acid-deficient	164	0.81±0.09 *, **, ***
Recovery	146	0.80±0.13 ***
Pair-fed control	123	0.72±0.15 **

* p<0.0001, ** p<0.0001, *** p=0.527.

Discussion

In the control and pair-fed control groups electron microscopy of the optic nerve confirmed that the optic nerve showed none of the histopathologic changes seen in the ascorbic acid deficient rats. Thus, changes in the ascorbic acid-deficient rats were not due to maldevelopment.

In the current study, the numbers of fibers and of myelin lamellae in the optic nerves were significantly lower in the ascorbic acid-deficient rats than in the control and pair-fed control rats. Even when ascorbic acid-deficient rats were supplemented with ascorbic acid, their optic nerves did not recover: the numbers of myelinated axons and lamellar layers of the myelinated nerve, and the thickness of myelin sheaths in optic nerves were not significantly different between the ascorbic acid-deficient and recovery rats. It appears that axons continue to degenerate after the resumption of a normal diet and water supplemented with sufficient ascorbic acid. This means that once the CNS is destroyed it never recovers.

Our series of studies on the effect of deficiencies of several trace elements showed similar results in the ascorbic acid-deficient study (Dake and Amemiya, 1991; Mishima, Dake, Amemiya et al, 1996; Gong and Amemiya, 1999; Gong and Amemiya, 2001). One of the assumed causes is a disturbance of superoxide dismutases which contain Zn, Cu, Mn and Mg. In the current study, however, Zn, Cu and Mg were not reduced in the ascorbic acid-deficient condition. Thus the effect of Zn, Cu and Mg on the optic nerve may be neglected in ascorbic acid deficiency.

Antioxidant systems of the CNS act in concert to protect cerebral tissue from oxidative damage. Ascorbic acid and glutathione act as a first defense line in this process, serving as redox buffers and free radical scavengers to limit the reactivity of radical intermediates generated by ascorbic acid metabolism (Meister, 1992). Both are effective scavengers of peroxyl and hydroxyl radicals, superoxide anion, and singlet oxygen (Nishikimi, 1975; Basaga, 1990). Through their action against radicals generated in the aqueous phase, ascorbic acid and glutathione peroxidase protect and recycle α-tocopherol and prevent membrane lipid peroxidation (Seregi, Schafer and Komlos, 1978; Vatassery, Smith and Quach, 1989). Since myelin is a lipid membrane (Trapp and Bershon, 1978), the disturbance of these preventive mechanisms by ascorbic acid deficiency may lead to decreased numbers of fibers and myelin lamellae in the optic nerve. Such actions of ascorbic acid on the myelinated nerve have not been reported yet. Activity of glutamatergic and dopaminergic neurons has been closely linked to changes in extracellular ascobic acid concentrations in the brain. Aspects of neural activity modulated by ascorbic acid concentrations include neurotransmitter membrane receptor synthesis and functions and neurotransmitter dynamics. Animal models and cell culture experiments indicate that ascorbic acid is an important factor in the developing nervous system, particularly for the growth and maturation of glial cells and myelin (Jacob, 1999). The optic nerve needs ascorbic acid for the maintenance of its cell structure.

There is a report on the possible involvement of ascorbic acid in the regulation of myelin gene activity in the CNS (Laszkeiwicz, Wiggins, Konat, 1992). But, to the best of our knowledge, it has not been reported that ascorbic acid is needed for the development of myelinated nerve fibers. The same disturbance due to ascorbic acid deficiency could occur in nerves other than the optic nerve.

REFERENCES

Amemiya T. Cytochemical and electron microscopic examination of the retina of rats with hypovitaminosis A. *Acta Soc Ophthalmol Jpn.* 1968;72:1074-1099.

Amemiya T. Effect of vitamin E deficiency on photoreceptor outer segment and pigment epithelium of the rat retina. *Acta Soc Ophthalmol. Jpn.* 1978;82:822-826.

Basaga HS. Biomedical aspects of free radicals. *Biochem Biol.* 1990;68:989-998.

Carter-Dawson L, Tanaka M, Kuwabara T, Bieri JG. Early corneal changes in vitamin A-deficient rats. *Exp Eye Res.* 1980;30:261-268.

Dake Y, Amemiya T. Electron microscopic study of the optic nerve in copper deficient rats. *Exp Eye Res.* 1991;58:277-281.

Dowling JE, Gibbons IR. The effect of vitamin A deficiency on the fine structure of the retina. In Smelser GK, ed. *The Structure of the Eye.* New York;Academic Press Inc;1961:85-99.

Fujikawa A, Gong H, Amemiya T. Vitamin E prevents changes in the cornea and conjunctiva due to vitamin A deficiency. *Graefes Ach Clin Exp Ophthalmol.* 2003;241:287-297.

Gong H, Amemiya T. Ultrastructure of retina of manganese-deficient rats. *Invest Ophthalmol Vis Sci.* 1996;37:1967-1974.

Gong H, Amemiya T. Optic nerve changes in manganese-deficient rats. *Exp Eye Res.* 1999;68:313-320.

Gong H, Amemiya T. Corneal changes in manganese-deficient rats. *Cornea.* 1999;18:472-482.

Gong H, Amemiya T. Optic nerve changes in Zn-deficient rat. *Exp Eye Res.* 2001;72:363-369.

Gong H, Takami Y, Kitaoka T, Amemiya T. Corneal changes in magnesium-deficient rats. *Cornea.* 2003;22:448-456.

Gong H, Takami Y, Amemiya T, Tozu M, Ohashi Y. Ocular surface in Zn-deficient rats. *Ophthalmic Res.* 2004;36:129-138.

Horio F, Ozaki K, Yoshida A, Makino S, Hayashi R. Requirement for ascorbic acid in a rat mutant unable to synthesize ascorbic acid. *J Nutr.* 1985;115:1630-1640.

Hoyt CS 3rd. Vitamin metabolism and therapy in ophthalmology. *Surv Ophthalmol.* 1979;24:177-190.

Jacob RA. The integrated antioxidant system. *Nutr Res.* 1995;15:755-766.

Jacob RA. Vitamin C. In Maurice E, Shils ME, Olson JA, Shike M, Ross AC ed. 9th ed. *Modern Nutrition in Health and Disease.* Philadelphia:Lippincott Williams & Wilkins;1999:467-483.

Kanazawa S, Kitaoka T, Ueda Y, Gong H, Amemiya T. Interaction of zinc and vitamin A on the ocular surface. *Graefes Clin Exp Ophthalmol.* 2002;240:1011-1021.

Kurata T. Ascorbic acid. In:Japan Vitamin Soc, ed. Handbook of Vitamin, *Water Soluble Vitamins.* Kyoto:Igaku Dojin;1989:171-191.

Laszkeiwicz L, Wiggins RC, Konat G. Ascorbic acid upregulates myelingene expression in C6 glioma cells. *Metab Brain Dis.* 1992;7:157-164.

May JM, Qu ZC, Whitesell RR, Cobb CE. Ascorbate recycling in human erythrocytes: Role of GSH in reducing dehydroascorbate. *Free Radic Biol Med.* 1996;20:543-551.

Meister A. On the antioxidant effect of ascorbic and glutathione. *Biochem Pharmacol.* 1992;44:1905-1915.

Mishima K, Dake Y, Amemiya T, Nishimura M. Electron microscopic study of optic nerves of macular mice. *Exp Eye Res.* 1996;63:85-90.

Niki E. Antioxidants in relation to lipid peroxidation. *Chem Phys Lipids.* 1987;44:227-253.

Mizushima Y, Harauchi T, Yoshizaki T, Makino S. A rat mutant unable to synthesize ascorbic acid. *Experientia.* 1984;40:359-361.

Nishikimi M. Oxidation of ascorbic acid with superoxide anion generated by the xanthine-xanthine oxidase system. *Biochem Biophys Res Comm.* 1975;63:463-468.

Rice ME, Lee EJ, Choy Y. High levels of the ascorbic acid , not glutathione , in the CNS of anoxia-tolerant reptiles contrasted with levels in anoxia-intolerant spieces. *J Neurochem.* 1995;64:1790-1799.

Robertson WG Jr, Kuwabara T, Bier JG. Vitamin E deficiency and the retina: Photoreceptor and pigment epithelial changes. *Invest Ophthalmol Vis Sci.* 1979;18:683-690.

Seregi A, Schafer A, Komlos M. Protective role of ascorbic acid content against lipid peroxidation. *Experientia.* 1978;34:1056-1057.

Sies H, Murphy ME. Role of tocopherols in the protection of biological systems against oxidative damage. *J Photochem Photobiol* B. 1991;8:211-224.

Sies H, Stahl W, Sundquist AR. Antioxidant functions of vitamins: vitamins E and C, β-carotine, and other carotenoids. *Ann NY Acad Sci.* 1992;669:7-20.

Takami Y, Gong H, Amemiya T. Riboflavin deficiency induces ocular surface damage. *Ophthalmic Res.* 2004;36:156-165.

Trapp BD, Bersohn J. Essential fatty acid deficiency and CNS myelin. Biochemical and morphological observations. *J Neurol Sci.* 1978;37:249-266.

Vatassery GT, Smith WE, Quach HT. Ascorbic acid, glutathione and synthetic anti-oxidants prevent the oxidation of vitamin E in platelets. *Lipids.* 1989;24:1043-1047.

Van Horn DL, Schutten WH, Hyndiuk RA, Kurz P. Xerophthalmia in vitamin A-deficient rabbits. Clinical and ultrastructural alterations in the cornea. *Invest Ophthalmol Vis Sci.* 1980;19:1067-1079.

Wefers H, Sies H. The protection by ascorbate and glutathione against microsomal lipid peroxidation is dependent on vitamin E. *Eur J Biochem.* 1988;174:353-357.

Xu DP, Washburn MP, Sun GP, Wells WW. Purification and characterization of a glutathione dependent dehydroascorbate reductase from human erythrocytes. *Biochem Biophys Res Commun.* 1996;221:117-121.

Chapter 13

INTERACTIONS BETWEEN VITAMIN AND ELEMENT AND BETWEEN VITAMINS

I. SIGNIFICANCE

In chemical reactions, a catalytic metal can be substituted by another one, e.g. Cu^{++} instead of Fe^{++}. Biochemical reactions also show such a catalytic substitution of an enzyme or co-enzymes in metabolic reactions. Such enzymes and co-enzymes might be metalloenzymes containing trace elements.

It is postulated that there are interactions in various ways among nutrients including vitamins and elements. The interactions are sometimes synergistic and sometimes antagonistic. The biological interaction of elements based on the physicochemical properties of their ions is that resemblance of ion's valence shell structures might be antagonistic to each other biologically (Hill and Matrone, 1970). Ganther et al (1972) suggested that interactions may be the result of a chemical combination of the ions. Effects include interactions at the absorptive sites, the excretory patterns and relation of a catalytic substitute for each other in enzyme structure in vivo and thereby changes or substitutions of enzymatic activity (Hill, 1975). Biological interactions occur between selenium and a number of other elements and is supposed that some of the interactions are caused by the formation of a compound by selenium and other elements, which has less affinity for active groups on biologically active compounds (Hill, 1975). The previously published studies are almost the exact biochemical basis of the interactions, which are data on serum levels, effects of absorption and excretion, weight gain, growth and mortality rate. However, morphological changes due to interactions have scarcely been reported.

It would be very interesting to know whether the effect of either of the two nutrient deficiencies can be prevented by supplementation of other nutrients. It is still unknown whether any interaction occurs between two micronutrients. The study on an interaction between micronutrients is expected to be useful as a preventive, therapeutic or auxilliary drug (Kanazawa, Kitaoka, Ueda et al 2002; Fujikawa, Gong and Amemiya, 2003).

In this chapter, two-nutrient-interactions are described morphologically with light and electron microscopes and from the view-point of synergistic action.

II. EXPERIMENTS FOR INTERACTIONS

i. Interaction Between Vitamins E and A

a. Relationship Between Vitamin A Deficiency and Vitamin E

The purpose of this experiment is to assess morphologically whether vitamin E can prevent changes due to vitamin A deficiency.

Materials and Methods

Normal male infant Wistar Kyoto rats from normal mothers were weaned 20 days after birth and divided into three groups: group 1, A(-) rats fed a vitamin A-deficient diet; group 2, A(-)E(+) rats fed a vitamin A-deficient diet and injected intraperitoneally with 15mg of vitamin E per week: group 3, fed a usual diet with vitamin A 8.80 IU/g and vitamin E 0.091mg/g diet as controls. The vitamin A-deficient solid diet was commercially prepared and obtained from Nippon Clea (Tokyo, Japan) (Reeves, Nielsen and Fahey, 1993). This diet contains less than 0.01mg of retinol per 100g diet and all other nutrients. The vitamin E was obtained from Eisai Co. (Tokyo, Japan). This solution is known as tocopherol acetate (2, 5, 7, 8-tetramethyl-2-(4, 8, 12-trimethyltridecyl) -6-chromanyl acetate). Distilled and deionized water was provided freely to both groups. All the rats (11 A(-) rats, 8 A(-)E(+) rats and 5 normal controls) were killed at 13 weeks of age.

The cornea, superior palpebral conjunctivae, retina and optic nerve were examined by light microscopy, transmission (TEM) and scanning (SEM) electron microscopy.

Clinical Features

A(-) rats had coarse hair and hair loss at 3 months of the experiment. However, A(-) rats supplemented with vitamin E showed inspectively slight coarsening of hair and almost no hair loss. Body weight: At 13 weeks of age the body weight of A(-) rats was significantly lower than that of A(-)E(+) rats (P=0.0372): A(-) rats, 207.7±32.0g (n=11); A(-)E(+) rats, 249.4±48.5g (n=8); control rats, 410±11.5g (n=5).

Serum vitamin A: At 13 weeks of age the serum vitamin A level was 25.6±18.4ng/ml (n=11) in A(-) rats and 30.1±18.8ng/ml (n=8) in A(-)E(+) rats (p=0.6023); this is not a statistically significant difference. In the control rats, the vitamin A level was 526.8±54.6ng/ml (n=5), significantly higher than in other groups ($p<0.0001$).

Serum vitamin E: At 13 weeks of age the serum vitamin E level was 0.67±0.11mg/dl (n=11) in A(-) rats and 1.43±0.56mg/dl (n=8) in A(-)E(+) rats. This difference is significant (p=0.0004). In control rats, the vitamin E level was 0.58±0.12mg/dl (n=5), significantly lower than in A(-)E(+) (p=0.0147).

b. Relationship Between Vitamin E Deficiency and Vitamin A

The purpose of this experiment is to assess morphologically whether vitamin A can prevent changes due to vitamin E deficiency.

Materials and Methods

Normal male infant Wistar Kyoto rats from normal mothers were weaned 20 days after birth and divided into three groups: group 1, E(-) rats fed a vitamin E-deficient diet; group 2, E(-)A(+) rats fed a vitamin E-deficient diet and injected intraperitoneally with 5,000 IU of vitamin A per 2 weeks; fed the same diet as controls. The vitamin E-deficient solid diet was commercially prepared and obtained from Nippon Clea (Tokyo, Japan). This diet contains less than 0.01mg of α -tocopherol per 100g diet and all other nutrients. Vitamin A is retinol palmitate obtained from Eisai Co. (Tokyo, Japan). All the animals were killed at 16 months, and corneas, conjunctivas, retinas and optic nerves were examined by transmission (TEM) and scanning (SEM) electron microscopy.

Clinical Features

E(-) rats and E(-)A(+) rats were smaller than control rats, but E(-) rats showed slight hair coarsening as well as hair loss. E(-)A(+) rats and control rats showed no hair coarsening with hair loss.

Body weight: At 16 months of age the body weight of E(-) rats was significantly lower than that of control rats ($p<0.0001$), but not significantly different from E(-)A(+) rats ($p=0.0686$): E(-) rats, 420±100.1g (n=9); E(-)A(+) rats, 552.5±130.5g (n=4); control rats, 757.8±105.0g (n=9). There was a significant difference in body weight between E(-)A(+) rats and control rats ($p<0.0001$).

Serum vitamin E: At 16 months of age the serum vitamin E level was less than 0.1mg/dl in E(-) rats (n=7) and E(-)A(+) rats (n=4) and 0.96±0.02mg/dl in control rats (n=3).

Serum vitamin A: At 16 months of age the serum vitamin A level was 199.1±21.1ng/ml (n=7) in E(-) rats and 288.8±28.7ng/ml (n=4) in E(-)A(+) rats, There is a significant difference ($p<0.032$). In the control rats, the vitamin A level was 297±7ng/dl (n=3), significantly higher than in E(-) rats ($p=0.019$), but not significant compared to E(-)A(+) rats ($p=0.8184$).

ii. Interaction Between Vitamin A and Zinc

Relationship Between Vitamin A Deficiency and Zinc

The purpose of this experiment is to assess morphologically the interaction between vitamin A and Zn in their effect on the ocular surface.

Materials and Methods

Three-week-old normal weanling Wistar Kyoto rats were divided randomly into five groups: 1.Group A(+)Zn(+) was fed a solid diet containing both vitamin A and Zn. Deionized distilled water was provided freely. 2.Group A(-) and group A(-)Zn(+) were fed a commercially prepared vitamin A-deficient solid diet obtained from Nippon Clea (Tokyo, Japan). This diet contains less than 0.01mg of retinol per 100g of diet and all other nutrients. Deionized distilled water was provided freely to group A(-) rats, while the A(-)Zn(+) group was given deionized distilled water with 30mg Zn/100g. 3.Group Zn (-) and group Zn (-)A(+) were fed a commercially prepared Zn-deficient solid diet and all other nutrients obtained from Nippon Clea. This diet contains 0.07mg Zn/100g of diet. Deionized distilled water was provided freely to both groups. Group Zn(-)A(+) rats received an intraperitoneal injection of vitamin A(3000IU retinol palmitate) once a week beginning 3 to 5 weeks after birth.

Corneas and palpebral conjunctivas from rats of groups A(-), A(-)Zn(+) and A(+)Zn(+) were examined in the 12th and 16th weeks of the experiments. Corneas and palpebral conjunctivas from group Zn(-), group Zn(-)A(+) and group A(+)Zn(+) were examined in the 1st, 2nd and 3rd weeks of the experiments. Zn-deficient rats rarely live more than 4 weeks on a Zn-deficient diet, and signs of deficiency appear rapidly and are severe. The changes in vitamin A deficiency, however, occur more slowly. Therefore the time of examination differs between the Zn and vitamin A deficiency experiments.

Corneas and palpebral conjunctivas were examined by transmission (TEM) and scanning (SEM) electron microscopy.

Table 13.3.1. Body weight (g) of rats in the five experimental groups. The number of animals in each group was five.

weeks after start of experiment				
Group	1	3	12	16
Group A(+)Zn(+)	77.0 ± 2.6^{a}	110 ± 2.0^{a}	350 ± 7.07^{c}	356 ± 11.4^{c}
Group A(-)	–	–	$288 \pm 14.8^{c,d}$	$298 \pm 13.0^{c,d}$
Group A(-)Zn(+)	–	–	$320 \pm 25.5^{c,d}$	$302 \pm 19.2^{c,d}$
Group Zn(-)	$51.3 \pm 1.1^{a,b}$	$56.0 \pm 1.0^{a,b}$	–	–
Group Zn(-)A(+)	$51.0 \pm 1.0^{a,b}$	$55.7 \pm 1.0^{a,b}$	–	–

a: There is s significant difference between group Zn(-) and group A(+) Zn(+) ($p<0.05$) and between group Zn(-) A(+) and group A(+) Zn(+) ($p<0.05$).
b: There is no significant difference between group Zn(-) and group Zn(-) A(+).
c: The difference is significant between group A(-) and group A(+) Zn(+) ($p<0.05$) and between group A(-) Zn(+) and group A(+) Zn(+) ($p<0.05$).
d: There is no significant difference between group A(-) and group A(-) Zn(+).

Clinical Features

The body weights of rats in groups A(-) and A(-)Zn(+) were lower than those of group A(+)Zn(+) rats. The difference was significant between groups A(-) and A(+)Zn(+) and between groups A(-)Zn(+) and A(+)Zn(+) ($p<0.05$). However, there was no significant difference in body weight between group A(-) and group A(-)Zn(+) (Table 13.3.1). Group A(+) Zn(+) rats were in normal health with no hair loss. Groups A(-) and A(-)Zn(+) had coarse hair and hair loss starting at 3 months of the experiment.

The body weights of rats in groups Zn(-) and Zn(-)A(+) were lower than those of group A(+)Zn(+) rats. There was a significant difference between groups Zn(-) and A(+)Zn(+) and between groups Zn(-)A(+) and A(+)Zn(+) ($p<0.05$); however, there was no significant difference between groups Zn(-) and Zn (-)A(+) (Table13.3.1). Groups Zn(-) and Zn(-)A(+) had coarse hair and hair loss starting in the 2nd week of the experiment.

Table 13.3.2. Serum vitamin A levels (ng/ml) of rats in the five experimental groups. The number of animals in each group was five.

weeks after start of experiment				
Group	1	3	12	16
Group A(+)Zn(+)	392±15.0[a]	360±37.4[a]	403±14.9	399±10.3
Group A(-)	–	–	<30*	<30*
Group A(-)Zn(+)	–	–	<30*	<30*
Group Zn(-)	216±25.4[a,b]	194±10.1[a,b]	–	–
Group Zn(-)A(+)	227±32.6[a,b]	208±17.8[a,b]	–	–

* The serum vitamin A levels in group A(-) and group A(-)Zn(+) are lower than 30ng/ml, the limit of assay.

a: There is a significant difference between group Zn(-) and group A(+)Zn(+) ($p<0.05$) and between group Zn(-)A(+) and group A(+)Zn(+) ($p<0.05$).

b: There is no significant difference between group Zn(-) and group Zn(-)A(+).

Serum vitamin A levels: In the 12th and 16th weeks of the experiments, the serum vitamin A level was significantly lower in group A(-) and group A(-)Zn(+) than in group A(+)Zn(+). The serum vitamin A level in groups A(-) and A(-)Zn(+) was lower than 30ng/ml, the limit of assay of serum vitamin A (Table 13.3.2).

Serum vitamin A levels were lower in group Zn(-) and group Zn(-)A(+) than in group A(+)Zn(+). There was a significant difference in serum vitamin A levels between groups A(-) and A(-)Zn(+) and between groups Zn(-) and A(+)Zn(+) ($p<0.05$) (Table13.3.2).

Table 13.3.3. Serum zinc levels (ng/ml) of rats in the five experimental groups. The number of animals in each group was five.

weeks after start of experiment				
Group	1	3	12	16
Group A(+)Zn(+)	106.5±7.9[a]	113.6±7.9[a]	109±7.0[c,d]	106±3.8[c]
Group A(-)	–	–	85±5.0[c,d]	80±3.3[c]
Group A(-)Zn(+)	–	–	106±4.2[c,d]	100±3.6[c,d]
Group Zn(-)	45.8±1.7[a,b]	39.3±1.7[a,b]	–	–
Group Zn(-)A(+)	42.0±1.8[a,b]	39.8±2.2[a,b]	–	–

a: There is a significant difference between group Zn(-) and group A(+)Zn(+) ($p<0.05$) and between group Zn(-)A(+) and group A(+)Zn(+) ($p<0.05$)

b: There is no significant difference between group Zn(-) and group Zn(-)A(+).

c: The difference is significant between group A(-) and group A(-)Zn(+) ($p<0.05$) and between group A(-) and group A(+)Zn(+) ($p<0.05$).

d: There is no significant difference between group A(+)Zn(+) and group A(-)Zn(+).

Serum Zn levels: The serum Zn level was significantly lower in group A(-) than in groups A(+)Zn(+) and A(-)Zn(+) ($p<0.05$) (Table13.3.3).

Groups Zn(-) and Zn(-)A(+) had significantly lower serum Zn levels than did groups A(+)Zn(+) ($p<0.05$) (Table13.3.3).

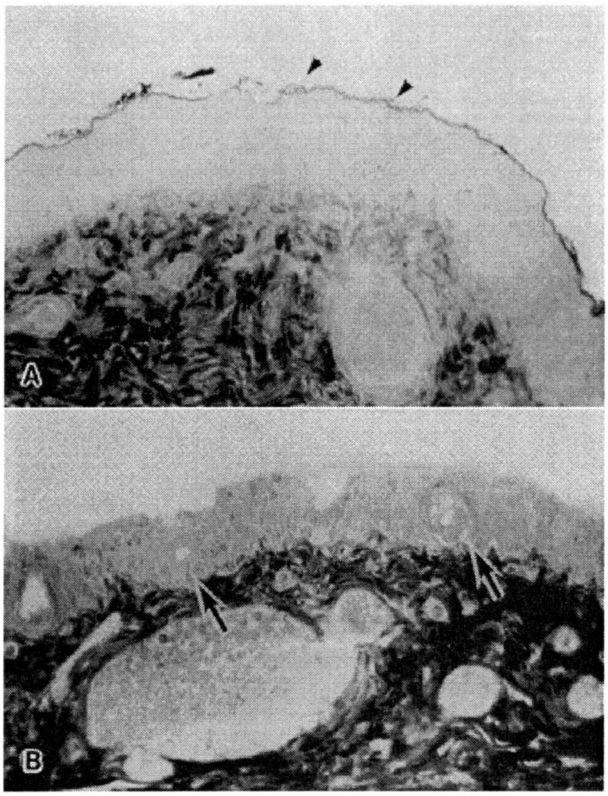

Fig. 13.1.1. Light micrographs of the conjunctiva of rats. (A) In an A(-) rat, the conjunctiva shows keratinization (arrowheads) of superficial epithelium and decreased goblet cells. (B) In an A(-)E(+) rats, the conjunctiva shows no keratinization and many goblet cells (arrows). Toluidine blue stain, × 200.

III. Results

i. Interaction Between Vitamins E and A

a. Relationship Between vitamin A Deficiency and Vitamin E

Light Microscopic Findings

The conjunctivae of A(-) rats showed severe keratinization and lack of goblet cells (Fig.13.1.1A), while the conjunctivae of A(-)E(+) rats had numerous goblet cells and no keratinization (Fig.13.1.1B). Normal rats had numerous goblet cells and no keratinization (Fig. 10.3.1A).

The corneas of A(-) rats showed severe keratinization. Some abnormal vessels were seen in the anterior stroma, and the basal cells had lost their columnar appearance (Fig.13.1.2A). The corneas of A(-)E(+) rats looked almost normal and had the columnar features of basal epithelial cells; they showed scarcely any keratinization (Fig.13.1.2B). The normal corneas had the columnar features of basal epithelial cells and no keratinization (Fig. 10.3.2A, 2B).

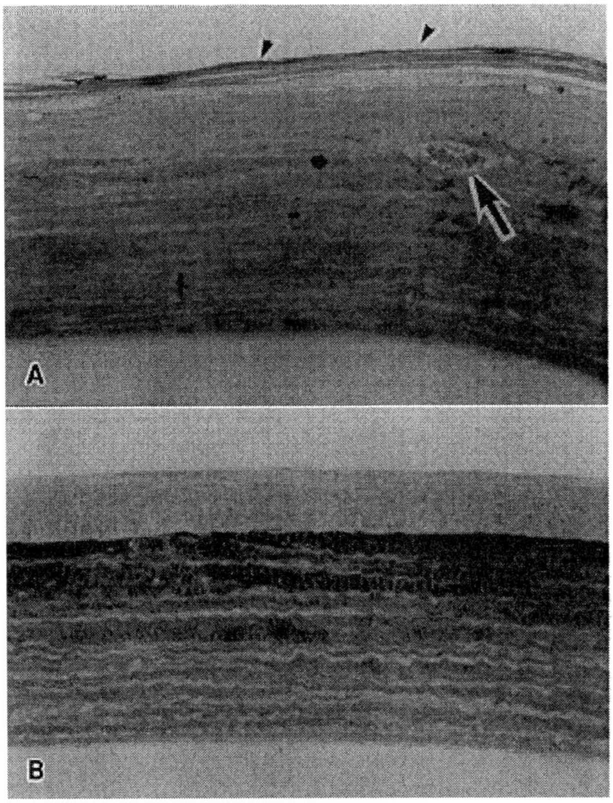

Fig. 13.1.2. Light micrograph of the cornea of rats. (A) An A(-) rat shows keratinization (arrowheads) of superficial epithelium and loss of columnar features in the basal epithelial cell. An abnormal blood vessel (arrow) is seen in the anterior stroma. (B) An A(-)E(+) rat shows no keratinization and normal columnar features of the basal cell. Toluidine blue stain, × 200.

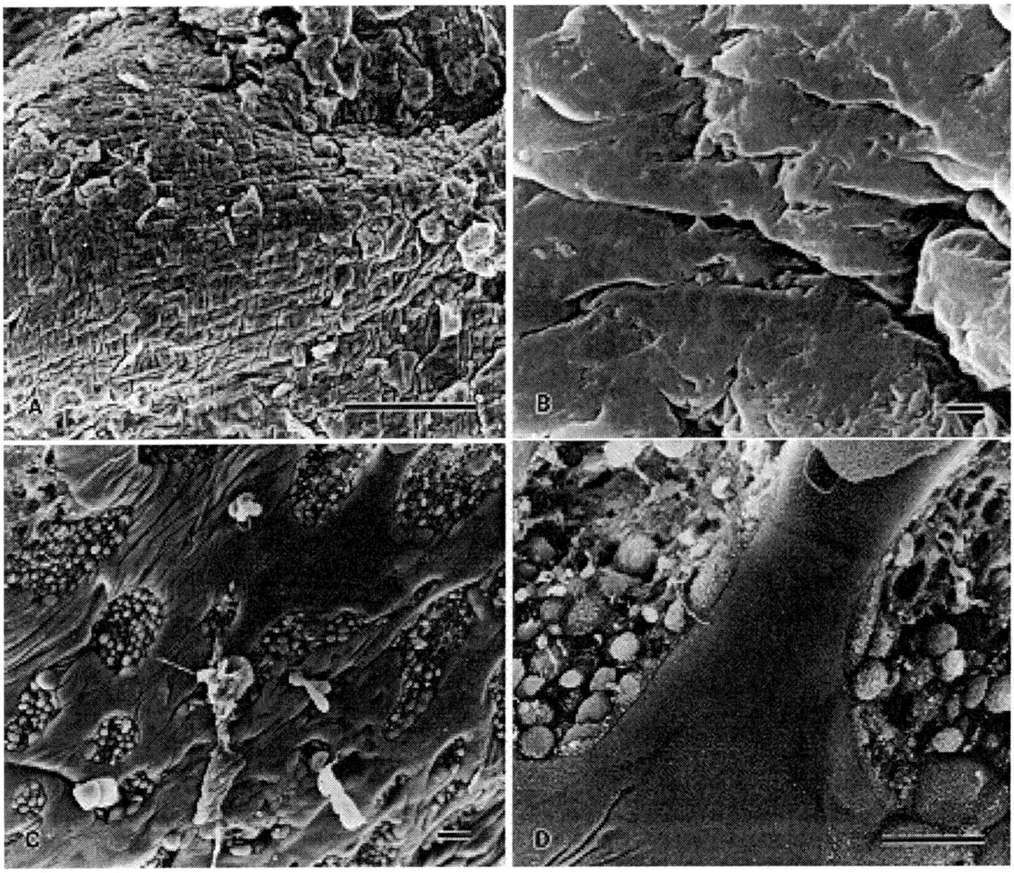

Fig. 13.1.3. SEM micrographs of the conjunctiva of rats. (A) In the conjunctiva of an A(-) rat, the surface shows severe keratinization and no goblet cells. (B) Higher magnification of the conjunctival surface of an A(-) rat, showing severe keratinization and no microvilli and microplicae. (C) The conjunctival surface of an A(-) E(+) rat shows many goblet cells. (D) Higher magnification of the conjunctival surface of a A(-)E(+) rat, showing well-developed microvilli and microplicae and many secretory granules in goblet cells. Bar: 100μm (A, C), 10μm (B), 1μm (D).

Electron Microscopic Findings

SEM Findings in the Conjunctiva

SEM showed many dark cells, keratinization and a lack of goblet cells at the conjunctival surface in A(-) rats (Fig.13.1.3A). In contrast, in A(-) E(+) rats the conjunctiva had many goblet cells (Fig.13.1.3C). High magnification showed only a few microplicae in A(-) conjunctivae (Fig.13.1.3B) and many microplicae in A(-)E(+) conjunctivae (Fig.13.1.3D). In normal rats the conjunctiva had many more densely arranged goblet cells and microplicae (Fig.10.3.1C) than in A(-)E(+) rats.

The differences between A(-)E(+) and A(-) rat conjunctivae were statistically significant: 5.0±8.3 goblet cells per standard field in A(-) rats, 51.0±16.0 in A(-)E(+) rats ($p<0.0001$), and 80.8±11.2 in controls (Table13.1.1).

Table 13.1.1. Number of goblet cells per 240,000 μm² standard field.

		(mean±SD)
Group	Number of fields examined	Number of cells per field
A(-)	8	5.0±8.3*,***
A(-)E(+)	8	51.0±16.0**,***
control	5	80.8±11.2*,**

* $p<0.0001$
** $p=0.0040$
*** $p<0.0001$.

TEM Findings in the Conjunctiva

TEM showed many keratohyalin granules, an absence of goblet cells and a loss of microvilli in A(-) conjunctivae (Fig.13.1.4A). In contrast, there were many goblet cells in A(-) E(+) rats, and they contained secretory granules (Fig.13.1.4B). Epithelial cells had well-developed microvilli (Fig. 13.1.4B) and no keratohyalin granules and keratinization.

Normal conjunctivae had many goblet cells rich in secretory granules (Fig. 10.3.1B).

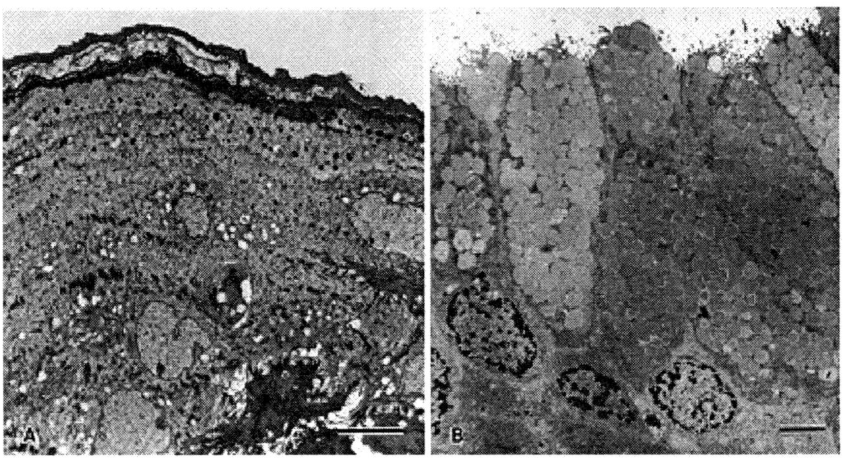

Fig. 13.1.4. TEM micrographs of the rat conjunctiva. In an A(-) rat, the conjunctival surface shows keratinization and epithelial cells contain numerous keratohyalin granules (A). Goblet cells are not seen (A). However, an A(-)E(+) rat conjunctiva has well-developed secretory granules in goblet cells (B). Bar: 5μm (A), 2μm (B).

SEM Findings in the Cornea

SEM revealed that A(-) rat corneas (Fig. 13.1.5A) had many more dark cells than A(-) E(+) rat corneas (Fig.13.1.5C). At high magnification, A(-) rat corneas showed very few microvilli and keratinization (a rough and uneven surface) (Fig.13.1.5B). In contrast, A(-)E(+) rat corneas had many dense microvilli and fine microplicae on the surface (Fig.13.1.5D). Normal cornea had many microvilli and microplicae on the surface (Fig. 10.3.2A,B).

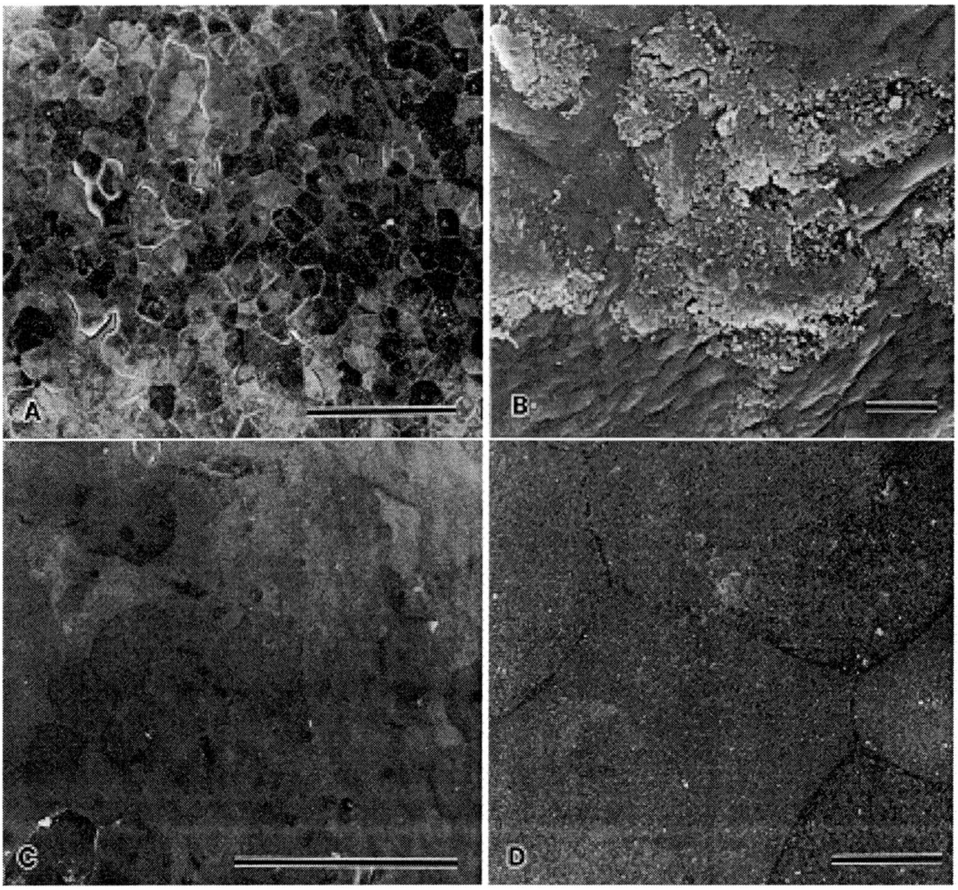

Fig. 13.1.5. SEM micrographs of the corneal surface of rats. In an A(-) rat, dark cells are numerous (A), and they have rough surface without microvilli and microplicae (B). In a A(-)E(+) rat, dark cells are in majority in the corneal surface (C). However, they have numerous, but undeveloped microvilli (D). Bar:100μm (A, C), 10μm (B, D).

Table 13.1.2. Ratio of light cell / light cells plus dark cells.

		(mean±SD)
Group	Number of fields examined	ratio
A(-)	6	0.04±0.03*,***
A(-)E(+)	7	0.11±0.06**,***
control	15	0.24±0.11*,**

* $p<0.0003$

** $p=0.0067$

*** $p<0.0343$.

In SEM micrographs of corneas, the ratio of light cells /light cells plus dark cells of A(-) rat corneas was significantly lower than that of A(-)E(+) rat corneas ($p=0.0343$). The ratio of light cells /light cells plus dark cells was highest in the control rat corneas (Table13.1.2). The epithelial cells of A(-) rat corneas were smaller than those of A(-) E(+) rat corneas because

A (-) rat corneas had more epithelial cells per 600μm^2 field on SEM micrographs than did A(-) E(+) rat corneas (p=0.0407) (Table13.1.3). SEM micrographs showed that control rat corneas had fewer and larger epithelial cells per 600μm^2 field than did the other groups (Table13.1.3).

Table 13.1.3. Number of epithelial cells per 600 μm^2 standard field.

		(mean±SD)
Group	Number of fields examined	Number of cells per field
A(-)	6	131.0±29.0*,***
A(-)E(+)	7	103.3±12.1**,***
controls	15	77.6±15.1*,**

* p<0.0001
** p=0.0008
*** p<0.0407.

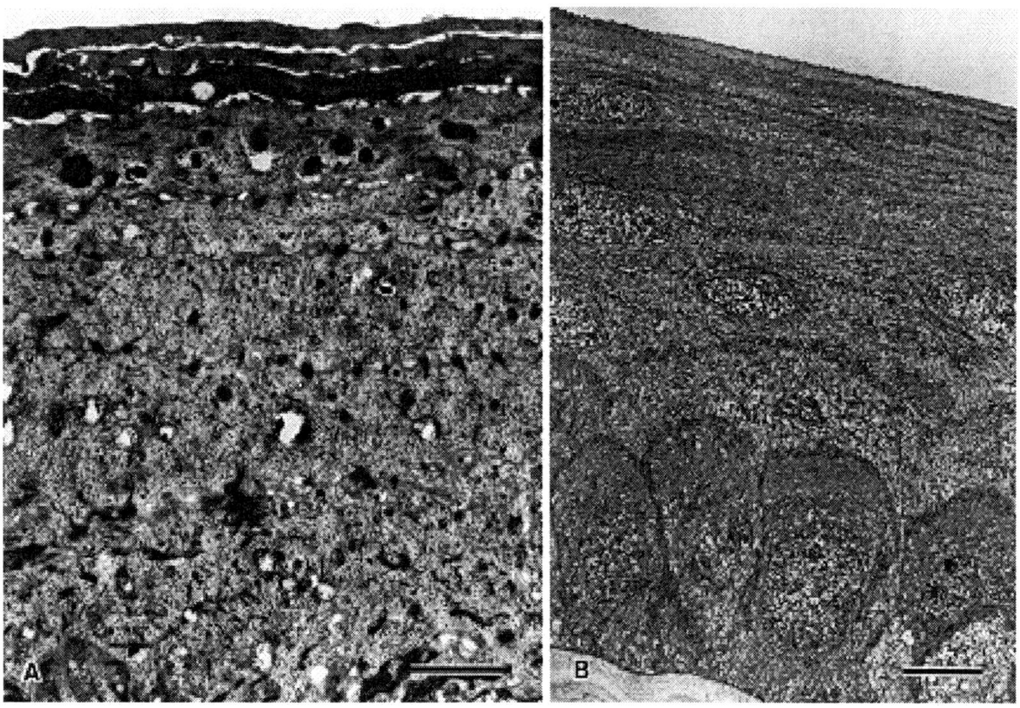

Fig. 13.1.6. TEM micrographs of the rat cornea. The cornea of a A(-) rat shows severe keratinization in the superficial epithelial layers and numerous keratohyalin granules (A). No microvilli are seen in the most superficial epithelial layer (A). However, the epithelium of a A(-)E(+) rat has many microvilli in the most superficial layer, but no keratohyalin granules (B). Bar: 1μm (A, B).

TEM Findings in the Cornea

In the A(-) rat corneas, there was severe keratinization in the superficial epithelial layer and epithelial cells contained numerous keratohyalin granules (Fig.13.1.6A). On the other hand, A(-)E(+) rats had no keratinization and keratohyalin granules in the epithelium (Fig.13.1.6B). The most superficial epithelial cells had many microvilli (Fig.13.1.6B). In A(-), A(-)E(+) and control rats, the cornea showed many hemidesmosomes and a continuous basement membrane in the basal cells and no abnormal dense bodies were seen in the subepithelial layer.

A(-) rat corneas had 0.78±0.77 microvilli per 1μm standard field, compared with 2.04±0.79 ($p<0.0001$) in A(-)E(+) rat corneas. Control rats had 2.83±0.52 microvilli per 1μm standard field (Table13.1.4).

Table 13.1.4. Number of microvilli per 1μm standard field.

		(mean±SD)
Group	Number of fields examined	Number of microvilli per field
A(-)	55	0.78±0.77*,***
A(-)E(+)	58	2.04±0.79**,***
control	12	2.83±0.52*,**

* $p<0.0001$
** $p=0.0015$
*** $p<0.0001$.

b. Relationship Between Vitamin A and Vitamin E Deficiency

1. The Cornea

SEM Findings

In the cornea of E(-) rats, the most superficial layer of the epithelium was occupied by dark cells (Fig.13.2.1A), and microvilli and microplicae were scarce (Fig.13.2.1B). In the cornea of E(-)A(+) rats, dark cells were less than in that of E(-) rats (Fig.13.2.1C) and seemed to be a little bit more or almost the same as in that of controls (Fig.13.2.1C). Microvilli and microplicae were numerous (Fig.13.2.1D), but fewer than in the cornea of control rats.

TEM Findings

E(-) rats showed decreased microvilli in the most superficial epithelial layer of the cornea (Fig.13.2.2A). Basal cells had irregularly invaginated nuclei (Fig.13.2.2A). Basal cells had lost their basement membranes and hemidesmosomes (Fig.13.2.2A). In the cornea of E(-)A(+) rats, many microvilli were present in the most superficial epithelial cells and epithelial cells had many fibrils, ribosomes and desmosome-like intercellular junctions (Fig. 13.2.2B), Basal cells showed no abnormalities: oval nuclei, many hemidesmosomes, normal basement membrane, no cellular debris and no subepithelial dense bodies (Fig.13.2.2C). The endothelial cells and Descemet membrane showed normal features.

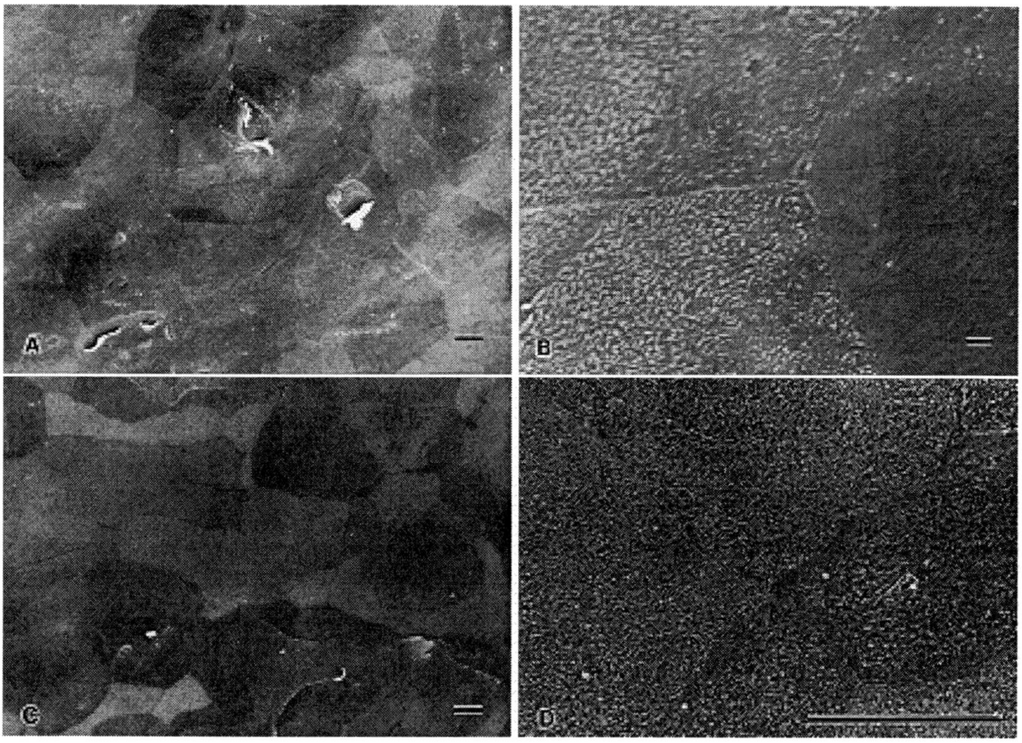

Fig. 13.2.1. SEM micrograph of the cornea of rats. In the cornea of an E(-) rat, there is a large number of dark cells in the most superficial epithelium(A), and microvilli and microplicae are scarce(B). In the cornea of an E(-)A(+) rat, dark cells are less than in an E(-) rat (C) and have numerous microvilli and microplicae(D). Bar: 10μm (A,C, D), 1μm (B).

2. The Retina

Light Microscopic Findings

In E(-) rats the retina had no photoreceptor outer and inner segments and nuclei (Fig. 13.2.3A) in 20% of E(-) rats, one line of photoreceptor cell nuclei (Fig. 13.2.3B) in 20% and 3-4 lines (Fig. 13.2.3C) in 60%. On the other hand, the retina kept more than 4 lines of photoreceptor cell nuclei with the outer and inner segments (Fig.13.2.3D) in 100% of E(-)A(+) rats.

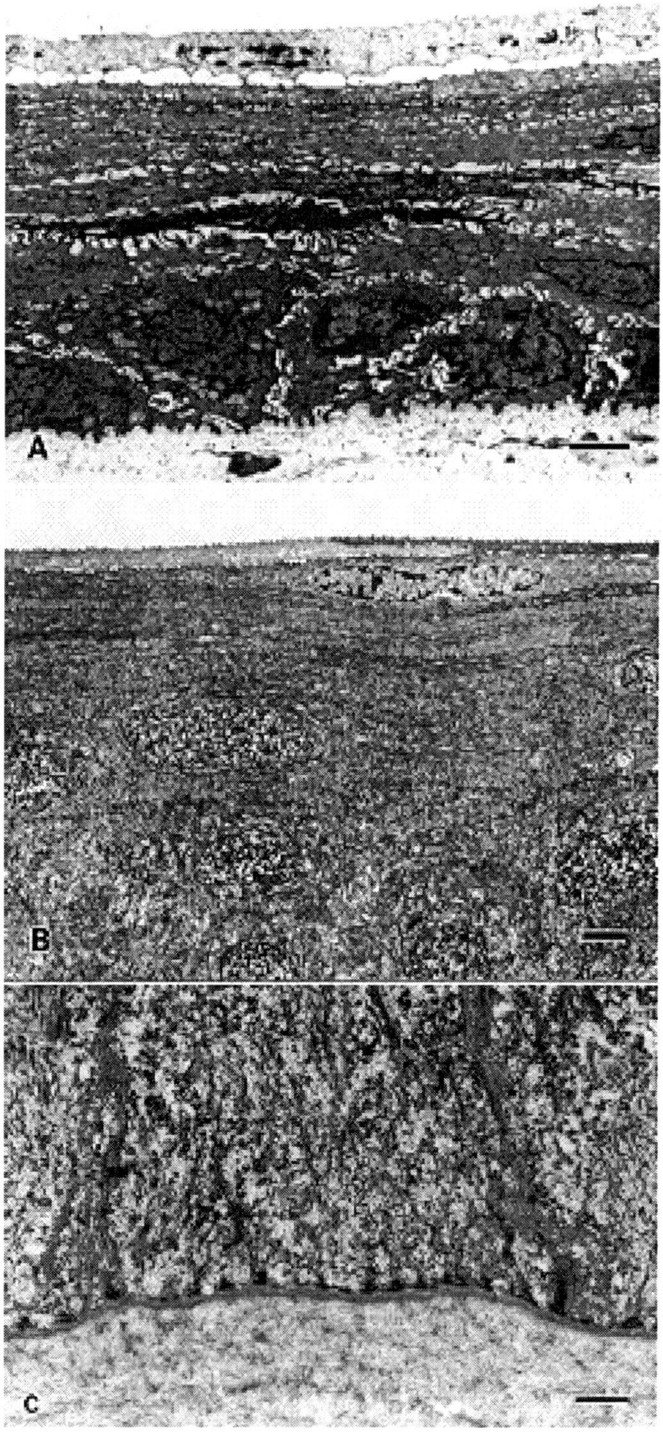

Fig. 13.2.2. TEM micrographs of the corneas of E(-) and E(-)A(+) rats. The cornea of an E(-) rat shows underdeveloped microvilli in the most superficial epithelial cells (A), but the cornea of an E(-)A(+) rat has many microvilli (B) Hemidesmosomes and basement membrane of an E(-)A(+) rat cornea look intact (C). Bar; 2μm (A, B), 500nm (C).

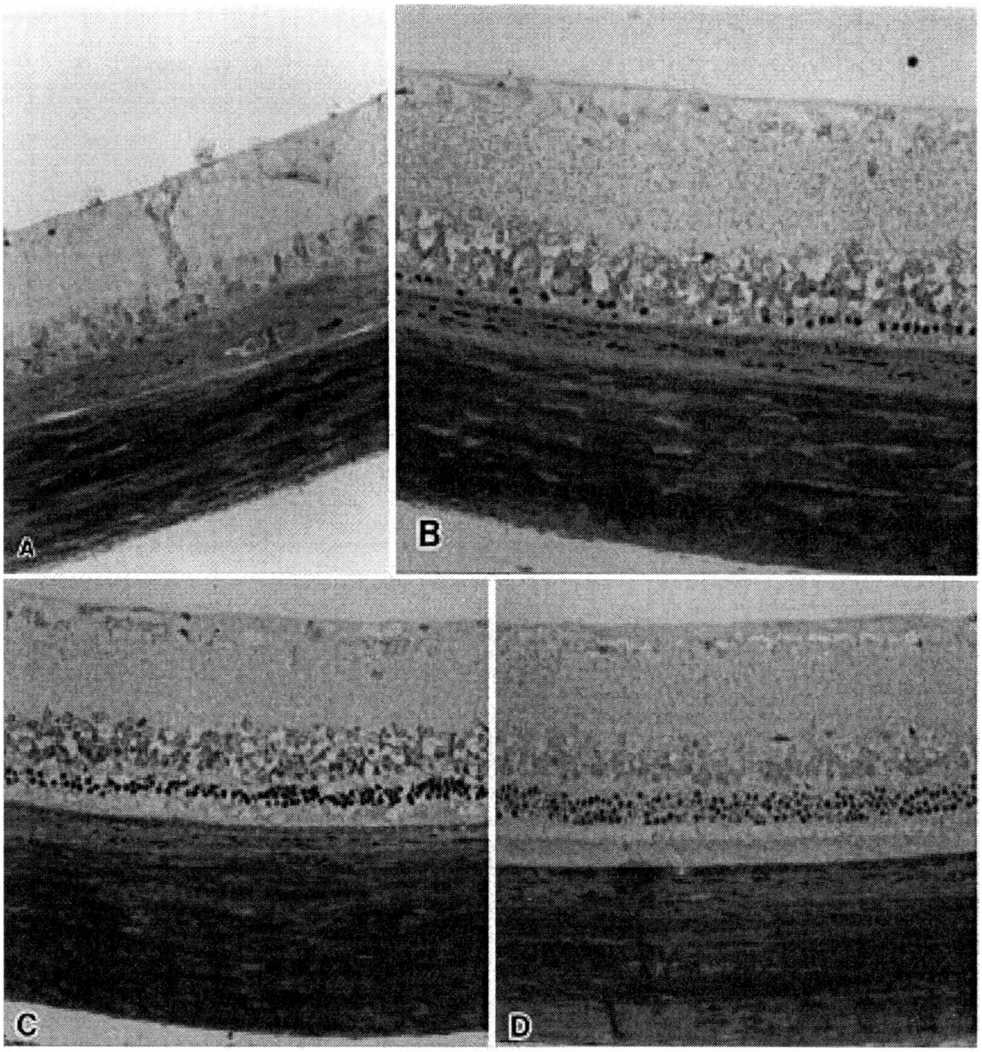

Fig. 13.2.3. Light micrographs of the retina of E(-) and E(-)A(+) rats. A. The retina of an E(-) rat has no photoreceptor cells from the outer segment to nucleus. B. The retina of an E(-) rat has one line of photoreceptor cell nuclei, but no outer and inner segments. C. The retina of an E(-) rat keeps 1-3 lines of photoreceptor cell nuclei and inner segments. A, B and C show the degeneration in the inner nuclear layer. D. The retina of an E(-)A(+) rat keeps 3 or 4 lines of photoreceptor cell nuclei and outer and inner segments. × 200 (A-D).

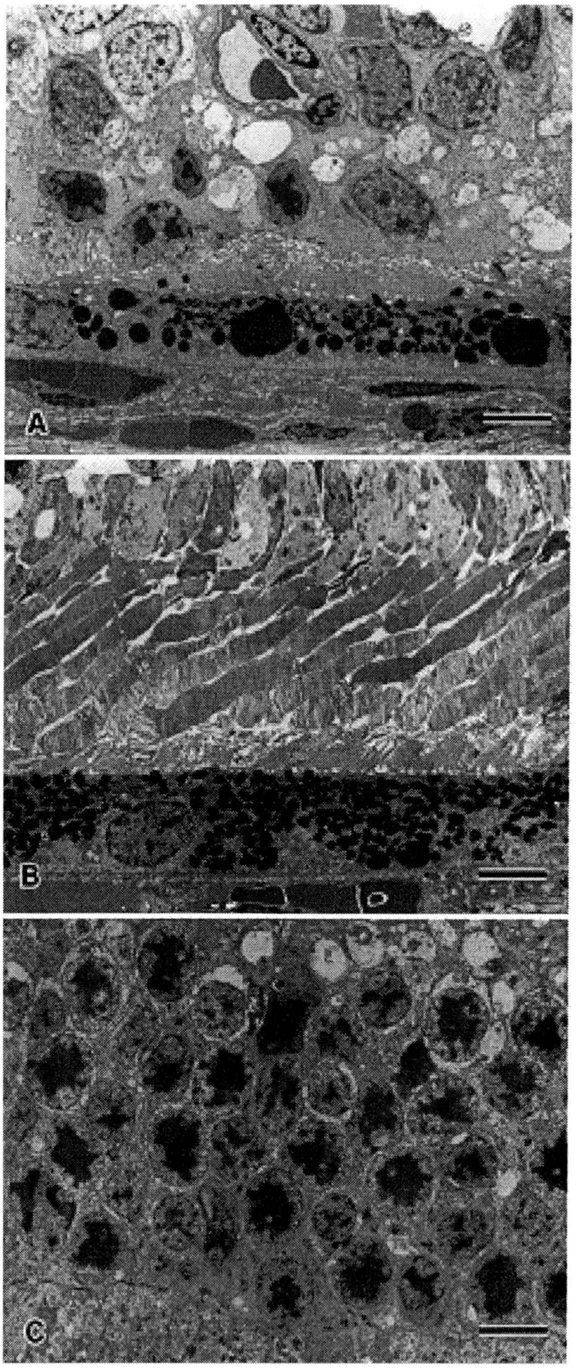

Fig. 13.2.4. TEM micrographs of the retinas of E(-) and E(-)A(+) rats. In the retina of an E(-) rat, the RPE contains a large number of lipofuscin granules and photoreceptor outer segments disappear (A). No photoreceptor cell nuclei are seen (A). Nuclei of the inner nuclear layer are also decreased to 2 or 3 lines and Müller cell processes are vacuolated (A). In the retina of an E(-)A(+) rat, the RPE have numerous lipofuscin granules. Photoreceptor outer segments are seen (B). Four or 5 lines of photoreceptor cell nuclei remain,and Müller cell processes look intact without vacuolation (C). Bar: 10μm (A – C).

TEM Findings

In E(-) rats, the retina was thin. The RPE contained numerous lipofuscin granules. In the most severely deficient rats, the photoreceptor cells including outer and inner segments and nuclei disappeared (Fig. 13.2.4A). The outer and inner nuclear layer nuclei were prominently decreased and cellular components were vacuolated among nuclei (Fig.13.2.4A). On the other hand, in the retina of E(-)A(+) rats photoreceptor outer and inner segments were present, but decreased (Fig.13.2.4B). Outer segment discs were irregular in electron density. Three to 4 lines of photoreceptor cell nuclei remained (Fig.13.2.4C) and Müller cell processes looked intact among nuclei of the outer nuclear layer (Fig.13.2.4C). The RPE had numerous lipofuscin granules (Fig.13.2.4B). The inner nuclear layer had 2-3 lines of nuclei , which contained vacuoles among nuclei, in E(-) rats (Fig. 13.2.5A). On the other hand, in E(-) A(+) rats the inner nuclear layer had 4 lines of nuclei which were compactly arranged without vacuolation (Fig. 13.2.5B).

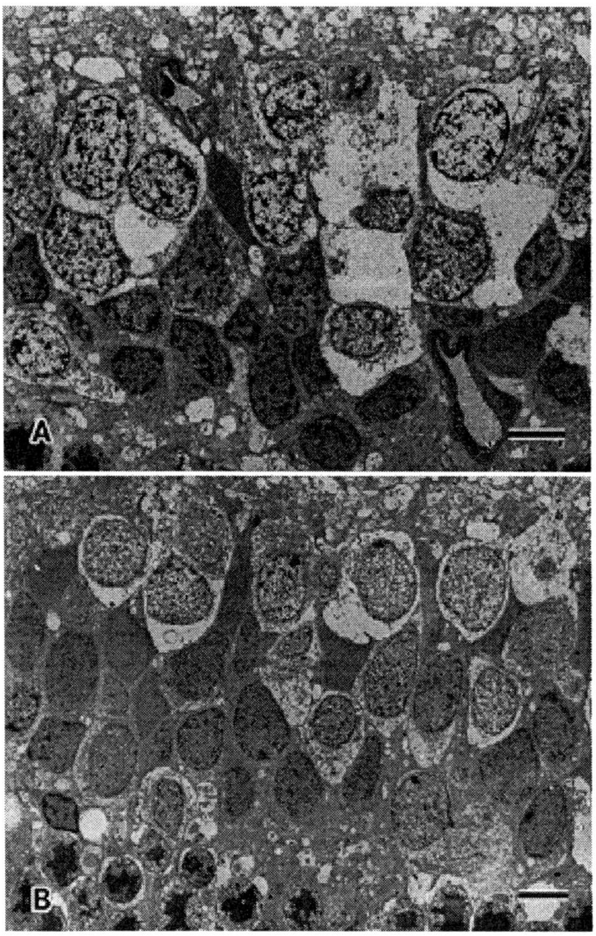

Fig. 13.2.5. Electron micrographs of the inner nuclear layer of the retina of E(-) and E(-)A(+) rats. An E(-) rat has 3-4 lines of inner nuclear layer nuclei and contains vacuoles anong nuclei (A). In an E (-) A(+) rat (B), The inner nuclear layer consists of 4 lines of nuclei which are compactly arranged and shows no degeneration. Bar: 5μm (A, B).

3. The Optic Nerve

Light Microscopic Findings

Light microscopy showed no significant difference in appearance between E(-) (Fig.13.2.6A) and E(-)A(+) (Fig.13.2.6B) rats: optic nerve fibers were sparse and the average diameter of the optic nerve was 0.62±0.082mm (n=3) in E(-) rats and 0.71±0.060mm (n=3) in E(-)A(+) rats (p=0.1993). However, there was no significant difference between the two groups (p=0.1993).

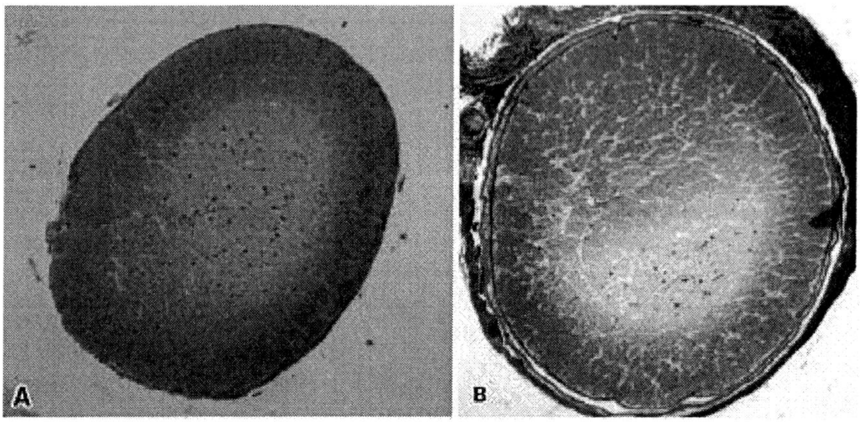

Fig. 13.2.6. Light micrographs of optic nerves of E(-) and E(-)A(+) rats. The optic nerve of an E(-) rat shows scarce optic nerve fibers, especially in the center (A), but is almost the same as that of an E(-) A(+) rat (B). Toluideine blue stain, ×10.

TEM Findings

In the optic nerve of an E (-) rat (Fig.13.2.7A), myelinated axons were decreased in number and degenerated. The myelin sheaths were thin and severely degenerated (Fig.13.2.7A, B). Axonal cytoplasmic components were destructed. Glial cells were proliferated (Fig.13.2.6A, B). In the optic nerve of E(-)A(+) rats, the appearance was almost the same as that of E(-) rats (Fig. 13.2.7C, D). The number of E(-)A(+) rat groups: 219.8±35.3/600μm^2 (n=23 fields examined) in E(-) group and myelinated axons showed a statistically significant difference between E(-) rat and 184.1±25.4/600μm^2 (n=24 fields examined) in E(-)A(+) group ($p<0.002$).

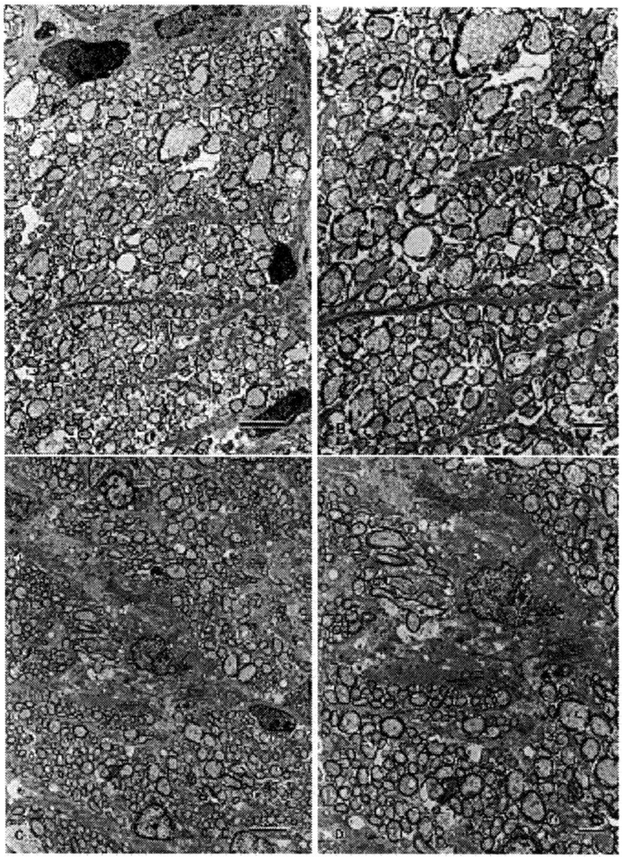

Fig. 13.2.7. TEM micrographs of optic nerves of E(-) and E(-)A(+) rats, In the optic nerve of an E(-) rat, myelinated axons are decreased and degenerated (A). Myelin sheaths are degenerated and irregular in shape. In axons, mitochondria and neurotubulus are destructed. Glial cells are proliferated (A and B). In E(-)A(+) rats, the optic nerve shows almost the same features (C, D). Bar: 5μm (A, C), 2μm (B, D).

Discussion

Corneal and conjunctival changes induced by vitamin A deficiency are quite different from those by vitamin E deficiency. That is, vitamin A deficiency causes keratinization and a decrease and loss of microvilli and microplicae in the most superficial epithelial cells of the cornea (Sommer, 1983; Kanazawa, Kitaoka, Ueda, et al, 2002; Fujikawa, Gong and Amemiya, 2003) and scarce goblet cells and keratinization in the conjunctiva (Fujikawa, Gong and Amemiya).

There are just a few studies on the contribution of vitamin E to the cornea and conjunctiva (Stephens, Negi, Skort et al, 1988). In vitamin E deficiency, the conjunctiva has scarce microvilli and microplicae and decreased or few goblet cells (Fujikawa, Gong and Amemiya, 2003). A few superficial layers of the epithelial cells lose desmosome-like intercellular junctions and are separated. The cornea also has decreased microvilli and microplicae and superficial layers are separated. However, no keratinization appears in the conjunctiva and cornea. The basal cells release cellular debris into the subepithelium. The current experiments showed that vitamin A or E deficiency could be compensated for by supplementation with vitamin E or A, although the compensation was incomplete. Main damages in vitamin A or E deficiency occur in the epithelium (Pfister and Renner, 1978; Van Horn, Schutten, Hyndiuk et al, 1980), which regenerates every 7-8 days. This may be the reason why conjunctival and corneal damages can be easily prevented despite of incompleteness. The most specific conjunctival and corneal change induced by vitamin A deficiency is keratinization and the appearance of keratohyaline granules which are never induced by vitamin E deficiency. Mechanism of keratinization is not clear, but vitamin A may stimulate the synthesis of glycoconjugates that may appear on the cell surface or be secreted as basement membrane components (Hatchell and Sommer, 1984; Ubels, Edelhauser and Austin, 1983). Since vitamin E could prevent keratinization caused by vitamin A deficiency, its action is probably related to some stage of the keratinization process.

With the exception of keratinization, decreased microvilli and microplicae and dark cell phenomenon in the epithelial cells were induced not only by vitamin A deficiency but also by vitamin E deficiency. Either vitamin could prevent such epithelial changes in some degree. Because vitamins A and E are related to the development, growth and maintenance of epithelial cells and are essential micronutrients (Anderson, Richard, Rock, 1993; Hatchell, Ubels, Stekiel et al, 1985, Sullivan, McCulley and Dohlman, 1973). However, differences in the degree of morphological prevention by vitamin A or E suggest that roles and mechanisms for the epithelial cell are delicately or clearly different according to vitamins, because the prevention of damages by one vitamin deficiency was incomplete by another vitamin.

The most specific changes induced by vitamin E in the retina was an accumulation of a large amount of lipofuscin granules which was neither prevented nor lightened by vitamin A. Lipofuscin granules in the RPE is the result of dysfunction of lysosomes over phagocytizing OS discs degenerated by peroxidation due to vitamin E deficiency. (Amemiya, 1978; Robison, Kuwabara and Bieri, 1979). Although vitamin A also has antioxidant actions such as quenching of singlet oxygen and other electrically excited molecules that are produced by photoexcitation reactions, vitamin A could not prevent a great amount of production of lipofuscin granules in the RPE due to vitamin E deficiency. According to these experiments, the activity of vitamin E as membrane stabilization and antioxidation may be stronger than that of vitamin A, although antioxidant mechanisms of both vitamins differ from each other. However, it may be due to prominently decreased production of OS discs as a result of vitamin A deficiency that no lipofuscin granules were found in the RPE (Dowling and Gibbons, 1961; Amemiya, 1968). That is, it is not due to stronger antioxidant action of vitamin E that no lipofuscin granules were accumulated under vitamin A deficiency in supplementation with vitamin E.

The common retinal changes in vitamin A deficiency or vitamin E deficiency are decrease and disappearance of photoreceptor cells, especially OS discs, and result from the vacuolation of OS discs. However the causes of OS changes are different each other. Vitamin A is contained in the photoreceptor cell, especially in OS disc membranes with fatty acids. Thus vitamin A deficiency leads to destruction and decreased production and reproduction of OS discs. These sequence results in no lipofuscin granules in the RPE (Dowling and Gibbons, 1961; Amemiya, 1968). On the other hand, deficiency of vitamin E which has strong membrane stabilization and antioxidation and is soluble in fatty acids leads to fragile OS discs and decrease and disappearance of OS discs (Amemiya, 1978, Robison, Kuwabara and Bieri, 1979). Thus the RPE at first overphagocytizes destructed OS disc membranes which are accumulated excessively in the RPE as lipofuscin granules. These never decrease with administration of vitamin E after its deficiency (Amemiya, 1981). Supplementation of vitamin A under vitamin E deficiency could not prevent retinal changes completely, but reduced changes. Vitamin A which is soluble in fatty acids, may enforce photoreceptor cell structures, especially OS discs and retinal membrane structures and may have a little bit or moderate antioxidant effects on lipid membranes.

In the optic nerve, the common changes in vitamin A deficiency and vitamin E deficiency were changes in the myelin sheath such as thinness, irregular arrangement of lamellae and deformity. Cytoplasmic components in axons were also destructed. In an interaction between vitamins A and E, however, supplementation of one vitamin seems to inhibit progressive changes in the cornea and retina in some degree under another deficiency. A series of the author's studies on a deficiency of single vitamin and trace element revealed that optic nerve changes always progress after recovery from deficiency (Amemiya, Kawata and Maekawa, 1987; Dake and Amemiya,1991; Mishima, Dake and Amemiya, 1996; Gong and Amemiya,1999; Gong and Amemiya,2001; Tsuda, 2002; Gong,Takami and Amemiya, 2003). Thus it is understandable that, while the cornea, a reproducible tissue, of E(-) rats can be preserved by interaction with another vitamin, the optic nerve and retina, non-reproducible tissues, might not be preserved. In E(-) and E(-)A(+) experiments, however, it is surprising that the retina, CNS, was rather well protected from vitamin E deficiency with supplementation of vitamin A. Vitamin A might have a stronger affinity to the retina than vitamin E.

In conclusion, preventive interactions occur in ocular tissues between vitamins A and E. Interactions appeared most prominently in the conjunctiva and cornea, moderately in the retina and least in the optic nerve.

ii. Interaction Between Vitamin A and Zinc

SEM Findings in the Conjunctiva

In group A(+)Zn(+), microvilli and microplicae were numerous and well-developed in the most superficial conjunctival epithelium and goblet cells with well-developed granules were seen frequently in the epithelium (Fig.13.3.1A). On the other hand, in group A(-) the surface of the conjunctiva showed no microvilli and microplicae but keratinization and desquamation of the superficial epithelium (Fig.13.3.1B). There were no goblet cells in the conjunctiva of group A(-) rats. Conjunctival microvilli and microplicae of group A(-)Zn(+) rats were fewer than in group A(+)Zn(+), but more numerous than in group A(-). In group A(-)Zn(+) rats, there were no goblet cells in the conjunctiva (Fig.13.3.1C). Group A(-)Zn(+) rats had more dark cells in the conjunctiva than did group A(+)Zn(+) rats, and the ratio of light cells to light and dark cells was significantly higher in group A(+)Zn(+) than in group A(-)Zn(+) ($p<0.05$) (Table13.3.4). However, the ratio in group A(-) could not be calculated because of extensive keratinization of the epithelial cells.

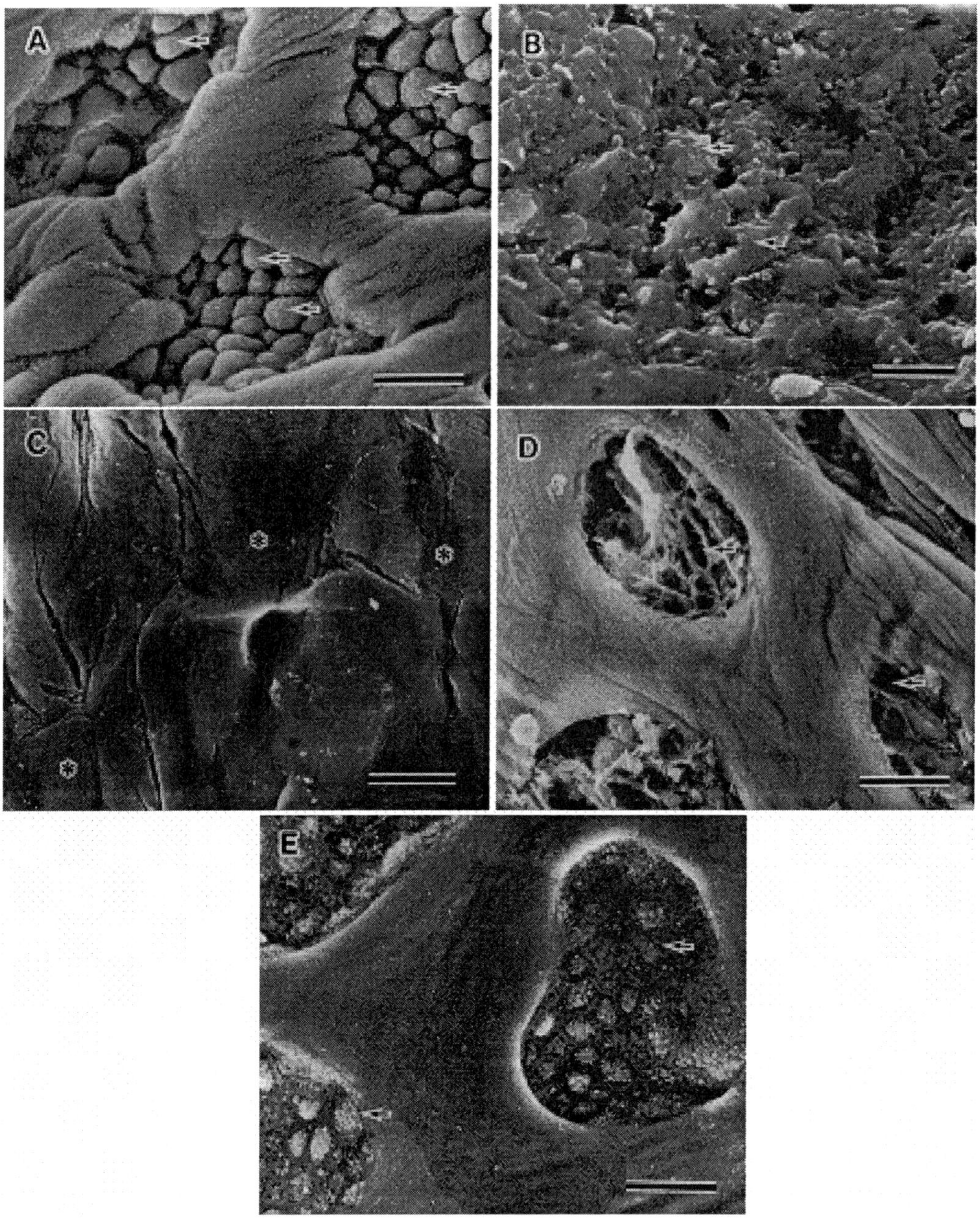

Fig. 13.3.1. SEM photographs of the conjunctival epithelium of rats: group A(+)Zn(+) (A), A(-) (B), A(-)Zn(+) (C), Zn(-) (D) and Zn(-)A(+) (E). A. A group A(+)Zn(+) rat shows numerous fine microvilli in the most superficial conjunctival epithelium and many goblet cells with well-developed granules (arrows). B. In a group A(-) rat, there are almost no microvilli, but keratinization (arrows) in the most superficial epithelium. C. In a group A(-)Zn(+) rat, the conjunctiva has light cells with numerous microvilli (asterisks) but no goblet cells. D. A group Zn(-) rat shows decrease in microvilli in the most superficial epithelium. The goblet cells show hole-like structures of granules (arrows). E In the conjunctiva of a group Zn(-)A(+) rat, goblet cells with granules (arrows) are seen. Bar: 10μm (A-E).

Table 13.3.4. Ratio of light cells to light and dark cells in the conjunctivas and corneas of the five experimental groups (n: number of fields examined).

Group	Conjunctiva (n=12)	Cornea (n=16)
Group A(+)Zn(+)	0.558±0.095[a]	0.645±0.059[b]
Group A(-)	*	0.447±0.098[b]
Group A(-) Zn(+)	0.486±0.095[a]	0.529±0.085[b]
Group Zn(+) A(+)	0.588±0.059[c]	0.675±0.089[d]
Group Zn(-)	0.417±0.05[c]	0.465±0.059[d]
Group Zn(-) A(+)	0.473±0.07[c]	0.577±0.054[d]

*: The ratio in group A(-) could not be calculated because of extensive keratinization of the epithelium.

a: There is a significant difference between group A(+)Zn(+) and group A(-)Zn(+) ($p<0.05$).

b: The difference is significant between group A(+)Zn(+) and group A(-)Zn(+) ($p<0.05$) and between group A(-)Zn(+) and group A(-) ($p<0.05$).

c: There is a significant difference between group A(+)Zn(+) and group Zn(-)A(+) ($p<0.001$) and between group Zn(-)A(+) and group Zn(-) ($p<0.01$).

d: There is a significant difference between group A(+)Zn(+) and group Zn(-)A(+) ($p<0.01$) and between group Zn(-)A(+) and group Zn(-) ($p<0.05$).

Table 13.3.5. Number of goblet cells in the conjunctiva. The number of fields examined in each group was ten.

Group	Number of goblet cells/$3\times10^4\mu m^2$
Group A(+)Zn(+)	17.9±1.287[a]
Group A(-)	*
Group A(-)Zn(+)	*
Group Zn(-)	12.1±1.912[a]
Group Zn(-)A(+)	15.5±2.461[a]

*: The number of goblet cells in groups A(-) and A(-)Zn(+) could not be counted because of epithelial keratinization.

a: There is no significant difference between group A(+)Zn(+) and group Zn(-)A(+) ($p<0.05$) and between group Zn(-)A(+) and group Zn(-) ($p<0.01$).

The conjunctiva of group Zn(-) demonstrated a decrease in microvilli in the superficial epithelial cells, while the conjunctivas of group Zn(-)A(+) had a certain decrease in microvilli but displayed more microvilli than did the conjunctiva of group Zn(-) rats. In the conjunctivas of group Zn(-) rats, goblet cells were decreased. The conjunctiva of group Zn(-)A(+) had more goblet cells than did those of group Zn(-) rats. However, the conjunctiva of group Zn(-)A(+) rats had less goblet cells than did those in group A(+)Zn(+). The number of goblet cells in the conjunctiva was significantly higher in the rats of group A(+)Zn(+) than in group Zn(-)A(+) ($p<0.05$), and the difference between group Zn(-)A(+) and group Zn(-) was also significant ($p<0.01$) (Table13.3.5). The goblet cells of group Zn(-) rats showed hole-like structures of granules (Fig.13.3.1D). The granules of goblet cells of rats in group Zn(-)A(+) (Fig.13.3.1E) were smaller and more shrunken than those of group A(+)Zn(+) rats. However, the goblet cells of group Zn(-)A(+) had more granules than did those of group Zn(-). The ratio of light cells to light and dark cells in the conjunctiva was significantly higher in group A(+)Zn(+) than in group A(-) Zn(+) ($p<0.001$) and the difference between group Zn(-) and group Zn(-)A(+) was also significant ($p<0.01$) (Table13.3.4).

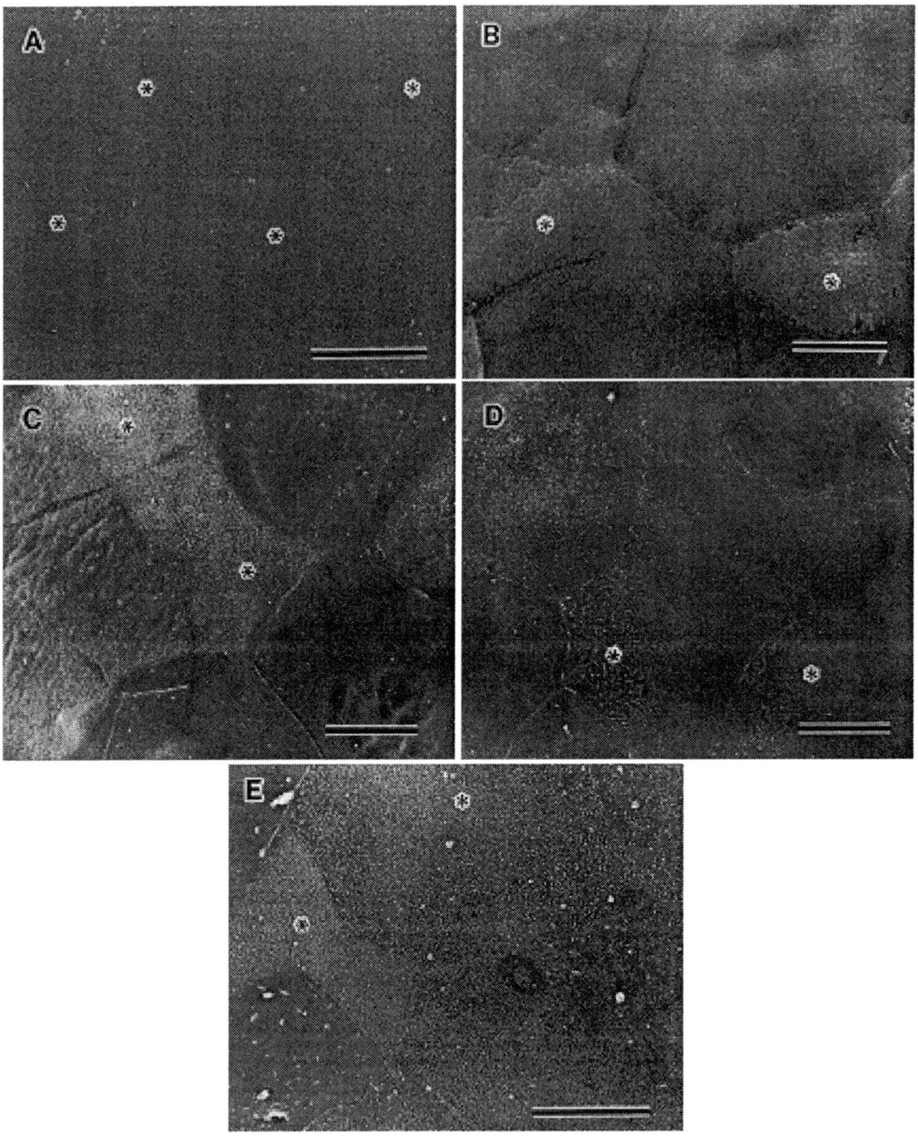

Fig. 13.3.2. SEM photographs of corneal epithelium of rats: group A(+)Zn(+) (A), A(-) (B), A(-)Zn(+) (C), Zn(-) (D) and Zn(-)A(+) (E). A. In a group A(+)Zn(+) rat, many light cells (asterisks) are seen in the most superficial corneal epithelium and have numerous microvilli and microplicae. B. In a group A(-) rat, the corneal epithelium shows an absence of microvilli and keratinization (asterisks). C. The superficial corneal epithelium of a group A(-)Zn(+) rat has a lower number of light cells (asterisks) and no keratinization. D. The most superficial corneal epithelium of a group Zn(-) rat shows many dark cells with scarce microvilli (asterisks). E. In a group Zn(-)A(+) rat, the microvilli and microplicae in the epithelium are less numerous than in a group Zn(+) A(+) rat, but more numerous (asterisks) than in a group Zn(-) rat. Bar: 10μm (A-E).

SEM Finings in the Cornea

There were many light cells on the corneal epithelium of group A(+) Zn(+) rats, which had a high density of microvilli and microplicae in the most superficial epithelial cells (Fig.13.3.2A). The corneal epithelium in groups A(-) and A(-)Zn(+) rats showed more dark cells than did those in group A(+)Zn(+) rats. In group A(-) rats (Fig.13.3.2B) there were more dark cells in the epithelium than in group A(-)Zn(+) rats (Fig.13.3.2C). In group A(-) rats microvilli were absent in the most superficial epithelial cells of the cornea (Fig.13.3.2B). The density of microvilli and microplicae was lower in the light cells of group A(-) rats than in those of group A(+)Zn(+) rats. On the other hand, the corneas of group A(-)Zn(+) rats (Fig.13.3.2C) had a certain decrease in microvilli, but exhibited more microvilli than did the corneas of group A(-) rats (Fig.13.3.2B). The corneas in group A(-) showed keratinization (Fig.13.3.2B), but those in group A(-)Zn(+) showed no keratinization (Fig.13.3.2C). The ratio of light cells to light and dark cells in the cornea was significantly higher in group A(+)Zn(+) than in group A(-) and group A(-)Zn(+) ($p<0.01$), and the difference between group A(-) and group A(-)Zn(+) was also significant ($p<0.05$) (Table13.3.4).

The corneas of group Zn(-) rats demonstrated an absence of microvilli in the most superficial epithelial cells (Fig.13.3.2D). The density of microvilli and microplicae in the light cells of group Zn(-) rats was lower than in those of group A(+)Zn(+) rats, while the corneas of group Zn(-) A(+) rats (Fig.13.3.2E) had a certain decrease in microvilli but showed more microvilli than those of group Zn(-) (Fig.13.3.2D).

In the corneas of groups Zn(-) and Zn(-)A(+), dark cells were more numerous on the surface than in those of group A(+)Zn(+). The ratio of light cells to light and dark cells in group Zn(-) was significantly different from that in group A(+)Zn(+) and group Zn(-)A(+) ($p<0.01$). There was a significant difference between group Zn(-) and group Zn(-) A(+) ($p<0.05$) (Table13.3.4).

TEM Findings in the Conjunctiva

In group A(+)Zn(+) rats, there were fine microvilli and goblet cells with well-developed secretory granules on the conjunctival epithelium (Fig.13.3.3A). Group A(-) rats demonstrated almost no microvilli and microplicae, but showed keratinization and epithelial cells containing keratohyalin granules. There were no goblet cells in group A(-) rats (Fig.13.3.3B). Group A(-) Zn(+) rats had a few microvilli but no goblet cells (Fig.13.3.3C).

In groups Zn(-) and Zn(-)A(+) rats, the conjunctivae demonstrated a decrease in microvilli in the superficial epithelial cells. The conjunctivae of group Zn(-)A(+) had some decrease in microvilli but had more microvilli than did those of group Zn(-). In group Zn(-) rats, granules of goblet cells were hard to find, buried under the superficial epithelial cells (Fig.13.3.3D). The conjunctivae of group Zn(-)A(+) rats had more goblet cells with granules than did those of group Zn(-) rats (Fig.13.3.3E). No epithelial cells exhibiting keratinization or containing keratohyalin granules were seen in the conjunctivas of group Zn(-) and group Zn(-) A(+) rats.

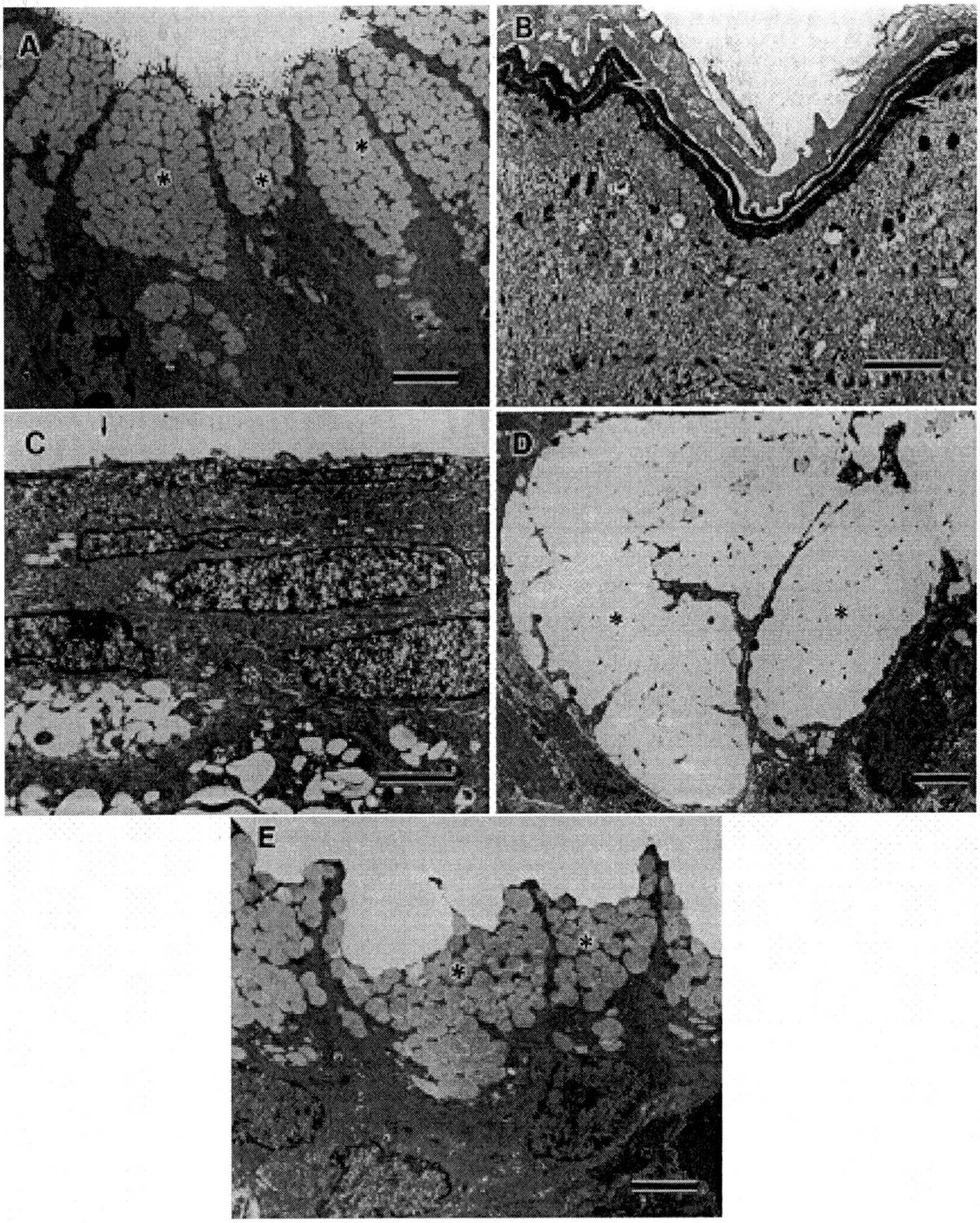

Fig. 13.3.3. TEM photographs of conjunctival epithelium of rats: group A(+)Zn(+) (A), A(-) (B), A(-)Zn(+) (C), Zn(-) (D) and Zn(-)A(+) (E). A. The conjunctiva of a group A(+)Zn(+) rat has microvilli and goblet cells with well-developed secretory granules (asterisks). B. A group A(-) rat has keratinization (arrows) and many keratohyalin granules in the epithelial cytoplasm. There are no microvilli or goblet cells. C. In a group A(-)Zn(+) rat, there are a few microvilli (arrows), but no goblet cell. Keratinization is not seen. D. In a group Zn(-) rat, granules of goblet cells are hard to find (asterisks). E. In a group Zn(-)A(+) rat, the conjunctiva has goblet cells with granules (asterisks) and shows no keratinization. Bar: 2μm (A-E).

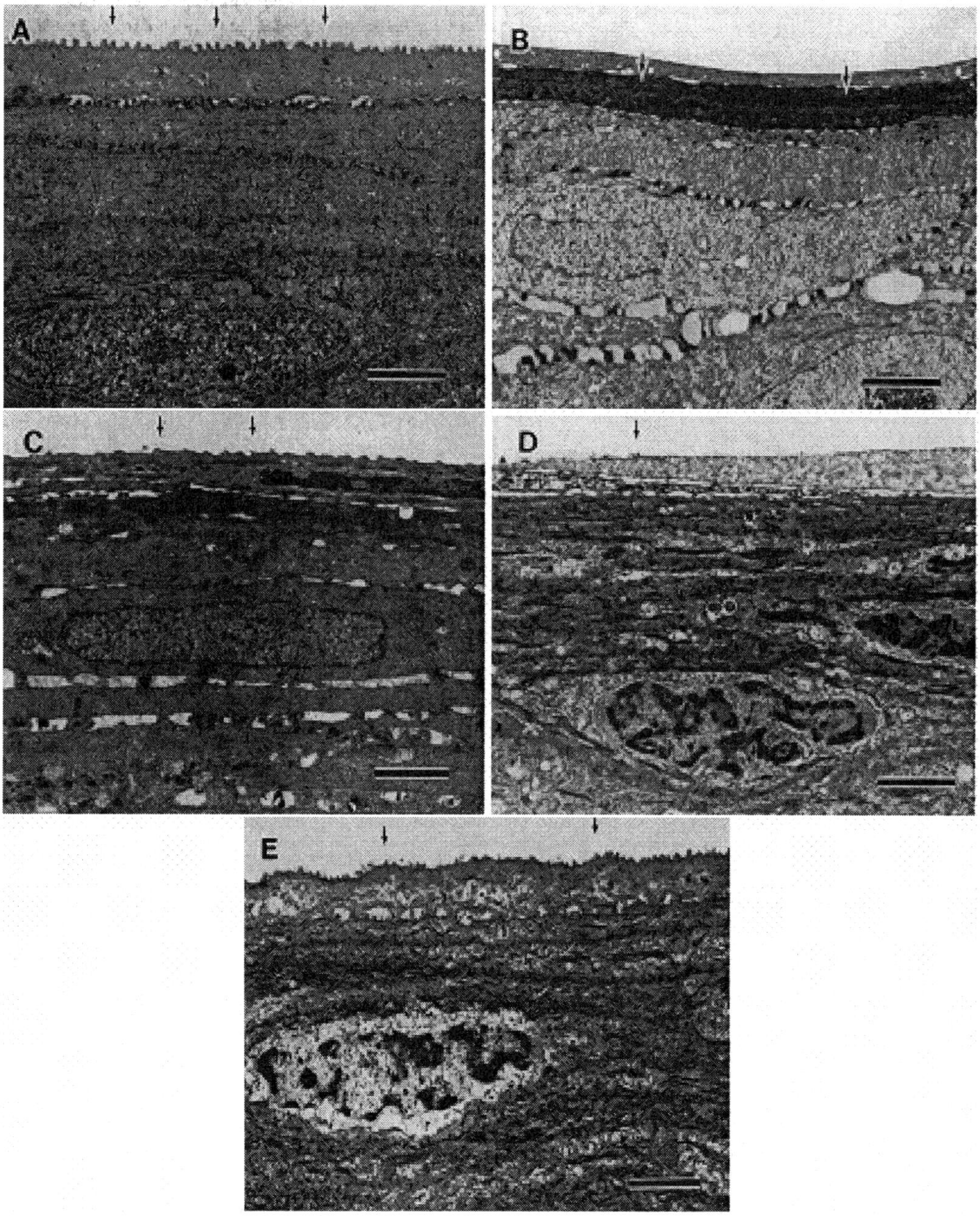

Fig. 13.3.4. TEM photographs of corneal epithelium of rats: group A(+)Zn(+) (A), A(-) (B), A(-)Zn(+) (C), Zn(-) (D) and Zn(-)A(+) (E). In a group A(+)Zn(+) rat, there are many microvilli (arrows) in the most superficial epithelium. B. A group A(-) rat cornea shows keratinization (arrows), but no microvilli in the epithelial cells. C. A group A(-)Zn(+) rat shows a slight decrease in the number of microvilli (arrows) in the superficial epithelial cells, but there is no keratinization in the cornea. D. The cornea of a group Zn(-) rat has few microvilli (arrows) in the superficial epithelial cells. E. In a group Zn(-)A(+) rat, the cornea shows some decrease in microvilli and no keratinization. Bar: 2μm (A-E).

TEM Findings in the Cornea

Group A(+)Zn(+) rats had a high density of microvilli and microplicae in the superficial epithelial cells of the cornea (Fig.13.3.4A). In the cornea of group A(-) rats, keratinization was present and microvilli and microplicae were not observed in the most superficial epithelial cells (Fig.13.3.4B). In the cornea of group A(-) rats, epithelial cells contained keratohyalin granules and thick dense membranes, indicating keratinization. Intercellular spaces were wide, but in spite of decreased desmosomes epithelial cells appeared as light cells because of decreased fibrils in the cytoplasm. Group A(-)Zn(+) rats had a slight decrease in microvilli in the superficial epithelial cells. The density of the corneal epithelial cell layer in group A(-)Zn(+) rats was less than that in group A(+)Zn(+), but more than that in group A(-) rats because of a slight increase of fibrils in the cytoplasm, although intercellular spaces were present. However, there was no keratinization in the cornea of group A(-)Zn(+) rats (Fig.13.3.4C).

In group Zn(-) rats, the cornea had few microvilli and microplicae in the superficial epithelial cell (Fig.13.3.4D). The corneas of group Zn(-)A(+) rats (Fig.13.3.4E) showed some decrease in microvilli. However, the corneal epithelium of group Zn(-)A(+) rats had more microvilli and microplicae than did those of group Zn(-) rats. No keratinization was found in the corneas of group Zn(-) and group Zn(-)A(+) rats.

Discussion

Generally speaking, a catalytic agent can be replaced by another agent in chemical reactions and an enzyme or trace element could be replaced by another in biochemical reactions. Biochemistry suggests an interaction between some vitamins, between some trace elements and between some vitamins and trace elements. There have been no studies showing that a deficiency of one nutrient can be compensated by supplementation with another nutrient. If such a compensation is shown morphologically, an interaction between some nutrients is easily proven. A series of corneal studies on deficiencies of vitamins and trace elements show that corneal observation with SEM can easily and clearly prove an interaction between two nutrients morphologically.

The author and his associates paid special attention to the similar abnormalities in deficiencies of vitamin A and Zn and easily obtained data with SEM. The current study showed a decrease in the plasma vitamin A concentration in Zn-deficient rats. An earlier review (Brown, Chan and Smith, 1976) reporting responses of vitamin A concentration in plasma and liver to experimental Zn deficiency have shown inconclusive evidence of an interaction between vitamin A and Zn, mainly because of inadequate control of the secondary effects of food and growth restriction in Zn deficiency in most animal studies. While in the rats with inadequate dietary Zn no change occurred in liver Zn and alcohol dehydrogenase (ADH) levels, the retina was more sensitive to lack of dietary Zn (Huber and Gershoff, 1975). Newly absorbed vitamin A is mobilized and utilized in preference to that previously stored in the liver of Zn-deficient rats (Carney, Underwood and Loerch, 1976). Injection of vitamin A in the group Zn(-) rats may be useful for preventing corneal and conjunctival change, because despite the fact that there was no significant difference in the plasma vitamin A and Zn levels between groups Zn(-) and Zn(-)A(+) in the current study, group Zn(-)A(+) showed some improvement in the ocular surface.

The interaction between vitamin A and Zn at various levels have been studied (Christian and West, 1998; Solomons and Russell, 1980). Biochemical studies have suggested that there are two common mechanisms to explain the potential dependence of vitamin A metabolism on Zn. One relates to the obligatory role of Zn on the synthesis of its carrier protein, retinol-binding protein (RBP). Zn maintains the serum vitamin A level and plays a role in the release of vitamin A from the liver, by influencing either the synthesis of RBP or the release of the RBP-vitamin A complex from the liver. Zn deficiency can depress the synthesis of RBP in the liver and lead to a lower concentration of RBP in the plasma (Mobarhan, Greenberg, Mehta et al, 1992; Smith, 1980; Smith, Brown and Smith, 1974). The other postulated mechanism for the interaction between Zn and vitamin A is explained by ADH. Zn is necessary for the oxidative conversion of retinol to retinaldehyde (retinal). ADH activity declines significantly and retinal oxidase activity increases significantly in Zn deficiency (Huber and Gershoff, 1975).

Although the corneas in group A(-) rats showed decreased microvilli and keratinization, group A(-)Zn(+) rats showed a slight decrease in microvilli but no keratinization. These results may be related to vitamin A metabolism. Zn deficiency may reduce ADH activity, thereby disturbing vitamin A metabolism. Thus, in vitamin A deficiency, excessive Zn may promote vitamin A metabolism by stimulating ADH activity to release liver stores of vitamin A. The replenishing of Zn in the group A(-) Zn(+) would cause the mobilization of remaining liver vitamin A, some of which would be used for preventing corneal and conjunctival changes. The decreased plasma Zn concentrations in group A(-) rats may impair the corneal wound healing effect of Zn. Supplementation of Zn may accelerate wound healing or delay the onset of corneal and conjunctival changes due to vitamin A deficiency in group A(-)Zn(+).

Studies at the cellular level showed that the effects of retinoic acid, the biologically active form of vitamin A in cells, are mediated by members of the superfamily of nuclear receptors. The retinoic acid receptor (RARs) and the retinoid X receptors (RXRs) bind to retinoid response elements on DNA, thereby controlling gene transcription (Giguere, Ong and Evans, 1987; Petkovich, Brand and Krust et al, 1987). Bossenbroek et al (1998) demonstrated the expression of RARs and RXRs in the rabbit cornea and conjunctiva. The DNA-binding domain of the RAR which contains zinc finger is susceptible to intercellularly relevant oxidizing agents (Casadevall and Sarkar, 1998). Zn plays a functional role in regulating DNA protein interactions of zinc finger proteins. In Zn deficiency the structure of these proteins could be abnormal, yielding a possible explanation for the resemblance of signs of Zn deficiency to those of vitamin A deficiency. The findings in the group A(-)Zn(+) rats in the current study showed that excessive Zn may prevent epithelial damage due to vitamin A deficiency. This may be related to the Zn finger of retinoic acid in the nucleus via the RARs and RXRs activated by excessive Zn supplementation. The concept of Zn finger proteins may explain the intriguing possibility of interaction between vitamin A and Zn.

There are reports suggesting a nutritional relationship between Zn and vitamin A in humans (Solomons and Russell, 1980). A positive association exists in malnourished populations, in which deficiencies of both micronutrients often coexist (Kozlowski, Taylor and Baer, 1987; Hustead, Greger and Gutcher, 1988; Coutsoudis, Coovadia, Broughton et al, 1991) Kraft et al (1987) examined electroretinogram (ERG) changes in both Zn^{-} and vitamin

A-deficient rats. Their report suggested that retinal function could be reserved with both vitamin A and Zn or with vitamin A, but not with Zn. In their light microscopic examination, Zn supplementation alone did not prevent ongoing retinal degeneration and corneal keratinization in several rats with both Zn and vitamin A deficiency. Udomkesmalee et al (1992) reported the findings of an interaction between vitamin A and Zn supplementation in Thai children with both Zn and vitamin A deficiencies. After 6 months of supplementation, the proportion of children with abnormal conjunctival impression cytology decreased significantly in the groups receiving Zn, vitamin A, and Zn plus vitamin A.

The current study showed that decrease and loss of microvilli in the superficial layer of the corneal and conjunctival epithelium could be prevented by vitamin A in Zn deficiency and by Zn in vitamin A deficiency. Although the effect of Zn is incomplete, it is surprising that Zn could prevent keratinization of the corneal and conjunctival epithelium in vitamin A deficiency. TEM also showed rather good, though incomplete, maintenance of the cytoplasmic organelles with supplementation of Zn or vitamin A.

In Zn deficiency excessive vitamin A may accelerate epithelial development to maintain the structure of microvilli. That is, there is an interaction between vitamin A and Zn. Since corneal and conjunctival epithelial cells are sensitive to deficiencies of vitamin A and Zn which cause similar easily observable changes, electron microscopic findings of the current experiment provides rather clear evidence of an interaction between vitamin A and Zn. Either vitamin A or Zn deficiency caused a decrease or loss of goblet cells in conjunctiva. These nutrients appear to be necessary for the maintenance of goblet cell structure and the production of mucous substances. Since the number of goblet cells was greatly decreased in groups A(-) and A(-)Zn(+), comparisons were very difficult. The role of vitamin A in goblet cell development and maintenance may be stronger than that of Zn.

In the current study, the author and his associates demonstrated that morphological impairment in rats with a deficiency of either nutrient could be compensated for by supplementation with the other nutrient, although the compensation was incomplete. Fluctuation in the status of one micronutrient can reasonably alter the metabolism of the other with functional consequences. Electron microscopic findings indicate a synergistic interaction between vitamin A and Zn for the maintenance of the corneal and conjunctival epithelium.

REFERENCES

Amemiya T. Cytochemical and electron microscopic examination of the retina of rats with hypovitaminosis A. *Acta Soc Ophthalmol Jpn*. 1968;72:1074-1099.

Amemiya T. Effect of vitamin E deficiency on photoreceptor outer segment and pigment epithelium of the rat retina. *Acta Soc Ophthalmol Jpn*. 1978;82:822-826.

Amemiya T. Effect of vitamin E administration on photoreceptor outer segment and retinal pigment epithelium of vitamin E deficient rats. *Int Vit Nutr Res*. 1981;51:114-118.

Amemiya T, Kawata T, Maekawa A. Ocular pathology of vitamin B_{12}-deficient rats. In Takaku H, Uchino H, ed. *Kyoto Symposium on Methyl B_{12}*. Tokyo:Kyodo Kikaku Tsushin; 1987:80-85.

Anderson JA, Richard NR, Rock ME. Requirement for vitamin A in long-term culture of human cornea. *Invest Ophthalmol Vis Sci*. 1993;34:3442-3449.

Bossenbroek NM, Sulahian TH, Ubels JL. Expression of nuclear retinoic acid receptor mRNA in the cornea and conjunctiva. *Curr Eye Res*. 1998;17:462-469.

Brown ED, Chan W, Smith JC Jr. Vitamin A metabolism during the repletion of zinc deficient rats. *J Nutr*. 1976;106:563-568.

Carney SM, Underwood BA, Loerch JD. Effect of zinc and vitamin A deficient diets on the hepatic mobilization and urinary excretion of vitamin A in rats. *J Nutr*. 1976;106:1773-1781.

Casadevall M, Sarkar B. Effect of redox conditions on the DNA-binding efficiency of the retinoic acid receptor zinc-finger. *J Inorg Biochem*. 1998;71:147-152.

Christian P, West KP Jr. Interactions between zinc and vitamin A: an update. *Am J Clin Nutr*. 1998;68:435-441.

Coutsoudis A, Coovadia HM, Broughton M, Salisbury RT, Elson I. Micronutrient utilization during measles treated with vitamin A or placebo. *Int J Vit Nutr Res*. 1991;61:199-204.

Dake Y, Amemiya T. Electron microscopic study of the optic nerve in copper deficient rats. *Exp Eye Res*. 1991;52:277-281.

Dowling JE, Gibbons IR. The effect of vitamin A deficiency on the fine structure of the retina. In: Smelser GK, ed. *The Structure of the Eye*. New York:Academic Press Inc;1961:85-99.

Fujikawa A, Gong H, Amemiya T. Vitamin E prevents changes in the cornea and conjunctiva due to vitamin A deficiency. *Graefes Arch Clin Exp Ophthalmol*. 2003;241:287-297.

Ganther HE, Goudie C, Sunde ML, Kopecky MJ, Wagner P, Oh SH, Hoekstra WG. Selenium. Relation to decreased toxicity of methylmercury added to diets containing tuna. *Science*. 1972;175:1122-1124.

Giguere V, Ong ES, Evans RM. Identification of a receptor for the morphogen retinoic acid. *Nature*. 1987;330:624-629.

Gong H, Amemiya T. Optic nerve changes in manganese-deficient rats. *Exp Eye Res*. 1999;68:313-320.

Gong H, Amemiya T. Optic nerve changes in zinc-deficient rats. *Exp Eye Res*. 2001;72:363-369.

Gong H, Takami Y, Amemiya T. Ultrastructure of the optic nerve in magnesium-deficient rats. *Ophthalmic Res*. 2003;35:84-92.

Hatchell DL, Ubels JL, Stekiel T, Hatchell MC. Corneal epithelial wound healing in normal and diabetic rabbits treated with tretinoin. *Arch Ophthalmol*. 1985;103:98-100.

Hatchell DL, Sommer A. Detection of ocular surface abnormalities in experimental vitamin A deficiency. *Arch Ophthalmol*. 1984;102:1389-1393.

Hill CH, Matrone G. Chemical parameters in the study of in vivo and in vitro interations of transition elements. *Fed Proc Fed Am Soc Exp Biol*. 1970;29:1474-1481.

Hill CH. Interrelationships of selenium with other trace elements. *Fed Proc*. 1975;34:2096-2100.

Huber AM, Gershoff SN. Zn deficiency affects the utilization of vitamin A as well as the catabolism of ethanol. Effect of zinc deficiency on oxidation and ethanol in rats. *J Nutr*. 1975;105:1486-1490.

Hustead VA, Greger JL, Gutcher GR. Zinc supplementation and plasma concentration of vitamin A pretern infants. *Am J Clin Nutr*. 1988;47:1017-1021.

Kanazawa S, Kitaoka T, Ueda Y, Gong H, Amemiya T. Interaction of zinc and vitamin A on the ocular surface. *Graefes Arch Clin Exp Ophthalmol*. 2002;240:1011-1021.

Kozlowski BW, Taylor ML, Baer MT. Anticonvulsant medication use and circulating levels of total thyroxine, retinol-binding protein, and vitamin A in children with delayed cognitive development. *Am J Clin Nutr*. 1987;46:360-368.

Kraft SP, Parker JA, Matuk Y, Raot AV. The rat electroretinogram in combined zinc and vitamin A deficiency. *Invest Ophthalmol Vis Sci*. 1987;28:975-984.

Mishima K, Dake Y, Amemiya T, Nishimura M. Electron microscopic study of optic nerves of macular mice. *Exp Eye Res*. 1996;63:85-90.

Mobarhan S, Greenberg B, Mehta R, Friedman H, Barch D. Zinc deficiency reduces hepatic cellular retinol-binding protein in rats. *Int J Vit Nutr Res*. 1992;62:148-154.

Petkovich M, Brand NJ, Krust A, Chambon P. A human retinoic acid receptor which belongs to the family of nuclear receptors. *Nature*. 1987;330:444-450.

Pfister RR, Renner ME. The corneal and conjunctival surface in vitamin A deficiency. *Invest Ophthalmol Vis Sci*. 1978;17:874-883.

Reeves PG, Nielsen FH, Fahey GC Jr. AIN-93 purified diets for laboratory rodents: final report of the American Institute of Nutrition ad hoc writing committee on the reformulation of the AIN-76A rodent diet. *J Nutr*. 1993;123:1939-1951.

Robison WG, Kuwabara T, Bieri JG. Vitamin E deficiency and the retina: Photoreceptor and pigment epithelial changes. *Invest Ophthalmol Vis Sci*. 1979;18:683-690.

Smith JE, Brown ED, Smith JC Jr. The effect of zinc deficiency on the metabolism of retinol-binding protein in the rat. *J Lab Clin Med*. 1974;84:692-697.

Smith JC Jr. The vitamin A-zinc connection: a review. *Ann NY Acad Sci*. 1980;355:62-75.

Solomons NW, Russell RM. The interaction of vitamin A and zinc: implications for human nutrition. *Am J Clin Nutr*. 1980;33:2031-2040.

Sommer A. Effects of vitamin A deficiency on the ocular surface. *Ophthalmology*. 1983;90:592-600.

Stephens RJ, Negi DS, Short SM, van Kuijk FJGM, Dratz EA, Thomas DW. Vitamin E distribution in ocular tissues following long-term dietary depletion and supplementation as determined by microdisection and gas chromatography-mass spectrometry. *Exp Eye Res*. 1988;47:237-245.

Sullivan WR, McCulley JP, Dohlman CH. Return of goblet cells after vitamin A therapy in xerosis of the conjunctiva. *Am J Ophthalmol*. 1973;75:720-725.

Tsuda Y. Optic nerve changes in ascorbic acid-deficient rats. *Acta Med Nagasaki*. 2002;47:161-166.

Ubels JL, Edelhauser HE, Austin KH. Healing of experimental corneal wounds treated with topically applied retinoids. *Am J Ophthalmol*. 1983;95:353-358.

Udomkesmalee E, Dhanamitta S, Shirisinha S. Effect of vitamin A and zinc supplementation on the nutrition of children in northeast Thailand. *Am J Clin Nutr*. 1992;56:50-57.

Van Horn DL, Schutten WH, Hyndiuk RA, Kurz P. Xerophthalmia in vitamin A-deficient rabbits. Clinical and ultrastructural alterations in the cornea. *Invest Ophthalmol Vis Sci*. 1980;19:1067-1079.

Chapter 14

SUMMARY OF ABNORMALITIES DUE TO NUTRITIONAL DEFICIENCIES

In the conjunctiva, deficiencies of vitamins A, B_2, C and E and of the trace elements Zn, Cu and Mn cause a decrease or loss of goblet cells and in the residual goblet cells secretory granules are scarce. In both conjunctival and corneal epithelium there are dark cells with scarce microvilli and microplicae. The resulting signs and symptoms are: tearing, foreign body sensation, dry eye syndromes, ulceration and infection, which have been described well in deficiencies of vitamins A, B_2 and zinc in humans. Only deficiency of vitamin A induces keratinization. Although vitamin E deficiency per se never causes keratinization, vitamin E administration can prevent the epithelial keratinization due to vitamin A deficiency. Vitamin E deficiency induces epithelial atrophy and detachment between epithelial cells by destabilizing their desmosome-like intercellular junctions. Thus, vitamin E plays a role in the maintenance of the epithelial structure. Vitamins A and B_2 and Zn also seem to influence the development and maintenance of epithelial cells. Vitamins A, C and E and the trace elements Zn, Cu and Mn have antioxidant activity which may play a role in lipid membrane stabilization in the conjunctiva and cornea.

In the retina, the photoreceptor outer segments first begin to degenerate and the degeneration extends to the inner segments and nuclei in deficiencies of vitamins A, C and E and of trace elements Zn, Mn and Cr. Vitamins A, C and E and Zn and Mn have a strong antioxidant action, and their deficiencies induce peroxidation of outer segment discs which have lipid membranes containing vitamin A and E and polyunsaturated fatty acids. After the degeneration of the outer segment discs, damage extends to the inner segments and nuclei. The disappearance of photoreceptor cells causes a decrease of the bipolar and horizontal cells. In the initial stage of degeneration of photoreceptor outer segment discs, phagocytized disc-like lamellar structures are increased in the retinal pigment epithelium in deficiencies of vitamin E, and trace elements Zn and Cr. Phagocytized lamellar structures are usually digested by lysosomes, but in vitamin E deficiency, they remain in many lipofuscin granules in the retinal pigment epithelium, probably because of lysosomal dysfunction. In vitamin A deficiency, the retinal pigment epithelium rarely contains lipofuscin granules. In the outer segment discs there are many vitamin A containing lipids, so vitamin A deficiency results in less renewal of discs. In the initial stages of Zn, Mg, Cr and vitamins B_2 and C deficiencies phagocytized lamellar structures in the retinal pigment epithelium are increased for 24 hours and disturb the circadian rhythm. The disturbance of antioxidant actions, such as that of superoxide dismutases, may be related to the degeneration of outer segment discs in Zn, Cu and Mn deficiencies. It is very interesting that the sensory retina comes into contact with the retinal pigment epithelium after the disappearance of the photoreceptor cell layer, so part of the sensory retina becomes rather thin, but retinal detachment never occurs. It is also interesting that the two-layer capillary networks in the retina are maintained even after the loss of photoreceptors and the outer plexiform layer.

In the optic nerve, myelinated nerve fibers are decreased and myelin lamellae become thin and deformed in deficiencies of vitamins A, B_2, B_{12}, C and E, and of Zn, Cu, Mn and Mg. These alterations may be explained by peroxidation of lipids in the myelin sheath due to weakened antioxidation caused by deficiencies of vitamin A, C and E, and Zn, Cu, Mn and Mg which are present in superoxide dismutases. Vitamin B_{12} also plays a role in lipid synthesis; its deficiency affects myelinated nerves and therefore ganglion cells and optic nerve, but not the photorecetpor cells, whereas a deficiency of vitamin A or E and of trace elements Zn and Mn, first causes degeneration of the photoreceptor outer segment then all the photoreceptor cells, the outer plexiform layer and inner nuclear layer. The result may be secondary retrograde degeneration of the optic nerve fibers. Mg deficiency causes focal necrosis in the optic nerve as well as in the retina and cornea.

In the rectus muscles, deficiency of vitamin B_{12} and E causes lipofuscin granules and lipid droplet-like material to appear in the sarcoplasm.

Since Se deficiency has been considered to have an antioxidant action through the glutathione peroxidase pathway, Se deficiency may cause almost the same damage to the conjunctiva, cornea, retina, optic nerve and rectus muscles. However, the abnormalities in the retina due to Se deficiency are quite different from those due to deficiencies of Zn, Cu, Cr, Mg and vitamin A, C and E. Se deficiency rarely causes degeneration in photoreceptor cells, especially outer segment discs, and no increase of lipofuscin granules, but a decrease of horizontal and amacrine cells, constituents of horizontal architecture, as a specific change. Thus, the antioxidant action of Se may be quite different from that of vitamin A, C and E as well as of trace elements Zn, Cu and Mn involved in superoxide dismutases.

INDEX

A

D

G

H

I

J

K

L

M

N

O

P

R

S

T

U

V

W

X

Y

Z